Sickle Cell Disease

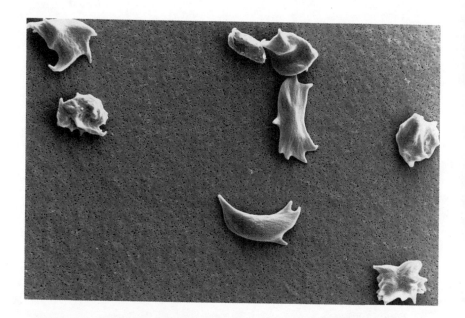

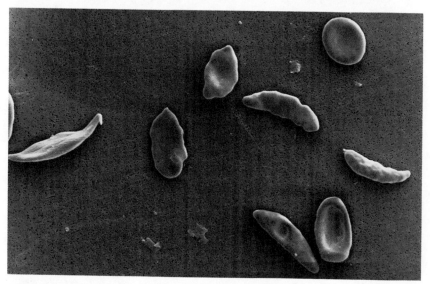

Reversibly and irreversibly sickled cells. These Hb SS cells were fractionated over a discontinuous Percoll/Renografin density gradient (50–70% Percoll). The cells were photographed with a Philips 525 scanning electron microscope at a magnification of 1,550. Top: Reversibly sickled cells prepared by gassing low-density cells (specific gravity < 1.108) with nitrogen for 15 minutes. Bottom: Irreversibly sickled cells obtained from a high-density fraction of the gradient (specific gravity >1.111). These cells were not deoxygenated with nitrogen.

SICKLE CELL DISEASE

Pathophysiology, Diagnosis, and Management

Edited by Vipul N. Mankad and R. Blaine Moore

PRAEGER

Westport, Connecticut
London

Library of Congress Cataloging-in-Publication Data

Sickle cell disease : pathophysiology, diagnosis, and management /
   edited by Vipul N. Mankad and R. Blaine Moore.
        p.   cm.
     Includes bibliographical references and index.
     ISBN 0–275–92503–X (alk. paper)
     1. Sickle cell anemia.   I. Mankad, Vipul N.   II. Moore, R.
Blaine.
     [DNLM: 1. Anemia, Sickle Cell—diagnosis.   2. Anemia, Sickle Cell—
physiopathology.   3. Anemia, Sickle Cell—therapy. WH 170 S56625]
RC641.7.S5S55 1992
616.1′527—dc20
DNLM/DLC
for Library of Congress   91–32168

British Library Cataloguing in Publication Data is available.

Library of Congress Catalog Card Number: 91–32168
ISBN: 0–275–92503–X

First published in 1992

Praeger Publishers, 88 Post Road West, Westport, CT 06881
An imprint of Greenwood Publishing Group, Inc.

Printed in the United States of America

The paper used in this book complies with the
Permanent Paper Standard issued by the National
Information Standards Organization (Z39.48–1984).

10 9 8 7 6 5 4 3 2 1

Dedicated to our families,
without whose support
this book could not have been developed—

Aparna, Mehul, and Raj;
Betty, Nicole, and Paul.

Contents

**Part III   PSYCHOSOCIAL ASPECTS OF SICKLE CELL
             DISEASE**

Preface

Sickle cell disease has been a subject of intense scientific inquiry. A bibliographic search of the period January 1966 to April 1992 1989 revealed 7,677 publications in the Index Medicus using the term *sickle cell* (1). Various aspects of this condition are reviewed periodically in biomedical journals. Monographs presenting clinical features, cultural anthropology, genetics, biochemistry, and medicine in various blends have also been published previously (2, 3). Proceedings of conferences that present reviews of ongoing research have also been published (4). Individuals interested in this disease look at the condition from different points of view. These may include a molecular and cellular perspective to understand the biochemical and physical processes involved in sickling, a clinical view of a disease with protean manifestations, a public health perspective of the affected populations, and a patient's view of coping with a disease that may alter his or her quality of life. While no single scientist, physician, or group of experts can have "complete knowledge" of a complex problem like sickle cell anemia, medical institutions frequently address such inadequacies by enlisting individuals with diverse interests. This book is an attempt by a multidisciplinary team to present recent information from the vantage points of various disciplines.

Medical students, residents, fellows in various subspecialities, nurses and other allied health professionals, basic scientists involved in fundamental investigations, public health workers, sociologists and social workers, epidemiologists and anthropologists, administrators and health policy planners all have an interest in sickle cell disease. While a single book cannot address all problems in equal depth to meet the needs of such a diverse group, we hope that an overall view will be helpful to anyone interested in the topic.

The first chapter presents the global nature of this genetic problem and discusses population genetics and epidemiology to demonstrate the international relevance of the study of sickle cell disease. The anthropological and genetic aspects are quite fascinating and are presented by an anthropologist and a clinical hematologist.

The chapters in Part I, on basic science, describe the effects of the genetic change on the physicochemical properties of sickle hemoglobin, the effects of hemoglobin polymerization on red cell metabolism and membrane changes which produce dense, irreversibly sickled cells, and cell–cell interactions in the blood vessels which produce rheological changes and decreased blood flow in various organs. The final chapter in this section describes the anatomical pathology of various organs affected by sickle cell disease. These discussions are presented by investigators with expertise in biochemical and pharmacological aspects of the pathophysiology of sickle cell disease. The chapter on organ pathology is presented by an individual who has collected a lifetime of experience in clinical and pathological correlations through autopsies and biopsies.

The clinical section presents diagnosis and screening, genetic counseling, general problems such as infections and pain, and organ-specific problems such as those affecting the brain, lungs, kidneys, and liver. Pathophysiology, clinical features, and management of these problems have been discussed by clinicians who provide care for them. Since the evaluation and management of patients with sickle cell disease usually requires interaction with radiologists, anesthesiologists and surgeons, several chapters review the role and functions of such consultants.

Any view of the sickle cell patient must include the interaction of the individual with the society and should address psychosocial dimensions. The chapter in the final section of the book discusses this aspect of sickle cell disease.

Numerous reviewers have read several chapters and provided valuable suggestions. These include Drs. Steve Goodman, John Harrington, Kouichi Tanaka, Robert Johnson, Robert Bookchin, Elizabeth Manci, Roy Martino, Michael Kirkpatrick, Wanda Kirkpatrick, Manuel Cepeda, Ching Nan Ou, and Audwin Anderson. Kathy Billingsley and Sandra Jowers provided secretarial assistance. The editors wish to express gratitude for the time and effort of all these individuals. This work was supported in part by grant #P60 HL38639 from the National Heart, Lung and Blood Institute.

We hope that this effort will improve the understanding of sickle cell disease and contribute toward a better quality of life for those who have the disease or are at risk.

REFERENCES

1. MEDLINE Search, BRS Colleague (Lapham, NY), April 1, 1991.
2. Serjeant GR: *Sickle cell disease.* Oxford: Oxford Medical Publications, 1985.
3. Edelstein S: *The sickle cell, From myths to molecules.* Cambridge, MA: Harvard University Press, 1986.
4. Nagel RL: *Pathophysiological aspects of sickle cell vaso-occlusion.* New York: Alan R. Liss, 1987.

1

Introduction: Epidemiology and Population Genetics of Sickle Cell Disease and the Sickle Cell Trait

Vipul N. Mankad and Charles Hoff

This chapter provides a brief overview of the genetics, epidemiology, and geographic distribution of sickle cell disease and sickle cell trait. In doing so, it examines the role of gene action in the expression of the molecular and clinical phenotypes and a delineation of the population genetics model explaining the maintenance of the sickle cell gene in various populations.

BASIC GENETIC PRINCIPLES

The adult hemoglobin molecule (Hb A) is composed of four heme and four globin chains. The globin moiety consists of a pair of alpha (α) and a pair of beta (β) chains which have significant structural similarities. The phenotypic expression of the alpha globin chains is under the control of a duplicated pair of genes (i.e., four alleles) at the alpha loci on chromosome number 16 while that of the beta globin is under the control of a single pair of genes (i.e., two alleles) at the beta locus on chromosome number 11 (Figure 1.1). Structural homology between the alpha and beta globin genes suggests that these genes arose by duplication of a single gene at an early point in evolution but have become separated on two different chromosomes through the development of millions of additional genes. Zeta globin gene is located near the alpha locus and the epsilon, Gγ, Aγ, and δ genes are located near the beta locus. Mutations at one or more of the globin loci account for more than 400 structural variants of hemoglobin. While the majority of these abnormal hemoglobins are not associated with clinical diseases, some of the mutant genes may have a direct and strong effect on the molecular and clinical phenotypes illustrated by the following selected hemoglobinopathies.

The hemoglobin variant responsible for sickle cell disease and trait, hemo-

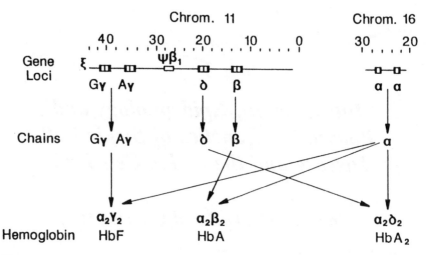

Figure 1.1 Diagram of globin genes, gene products, and major hemoglobins: Two alpha
loci on chromosome 16 and the beta globin gene cluster on chromosome 11
are shown. The scale is in kilobases (kb = 100 nucleotide base pars).

globin S (Hb S), is the result of a mutation in the codon for the sixth amino acid in
the beta globin gene (from GTG to GAG). This mutation results in the substitution
of the amino acid valine for glutamic acid in the sixth position of the beta globin.
The polymerization of Hb S at low oxygen tensions causes altered shape and physicochemical abnormalities of the red cells. Sickle cell anemia (SS) is the result of
Hb S alleles existing in a double dose (homozygous state), and sickle cell trait is
due to the presence of a single Hb S allele (heterozygous state). Sickle cell disease
is a generic term generally used to describe symptomatic disorders related to Hb S
and usually does not include sickle cell trait (which is a relatively healthy, but not
completely asymptomatic, condition).

Other common hemoglobinopathies are also due to point mutations in alleles
at the beta globin locus. One of the most prevalent of these is Hb C (lysine
replaces glutamic acid at position number 6), which is found in high frequency
among black Americans, who also have a high probability of carrying the Hb
S mutation. Since the Hb S and Hb C are allelic (caused by mutations of the
same gene), heterozygotes expressing both Hb S and Hb C are encountered in
populations with both alleles.

Thalassemias are a group of disorders characterized by a decreased rate of
synthesis of globin chains. Beta thalassemias due to either an absence of beta
globin production (beta zero thalassemia) or a quantitative decrease in the beta
globin production (beta plus thalassemia) occur due to mutations in the beta
globin cluster. Since genetic changes causing beta thalassemia are allelic to the
Hb S gene, they are usually not found on the same chromosome, but heterozygous

Table 1.1
Probability of Reproductive Outcome

Matings	Zygotes
AA x AA	100% AA
AA x AS	50% AA, 50% AS
AA x SS	100% AS
AS x AS	25% AA, 50% AS, 25% SS
AS x SS	50% AS, 50% SS

conditions expressing both genes on separate chromosomes are common (e.g., sickle beta thalassemia). The genes for the beta-hemoglobinopathies and the alpha thalassemias are not allelic. Since both influence the expression of the hemoglobin molecule, individuals expressing both Hb S and one of the varieties of alpha thalassemia are found in populations where both mutant alleles exist in appreciable frequencies. The presence of the alpha thalassemia gene in an individual with homozygosity for Hb S ameliorates some of the manifestations of sickle cell anemia by decreasing the concentration of hemoglobin S.

Symptomatic disorders containing sickle hemoglobin (i.e., sickle cell disease) include (1) sickle cell anemia (SS), (2) sickle-hemoglobin C disease, (3) sickle-beta$^+$ thalassemia and (4) sickle-beta$^\circ$ thalassemia. Mutations also exist at the gamma and delta globin loci which are involved in the production of other hemoglobinopathies.

GENETICS OF SICKLING DISORDERS

In populations possessing both the Hb A and Hb S alleles, three different genotypes are possible. They are the homozygotes for Hb A (AA), heterozygotes for both Hb A and Hb S (designated as AS and not SA, which is generally used to denote sickle beta thalassemia), and homozygotes for Hb S (SS). Thus, the abbreviations SS (for sickle cell anemia), AS (for sickle cell trait), and AA (for normal individuals) are used in this chapter to describe the genotypes and the Hb S and Hb A alleles are referred to as S and A alleles, respectively.

When sexual partners are chosen at random (i.e., regardless of their Hb genotype), the probability of the types of zygotes being formed are predictable according to Mendelian principles (Table 1.1). In the population genetics model for sickle cell trait and disease, random mating is assumed for the AA, AS, and SS genotypes. In reality, the mating may not be totally random but rather may be influenced by education, screening, and counseling. Moreover, the proportion of genotypes among neonates born of AS × AA, AS × AS, and AS × SS

Table 1.2
Molecular and Clinical Expressions of Genotypes

	Molecular Phenotype				Clinical Phenotypes		
	Presence of		Proportion of				
Genotype	Hb A	Hb S	Hb A	Hb S	Sickling Crises	Associated Anemia	Associated Pyenonephritis
AA	+[1]	-[2]	>95%	0%	-	-	-
AS	+	+	60-75%	25-40%	- or +	- or +	- or +
SS[3]	-	+	0%	80-95%	+	+	+

[1]Phenotype is absent = −.
[2]Phenotype is present in varying degress = +.
[3]A small proportion of SS individuals do not manifest any clinical signs of sickle cell disease. (See text for explanation.)

matings may not follow Mendelian patterns because of differential mortality in utero which may result from the genotypic status of either or both the fetus and the mother.

There are different levels of phenotypic expression among AS and SS individuals. This starts with the effect of the abnormal gene on the synthesis of the hemoglobin molecule and proceeds through succeeding phenotypic levels resulting from the direct and indirect influence of Hb S on the red cells, interaction of the red cells with other cells and the vasculature, rheologic abnormalities caused by such interaction, and organ damage which ultimately causes the signs and symptoms of sickle cell trait and disease. The gene action is strongest at the molecular level with a tendency for other genetic and environmental factors to have an increasing influence on the phenotype the greater the "metabolic distance" of a given phenotype from the site of the original gene action. Depending on which phenotype level is examined, the A and S alleles can be used as examples of a variety of genetic phenomena. For example, some of these phenomena are codominance, intermediateness, variable expressivity, pleiotropy, epistasis, and multifactorial action.

The A and S alleles are codominant in expression at the molecular level, since red cells carrying Hb A and Hb S both occur in heterozygote AS individuals. The alleles are also intermediate in expression since the circulating levels of Hb S in the erythrocytes are intermediate, that is, usually about 25–40 percent of the values for the homozygotes (i.e., SS patients). Moreover, the variation in the proportion of Hb S found among AS and SS individuals is associated with the variable expressivity in clinical phenotypic expression observed in these individuals (Table 1.2). The action of the S allele is also pleiotropic since it may affect more than one organ, for example, the hematologic, renal, hepatic, splenic, cardiovascular, or neurologic systems.

Phenotypic variation among AS individuals can result from differences at other gene loci which influence the expression of the S allele and environmental factors which also influence the action of the S allele, or both. One study among black × white hybrids in Brazil found that the greater the degree of white ancestry among AS individuals, the greater the likelihood of having higher levels of Hb S and manifesting subclinical signs of sickle cell disease (1). These findings suggest that polygenic complexes regulate Hb S/Hb A production and that, on the average, black AS heterozygotes possess more genes favoring Hb A production over Hb S than whites. The reasons for slightly increased Hb A and slightly decreased Hb S production in AS phenotypes are not clarified by studies at the molecular level. In this instance, the expression of Hb A/Hb S ratios are a case of multifactorial action. Concerning environmental factors, it is well known that hypoxemia resulting from exercise and exposure to high altitude increases the likelihood of a sickling crisis and of the manifestation of some of the clinical signs of sickle cell disease among AS individuals (2).

Variable expressivity of the clinical phenotypes among SS individuals is also well known. Some individuals have a large number of sickling crises and extensive renal, hepatic, splenic, cardiovascular, and cerebral pathology, while others have less severe signs and symptoms. The reasons for variations in the severity in SS individuals are of great interest to investigators in understanding the gene action as well as to clinicians in prognostic counseling and diagnostic and therapeutic investigations. Variation in the amount of fetal hemoglobin among SS individuals is the most plausible explanation for the variable clinical course because fetal hemoglobin has a high affinity for oxygen and ameliorates sickling. The coexistence in an individual of the allele for the hereditary persistence of fetal hemoglobin (HPFH) and the S allele causes a double heterozygous state (S-HPFH) and produces a mild clinical course (3). Individuals with this condition rarely have pain crises. However, SS individuals who do not have the gene for HPFH also vary in the amounts of fetal hemoglobin in their erythrocytes as a result of poorly understood genetic factors.

To summarize, the clinical expression of the S allele in both the heterozygous and homozygous states is subject to modification by environmental and other genetic factors. This is a point not often appreciated, since some genetic texts still treat the combination of A and S alleles as classic examples of dominance/recessiveness or codominance in phenotypic expression when, in fact, it is necessary to define the phenotypic level that the allele(s) are influencing.

DISTRIBUTION

The sickle cell beta-globin (S) allele may be found in populations inhabiting many areas of the world, and high prevalence rates are not necessarily restricted to black populations. The allele is found in regions of West Africa, parts of equatorial Africa, southern Italy, northern Greece, southern Turkey, eastern and western provinces of Saudi Arabia, and in the tribal populations in India. Furthermore, it is found in countries of North and South America among populations derived from areas of the Old World where there is a high prevalence of the allele (Figure 1.2).

To summarize, it is widely accepted that the present distribution of the S allele is caused by several factors, including (1) the prevalence of malaria and balancing selection for the mutant S allele because of the protection afforded heterozygous individuals (sickle cell trait) against falciparum malaria, (2) migrations of populations in which there is a high prevalence of the S allele to other regions of the world, and (3) gene flow from populations with the allele to those without it.

Single versus Multiple Mutations

Lehmann suggested that the S allele first appeared in the proto-Veddoid populations in Arabia and then traveled to Africa and the Indian subcontinent. This suggestion was based on observations of a high prevalence of sickle cell trait in the Veddoid populations in southern India (4). However, information that has been accumulated over recent years clearly supports the hypothesis that the gene arose by mutation within multiple geographic locations.

Blood group marker analysis generally supports the multiple mutation hypothesis but takes into account the migration of populations as well. For example, the selectively neutral, African blood group marker, cDe is uncommon in the Veddoid population, suggesting that there has not been a significant gene flow between the Veddoid and African gene pools (5). Gelpi and King showed that the silent Duffy blood group phenotype common in Africa, Fy(a − b−) was also found in Saudi Arabian individuals with the sickle cell trait (6). They hypothesized that African slaves brought to Western Saudi Arabia carried the S alleles and Fy(a − b−) and that these genes passed into the local population by admixture (gene flow). Subsequently, since the Fy(a − b−) phenotype provides protection against P. vivax and sickle cell trait against P. falciparum and since both types of malaria occur in Saudi Arabia, both genes were, and are, maintained at high frequencies by the combined presence of two different forms of malaria (6). This hypothesis is consistent with theoretical and observed population genetics models.

In areas where the S allele is prevalent, sickle cell trait or disease is not common among the groups that arrived late in those regions. For example, populations of ''Dravidians'' and ''Aryans'' who arrived in India after the Veddoids do not carry the S allele. Similarly, Bedoins and Jews in the Middle East do not have a high prevalence of the allele. Several tribes in Africa that live in the areas where the S allele and malaria are found do not have the S allele, also suggesting that these tribes recently migrated into these areas.

Restriction endonuclease analyses of the DNA in various populations suggest

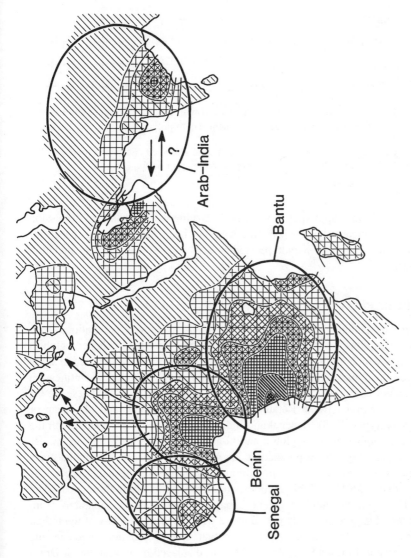

Figure 1.2. Distribution of major haplotypes of the sickle gene in Africa and Asia.

Source: A Ragusa, M Lombardo, G Sortino, et al. Betaˢ gene in Sicily is in linkage disequilibrium with the Benin haplocyte: Implications for Gene flow. *Am J Hematol* 27 (1988): 140. Reproduced with permission.

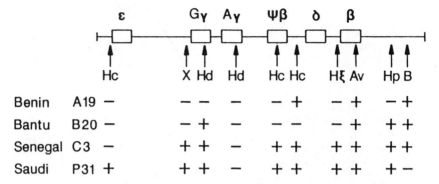

		Hc		X Hd	Hd	Hc Hc	HΣ Av	Hp B
Benin	A19 −		− −	−	− +	− +	− +
Bantu	B20 −		− +	−	− −	− +	+ +
Senegal	C3 −		+ +	−	+ +	+ +	+ +
Saudi	P31 +		+ +	−	+ +	+ +	+ −

Figure 1.3. Classification of haplotypes associated with sickel cell disease and based on restriction endonuclease fragment length polymorphism.

Source: GR Serjeant: Geography and the clinical picture of sickle cell disease: An overview. *Ann New York Acad Sci* 565 (1989): 111, Fig. 1. Reproduced by permission.

at least four major haplotypes in the world carrying the S allele (see discussion below). Since clear migration patterns have not been shown among these four distinct populations, the haplotype studies also support the multiple mutation hypothesis.

MAJOR HAPLOTYPES CARRYING THE S ALLELE

Restriction endonuclease analysis of the DNA in various populations demonstrates variations (mutations other than the specific gene for sickle hemoglobin) in the DNA which are inherited in a Mendelian manner and can be used to study anthropological questions. Such polymorphisms have permitted the identification of four major haplotypes associated with the S allele (Figure 1.3). These are (1) Benin, (2) Central African Republic or Bantu, (3) Senegal, and (4) Asian or Indian haplotypes (7, 8). Senegal and Indian haplotypes are associated with the presence of high fetal hemoglobin and G-gamma globin chains and are milder in clinical severity. Since populations in Africa in the above-mentioned areas have not witnessed large-scale migrations and have separate haplotypes, it is believed that the S beta globin mutations occurred separately in those areas. The Indian haplotype is found in several tribal populations living separately from each other which are generally not admixed with the large majority of the Indian population. Therefore, it is hypothesized that these populations lived in one location several thousand years ago and were displaced by migrations of Dravidian and Aryan populations. In this way, the Indian haplotype carrying the S allele was transmitted to remote parts of India and eastern Saudi Arabia. In the United States, sickle cell anemia in black populations consists of various combinations of haplotypes, that is, either homozygous for Bantu, Benin, or Senegal or double heterozygous for any of the two African haplotypes (9). Variation in the severity of the disease among patients with sickle cell anemia may be explained in part by these haplotypes and by the influence such mutations have on the production of fetal hemoglobin, G-gamma globin chains, and, possibly, other factors.

MALARIAL HYPOTHESIS

There is indirect evidence that the allele responsible for the production of hemoglobin S is maintained at a high frequency in tropical Africa because of the biological advantage it confers on the heterozygotes through partial protection from P. falciparum malaria. This evidence comes from several different lines of investigation. First, there is the well-documented correlation between the prevalence of the S allele and the worldwide distribution of endemic malaria (10–14). Second, among African populations where malaria is hyperendemic, both morbidity and mortality are reduced in trait individuals (AS heterozygotes) compared to both AA and SS homozygotes. In several studies the prevalence of malaria was found to be significantly lower in children with sickle cell trait than in normal controls (15–17), and parasite loads were lower in trait children (17). Demographic studies have also shown that the proportion of trait individuals increases with age relative to Hb A/Hb A individuals, resulting from differential mortality among the latter (18). Furthermore, higher mean fertility rates have been observed among females with trait (AS) compared to those who are AA (19).

THE MECHANISM OF PROTECTION AGAINST MALARIA

The apparent selective advantage of having the sickle cell trait in a malarial environment results from the lower malarial parasite load. Two different mechanisms have been proposed to explain why the malarial parasite does not survive as well in the trait individual. First, it has been hypothesized that there is a lower available oxygen supply for malarial parasites due to binding characteristics of Hb S. Presumably, this may limit the number of parasites able to survive in the host. Second, when a parasite attached to a red cell with Hb S consumes oxygen, the cell sickles. Phagocytic destruction of both the parasite and the red blood cell results, breaking the malarial cycle (20, 21). Quite likely, both mechanisms result in lower parasitemia.

THE POPULATION GENETICS MODEL

The mathematical population genetics model which explains the maintenance of the S allele is developed below. The underlying assumption of this model is that mating between individuals occurs at random. That is, people choose mates

Table 1.3
Changes in Genotype Frequency After Selection in a Random Mating Population

Genotype	Phenotype	Frequency Before Selection	Frequency Value	Frequency After Selection
AA	Hb A/Hb A	p^2	$W_1 < 1$	$p^2 W_1 < p^2$
AS	Hb A/Hb S	$2pq$	$W_2 = 1$	$2pq = 2pq$
SS	Hb S/Hb S	q^2	$W_3 \approx 0$	$q^2 (0) \approx 0$

Notes:
p = frequency of the A allele.
q = frequency of the S allele.

independent of their genetic hemoglobin status. On the basis of this assumption, the proportion of AA, AS and SS genotypes created at conception would follow a Hardy-Weinberg distribution (Table 1.3 and reference 22).

In malarial environments in Africa, the AA genotype has, on the average, a reduced survivability and fertility compared to the AS trait genotype. This results in a lowered realized fertility (production of viable offspring) by individuals with the Hb A/Hb A genotype. On the other hand, the SS genotype usually does not survive to the reproductive period. When this does occur, fertility is usually sufficiently impaired that there is a very low likelihood of producing viable offspring. In population genetics models it is customary to assign a fitness value equal to one to the genotype producing the maximum number of offspring or, conversely, a selection value of zero (since $W_1 = 1 - S_1$). As a result, the respective fitness values in the "malarial–sickle cell" model above are a value less than one for the AA genotype (depending on the fertility and mortality of this genotype in a given environment), a value of one for the AS heterozygote, and a value of zero for the SS genotype.

This classic "balancing selection" model in which an equilibirum frequency of the S(q) and A(p) alleles will be achieved if there are no changes in fitness ($\Delta W = 0$) values. That is, no change in gene frequency will occur from generation to generation as a result of the interplay of selection pressures. The equilibrium q may be found by taking the derivation of the average fitness ($\bar{W}$) of the population with respect to q ($d\bar{W}/dq$), setting the resultant equation to zero and solving for q in terms of the fitness values (W_1, W_2, W_3). When $d\bar{W}/dq = 0$, there is no further change in gene frequency from generation to generation and, by definition, equilibrium q has been reached (22).

Average Fitness: $\bar{W} = p^2 W_1 + 2pq W_2 + q^2 W_3 = (1 - q)^2 W_1 + 2(1 - q)q,$

since $W_2 = 1$, $W_3 = 0$, and $p = (1 - q)$

Derivation: $d\bar{W}/dq = (- 2 + 2q) W_1 + 2 - 4q$,

and, setting this equation $= 0$ and solving for q,

Equilibrium: $\hat{q} = (1 - W_1)/(2 - W_1)$

For example, a 20 percent reduction from the ideal fitness value ($W = 1$) of the AA genotype as a result of malaria associated morbidity and mortality ($W_1 = 0.8$) would result in any equilibrium frequency $q = 0.167$ (and $p = 0.833$). Those interested in a further discussion of population genetics models should consult the excellent text by C. C. Li (22).

SUMMARY

The population genetics of hemoglobinopathies characterized by the presence of sickle hemoglobin and causing symptomatic as well as asymptomatic conditions has been discussed. The mutant gene for sickle hemoglobin interacts with various other genes and with internal and external environmental factors to produce molecular and clinical phenotypes of a wide variety.

REFERENCES

1. Nance WE, and Grove J: Genetic determination of phenotypic variation in sickle cell trait. *Science* 177 (1972): 716–718m.
2. Sears DA: The morbidity of sickle cell trait: A review of the literature. *Am J Med* 64 (1978): 1021–1036.
3. Horger ED: Hemoglobinopathies. In D Kitay ed.: *Hematologic problems in pregnancy*, pp. 116–129. Oradell, NJ: Medical Economics Books, 1987.
4. Lehman H: Distribution of the sickle cell gene. *Eugen Rev* 46 (1954): 101–121.
5. Choremis E, Ikin EW, Lehman H, et al.: Sickle cell trait and blood groups in Greece. *Lancet* no. 12 (1953): 909–911.
6. Gelpi AP, and King MC: Association of Duffy blood groups with sickle cell trait. *Human Genet* 32 (1976): 65–68.
7. Nagel RL, Fabry ME, Pagnier J, et. al: Hematologically and genetically distinct forms of sickle cell anemia in Africa. *N Engl J Med* 312 (1985): 880–884.
8. Labie D, Srinivas R, Dunda O, et al.: Alpha and beta globin haplotypes in southern Indians bearing the sickle gene: Evidence for the unicentric origin of the beta S mutation in pre-Aryan populations of India. (personal communication), April 1989.
9. Hattori Y, Kutlar F, Kutlar A, et al.: Haplotypes of beta S chromosomes among patients with sickle cell anemia from Georgia. *Hemoglobin* 10, no. 6 (1986): 623–642.
10. Nagel RL: The origin of the hemoglobin S gene. *Einstein Quart J Biol Med* 2 (1984): 53–62.

11. Allison AC. Protection afforded by sickle cell trait against subterrian malarial infection. *Br Med J* 1 (1954): 290–294.
12. Motulsky A: Metabolic polymorphisms and the role of the infectious diseases in human evoluation. *Human Biol* 32 (1960): 28–62.
13. Wiesenfeld SL: Sickle cell trait in human biological and cultural evolution. *Science* 157 (1967): 1134–1140.
14. Allison AC: Malaria in carriers of the sickle cell trait and in newborn children. *Exper Parasitol* 6 (1957): 418–447.
15. Livingstone FB: Malaria and human polymorphisms. *Ann Rev Genet* 5 (1971): 33–64.
16. Cornille-Broger R, Fleming AF, Kagan I, et al.: Abnormal Haemoglobins in the Sudan savanna of Nigeria. *Ann Trop Med Parasitol* 75, no. 2 (1979): 161–172.
17. Vandepitte J, and Delaisse J: Sicklemie et Paludisme. *Ann Soc Belge Med Trop* 37 (1957): 703–735.
18. Lambotte-Legrand J, and Lambotte-Legrand C: Notes complementaires sur la D drepanocytose. I: Sicklemie et malaria. *Ann Soc Belge Med Trop* 38 (1958): 45–53.
19. Weiss ML, and Mann AF: *Human biology and behavior,* 4th ed. Boston: Little, Brown, 1985.
20. Luzzato L, et al.: Increased sickling of parasitized erythrocytes as mechanisms of resistence against malaria in the sickle cell trait. *Lancet* no. 1 (1970): 319–322.
21. Roth EF, et al.: Sickling rates of human AS red cells infected in vitro with plasmodium falciparum malaria. *Science* 202 (1978): 650–652.
22. Li CC: *First course in population genetics.* Pacific Grove, CA: Boxwood Press, 1978.

Part I

BASIC SCIENCE ASPECTS OF SICKLE CELL DISEASE

2

Molecular Aspects of the Polymerization of Hemoglobin S

A. Seetharama Acharya

define single pt

Sickle cell disease is a consequence of a single point mutation Glu-6(β)$\rightarrow$ Val in the hemoglobin molecule. This mutation in the A helix of the β-chain endows this segment of the molecule with a new *quinary structural memory* which enables the deoxy Hb S to polymerize. The kinetic and the equilibrium studies of the polymerization of deoxy Hb S have lead to the postulation of a nucleation-dependent polymerization mechanism which requires the formation of a critical nucleus of n molecules. Polymerization appears to be initiated by homogeneous nucleation—the formation of individual critical nuclei, and proceeds with the fiber growth and heterogeneous nucleation—the formation of nuclei on the surface of existing polymerized hemoglobin fiber. The quinary structure of deoxy Hb S fibers has been investigated by the crystallographic analysis of deoxy Hb S crystals and the electron microscopic studies of Hb S fibers, leading to the identification of a number of intermolecular contact regions of deoxy Hb S.

The intermolecular contact regions of deoxy Hb S are classified into three groups: (1) intra-double strand lateral contacts, (2) intra-double strand axial contacts, and (3) inter-double strand contacts. Polymerization studies of hybrid Hb S with additional mutations have confirmed the identity of many contact residues. Nearly 60 mutations of Hb S are known to date that influence the fiber formation. Both the equilibrium and the kinetic properties of deoxy Hb S polymerization are influenced by the perturbation of the intermolecular contact regions. These perturbations of the contact regions are achieved through elegant molecular engineering approaches such as the mutation of a contact residue by site directed mutagenesis/semisynthesis or by the selective chemical modification of a functional group of the contact regions. Though many such approaches have been advanced, and many modified forms of Hb S have been prepared, none of these, so far, has been able to completely neutralize the polymerization influence

of β6 mutation. Studies of the additivity/synergy of the antipolymerizing influence of the simultaneous perturbation of two or more intermolecular contact
regions, as well as studies of the progress curve of the polymerization through
structural probes selectively placed at the preselected contact region (achieved
through various genetic as well as chemical protein engineering approaches)
could conceivably provide new information about the mechanistic aspects and
the energetics of deoxy Hb S fiber formation. The discussions presented here
clearly demonstrate that though Glu–6(β) appears to be inert, in terms of the
oxygen affinity of the protein, this residue plays a very crucial role in keeping
the deoxy Hb A in solution at the high protein concentration that one finds under
physiological conditions. If nature had not provided us with this molecular
variant, namely Hb S, it would not have been easy, if not impossible to recognize
this 'crucial structural role of Glu–6(β) in the overall architecture of the hemoglobin molecule.

INTRODUCTION

The term _molecular disease_ was first introduced by Pauling and his associates
to describe the abnormality of the hemoglobin of patients with sickle cell disease
(1). Since then, significant progress has been made in understanding the structure-
and-function relationship of this mutant hemoglobin molecule and the primary
pathophysiological consequences of the sickle cell anemia at the molecular level
(2–5). The hemoglobin of patients with sickle cell disease, hemoglobin S, po-
lymerizes in the venous blood, namely, in the deoxy conformation of the protein.
Consequently, the red blood cells of patients with sickle cell disease with the
polymerized deoxy Hb S take the shape of a sickle; hence, the name _sickle cell_
disease. This chapter concentrates on the concept that the intracellular polymerization of the deoxy Hb S is the primary pathophysiological event in sickle
cell anemia. In this context, the molecular aspects of the polymerization have
been discussed here specifically as a systematic intracellular macromolecular
assembly process. The primary emphasis here has been the discussion of the _in_
vitro studies of the polymerization reaction of deoxy Hb S and the studies of
the intermolecular contact regions of the protein.

Hb S is the product of a single point mutation of the β-globin gene (6). This
single base mutation from A to T in the triplet codon for the sixth amino acid
residue of the β-globin chain results in the substitution of a negatively charged
glutamic acid (the normal state) for a hydrophobic valine residue (Figure 2.1).
The molecular defect of this mutant Hb is the sole structural factor responsible
for the intracellular polymerization and the formation of fibers. As a consequence
of the polymerization reaction within the erythrocytes, a significant reduction in
cell deformability occurs (3–5). This results in a distortion of the shape of the
red blood cell (sickling). These sickled cells obstruct the flow in the microcirculation. The severity in the vaso-occlusive manifestations of sickle cell disease
in a given patient is primarily dependent on the intracellular concentration of

1 10

β^A Val-His-Leu-Thr-Pro-<u>Glu</u>-Glu-Lys-Ser-Ala

β^S Val-His-Leu-Thr-Pro-<u>Val</u>-Glu-Lys-Ser-Ala

Figure 2.1. Chemical differences between the β chains of Hb A and Hb S. The amino acid sequences of the amino terminal 10 residues of the β^A and β^S chains are presented.

deoxy Hb S as well as the kinetics of the polymerization reaction. The chemical and/or genetic manipulation of these aspects of the polymerization reaction forms the basis of many of the current therapeutic approaches to decrease the severity of the disease (2–5, 7).

Normal adult Hb A is composed of four polypeptide chains which form the hemoglobin tetramer. Each polypeptide chain contains the prosthetic group, heme, which is the oxygen-carrying center of the protein. Two of these chains, containing 141 amino acid residues, are referred to as α-chains, and the other two chains, each with 146 amino acid residues, are referred to as β-chains (3). The net difference between Hb A and Hb S lies on only 2 (1 residue per β-chain) of the total 514 amino acid residues of Hb. This small difference is sufficient to cause this mutant Hb to polymerize in the deoxy conformation. This clearly reflects the crucial structural role played by Glu-6(β) in maintaining the deoxy Hb A in an unpolymerized state under physiological conditions.

It is now very well recognized that the overall structure and function of Hb S is similar to that of Hb A, specifically with reference to its oxygen-affinity. The liganded Hb S examined by low-resolution x-ray crystallography was found to be isomorphous with liganded Hb A (2). Consistent with the overall similarity in the structure of Hb A and Hb S, the solubilities of oxygenated Hb A and Hb S are nearly the same. Moreover, the oxygen affinity of Hb A and Hb S in dilute solutions are also the same. However, if the oxygen affinity of the protein is studied as a function of protein concentration, Hb A shows a monophasic behavior and the P_{50} increases with the concentration of Hb A in a linear fashion. The oxygen affinity of Hb S, on the other hand, shows a biphasic behavior: The point of inflection in a plot of P_{50} versus the protein concentration corresponds to that of the solubility of Hb S (Figure 2.2). With new molecular variants of Hb S and chemically modified derivatives of Hb S with increased solubility, the point of inflection is at a higher protein concentration. Thus, the influence of Val–6(β) mutation on the oxygen-affinity is indirect, a consequence of the polymerization reaction. This approach has been, in fact, used as a procedure for the determination of the minimum gelling concentration of many chemically modified forms of Hb S as well as many of the molecular variants of Hb S prepared *in vitro* (8).

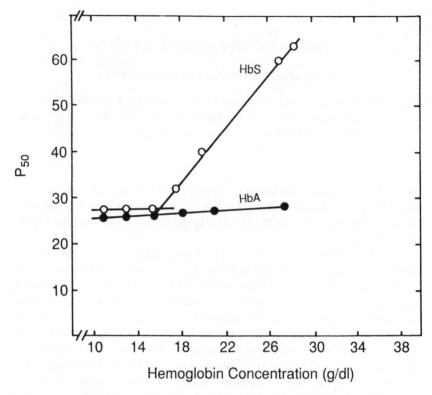

Figure 2.2. O_2 affinity of Hb A and Hb S as a function of protein concentration.

In spite of the close similarity in the crystal structure of Hb A and Hb S, the nuclear magnetic resonance (NMR) spectroscopic studies (9) and circular dichroic measurements (10) do indicate some subtle differences in the conformation of the two oxygenated Hb species. In solution, fully oxygenated Hb S has been found to be more susceptible to denaturation by mechanical shaking than Hb A. These observations reflect the increased flexibility of some of the segments of the Hb S molecule.

STRUCTURAL STUDIES OF Hb S POLYMERS

Though the overall conformation of oxy Hb A and oxy Hb S are nearly the same in dilute solution, the solubility of deoxy Hb S is significantly lower than that of deoxy Hb A. Deoxy Hb S at concentration levels found in the erythrocytes organizes itself into large polymers. These polymers align themselves into paracrystalline gel and have been examined by polarizing microscopy, fiber x-ray diffraction, and electron microscopy. These studies have suggested that in the

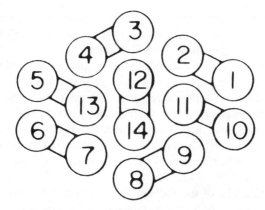

Figure 2.3. Section through the 14-strand model of deoxy Hb S fiber showing the possible pairing of tetramers into the double strand in the crystal.

polymer, Hb S tetramers are wound around a vertical axis, so that if viewed from one end, the polymers resemble the rings of Hb tetramers stacked on one another (11, 12).

Crystallographic analyses of crystals of deoxy Hb S have now established the orientation of the tetramers toward the polymer axis. These data have indeed permitted the identification of the contact regions between the neighboring tetramers. Some of these contacts are between the Hb tetramers lying side to side in the ring of the polymers while others are the contacts between the tetramers stacked on one another along the vertical axis (12).

X-ray diffraction and electron microscopic studies have shown that both the Hb S fiber and crystal are constructed from a similar structural motif, the Wishner-Love double strand. The double strand consists of two parallel rows of Hb S molecules arranged as half staggered pairs. Electron microscopic studies have established that the Hb S fiber consists of seven double strands of Hb S (Figure 2.3) twisting around a common axis (11–16).

The x-ray diffraction as well as electron microscopic studies have identified a number of regions of the Hb S molecule that are indeed contact regions between the tetramers in the polymer. These intermolecular contact regions of deoxy Hb S contribute to the stabilization of the fiber. Detailed knowledge of the intermolecular contact regions and the mechanistic aspects of their integration during polymerization is a necessary element to rationally design antisickling agents. The current challenge in this area of research remains the understanding of (1) the relative roles of intermolecular interactions between the deoxy Hb S molecules in the Hb S fiber as well as in the assembly process, (2) the energetics of these interactions, and (3) the driving forces responsible for the fiber formation.

The various intermolecular contact regions of Hb S have been grouped into three classes. These are: (1) intra-double strand axial contact regions, (2) intra-double strand lateral contact regions, and (3) inter-double strand contact regions.

The identity of intra-double strand lateral contacts and intra-double strand axial contacts have been mostly made available by the deoxy Hb S crystal structure and electron microscopic analysis of Hb S fiber.

The interactions within each strand are called axial contacts and the interactions between the strands are referred to as lateral contacts. Val-6(β) of one tetramer makes a lateral contact with the acceptor pocket generated by the Phe-85(β) and Leu-88(β) of the tetramers of the complementary strand. Only one of the Val-6(β) of a given tetramer makes such a contact (Figure 2.4). The interaction appears to be possible only in the deoxy conformation of the protein. The other important lateral contact appears to be between Asp-73(β) and Thr-4(β) of the complementary strand (11, 12).

Glu-22 and Glu-121 of the β-chain are involved in the axial contacts with residues of an α-chain on the adjacent molecule of the same strand; these represent only two of the many axial contacts. Besides many lateral and axial contacts, interactions between the parallel as well as the antiparallel double strands are also involved in the polymerization reaction, and these are primarily α-chain contacts. Padlan and Love have recently found that the only significant difference between deoxy Hb S and deoxy Hb A is in the amino terminal A-helix of the β-chain, namely the segment of the residues 4 to 18 of the β-chain (12). In the deoxy Hb S, although this A-helix remains intact as in Hb A, it undergoes a hinge-like displacement, allowing Val-6(β) and Thr-4(β) of the chain to make contact with the amino acid residues of the acceptor pocket.

KINETICS OF HEMOGLOBIN S POLYMERIZATION

Polymerization of Hb S can be induced in a concentrated solution of the protein by rapid deoxygenation. Gelation of Hb S is an endothermic, temperature-dependent process. Accordingly, the gelation can also be induced by a sudden increase in the temperature of the deoxygenated Hb S. The polymerization process by itself can be studied by a number of physical methods such as light-scattering measurements (17), birefringence (18), calorimetry (18), viscocity (19, 20), and nuclear magnetic resonance spectroscopy (21–23). When the polymerization reaction is studied by any one of the above methods, one observes a delay between the time of deoxygenation, or the temperature jump, and the onset of the Hb S polymerization (24–26). The results of all the physical methods appear to be complementary to one another. A reasonable physical model for such a sequence of events is that the delay period in the polymerization reaction represents a nucleation phenomenon wherein deoxy Hb S tetramers associate with one another to form many multimeric species of the parent tetrameric molecule namely, deoxy Hb S. Each of these multimeric (di, tri, tetra, or penta) species of the deoxy Hb S tetramer is in a thermodynamically unstable state compared to the parent tetrameric deoxy Hb S. At some aggregate size of n molecules, a critical nucleus is formed. At this stage, further addition of Hb S molecules into this macromolecular nucleated structure (i.e., the assembly pro-

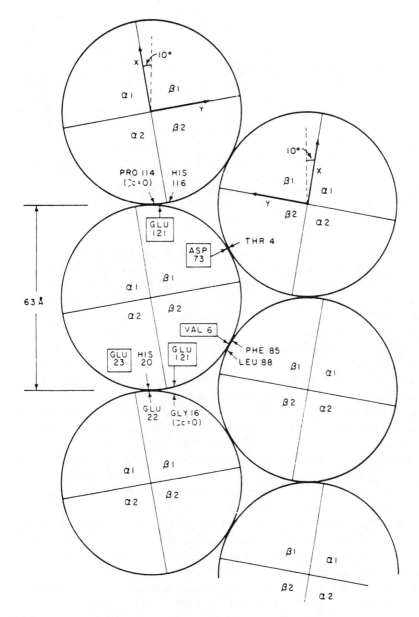

Figure 2.4. Structure of deoxy hemoglobin S depicting the arrangement of Hb S tetramers in the double-stranded structure determined by crystallographic analysis.

Source: KB Wishner, WC Ward and EE Lattman, Crystal structure of deoxyhemoglobin at 5 A° resolution, *J Mol Biol* 98 (1975): 179–194, Figure 8. Reprinted with permission.

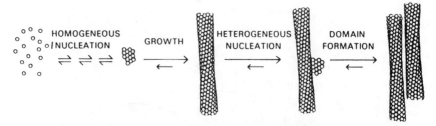

Figure 2.5. A Model for the polymerization of deoxy Hb S homogeneous and heterogeneous nucleation for the formation of Hb S fiber.

Source: Adapted, with permission, from CT Noguchi and AN Schechter, Sickle cell hemoglobin polymerization in solution and cells, *Ann Rev Biophys Chem* 14 (1983): 247, Fig. 3.

cess) becomes energetically favorable. In this physical model, the nucleation process represents the rate-limiting step of the polymerization reaction. The subsequent growth phase represents a relatively rapid addition of free deoxy Hb S units to the nucleus to form the long polymer. Depolymerization, either by the addition of oxygen or by the lowering of the temperature, takes place rapidly and exhibits no lag phase.

The kinetic scheme for the polymerization of Hb S discussed above predicts the existence of aggregates of some intermediate size between the deoxy Hb S tetramer and the fiber. The polymerization is a concerted process, and accordingly, these intermediates are in very low concentrations and, hence, are difficult to detect. However, the existence of such intermediates has been demonstrated by a number of physical techniques such as light scattering (27, 28), viscocity (29), and NMR spectroscopy (30), as well as electron spin resonance spectroscopic studies (31). Many estimates of the number of tetramers present in the nucleating structure have been advanced, and the size of the nucleating structure appears to decrease in the high phosphate buffer polymerizing system.

The early detailed kinetic studies on the polymerization of deoxy Hb S from concentrated solutions of deoxy Hb S has been interpreted in a simple model of homogeneous nucleation followed by fiber growth. On the other hand, the kinetics of the polymerization of Hb S from a less concentrated solution of deoxy Hb S presumably involves the initial homogeneous nucleation followed by a heterogeneous nucleation on the surface of the existing polymer (Figure 2.5). However, there is very little information about the mechanistic aspects of polymerization, particularly with respect to the structural/conformational aspects of intermolecular contact regions of the intermediates involved in the integration of "structural information" resident in each of the intermolecular contact regions. A fundamental question that needs to be addressed is whether the nucleation and growth phases of the polymerization reaction recognized by the kinetic studies are dominated by the integration of intrafiber axial contacts, intrafiber lateral contacts, or interfiber contacts and whether a hierarchy exists in the integration of the intermolecular interactions during the polymerization reactions. It is conceivable that the intermediates of the polymerization reaction are comparable to the *molten globule* state invoked in the protein-folding reactions in which a high flexibility is associated with the integrated structural elements. Studies with new molecular variants of Hb S which have structural/conformational probes strategically placed at a contact region in each class of intermolecular contact regions should provide new insights into these complex, but nonetheless interesting, architectural aspects of the polymerization reaction.

RHEOLOGY OF SICKLE CELL HEMOGLOBIN

The conversion of the solution of deoxy Hb S to a gel form results in a dramatic increase in its viscosity. The viscoelastic properties of the gel of sickle cell Hb reflects the density and the rigidity of the component fibers. Therefore, rheological measurements of the deoxy Hb S gels were expected to provide new insights into the structure of the gel. The rheological consequences of polymerization are also anticipated to have clear-cut implications for the deformability of sickle erythrocytes *in vivo*. The rheological properties of the deoxy Hb S gels are considered as the most immediate cause of vaso-occlusive manifestations in sickle cell disease. The viscosity of the deoxy Hb S above its minimum gelling concentration has been shown to increase precipitously. Briehl (32, 33) has shown that the gels of deoxy Hb S are not viscous; rather, they exhibit a solid-like behavior. However, if these gels are sheared they start becoming viscous, and the extent to which they become viscous depends on the shear strength. The shear apparently breaks up the polymer and, hence, lowers the viscosity. The disruption of the polymer significantly shortens the delay time (17, 29, 33, 34), apparently by creating more nucleation sites for the polymer growth. Erythrocytes containing the polymerized Hb S are subjected to different degrees of shearing during circulation, which could have contrary effects on intracellular polymerization. On one hand, shearing will decrease the risk of vaso-occlusion by making the intracellular polymerized gel more viscous rather than solid-like. The aggravation of vaso-occlusion by shearing is also conceivable as a consequence of shortening the delay time. These aspects have been the subject of intensive investigations in recent years.

DELINEATING THE INTERMOLECULAR CONTACT REGIONS IN THE DEOXY Hb S POLYMER BY PREPARING MOLECULAR VARIANTS OF THE PROTEIN

As discussed earlier, the crystallographic as well as the electron microscopic studies of deoxy Hb S crystals and polymers have implicated a number of regions of the Hb S molecule, besides the Val-6(β), that are proximal in a stereospecific fashion in the quinary structure of the protein for the generation of noncovalent interactions. Early studies by Allison (35) and Murayama (36) demonstrated that the polymerization of Hb S involves hydrophobic interactions. Subsequent studies have shown that electrostatic interactions also play a crucial role in the polymerization reaction (37). Thus, the polymerization of deoxy Hb S is a very complex phenomenon involving various types of noncovalent interactions. Quite understandably, these interactions also provide the stabilization energy needed to facilitate the polymerization reaction.

The direct evidence for the participation of the implicated intermolecular contact regions in the polymerization reaction comes from chemical studies wherein one or more of the intermolecular contact regions (other than Val-6([β]) are perturbed (i.e., having a mutation at the contact site). Indeed, the demonstration of the participation of regions of Hb S other than that involving the Val-6(β) was made by Bookchin, Nagel, and Ranney (38, 39) much before the results of the crystallographic analysis of deoxy Hb S were available. In this era of genetic engineering, studies of protein structure and function relationships predominantly involve the preparation of molecular variants. It may be pointed out that investigations of intermolecular contact regions of deoxy Hb S were indeed one of the early protein structural problems to be tackled by this molecular approach, thus demonstrating the power of molecular engineering studies in structural biology. The major difference at this stage is that in the earlier studies of contact regions of deoxy Hb S, only the naturally occuring molecular variants of α- and β/$β^S$-chains could be used due to the lack of precise methods for preparing other molecular variants. The genetic methods have increased the flexibility of preparing the molecular variants for such structural studies.

The polymerization studies with deoxygenated mixtures of S and non-S Hb have also provided valuable information about the regions of intermolecular contact by deoxy Hb S. The non-S Hb could influence the solubility (polymerization) of deoxy Hb S in three ways (40–46). First, non-S Hb will affect the chemical activity of deoxy Hb S by excluded volume effect even though the non-S Hb may not enter the polymer to any significant amount (44–45). The other possibility is that the non-S Hb may itself copolymerize to a limited extent with Hb S (42, 45–47). The third possibility is that mixed hybrids of Hb S and non-S Hb could be generated *in situ* (48), which will have significantly different tendencies to enter into the polymer phase compared to the parent Hb. By careful manipulation of the experimental protocols it is possible to dissect out the three different aspects by which the test non-S Hb could influence the polymerization of Hb S.

The investigation of Singer and Singer (49) established that Hb F increases the minimum gelling concentration of Hb S. However, Hb F failed to participate in the sickling phenomenon. On the other hand, mixtures of Hb A and Hb C gelled at a considerably lower concentration than comparable mixtures of Hb S and Hb F. Thus, these two hemoglobins apparently participate in the polymer formation. Bookchin, Nagel, and colleagues (38, 50) have extended this mo-

Table 2.1
β-Chain Intermolecular Contact Regions of Deoxy Hb S

Position	Structure	Influence on Inhibits	Polymerization Potentiates
β^{16}	Glu → Asp	+	
β^{17}	Lys → Glu	+	
β^{19}	Asn → Lys	+	
β^{22}	Glu → Ala		+
β^{66}	Lys → Glu	+	
β^{73}	Asp → Asn	+	
β^{80}	Asn → Lys	+	
β^{83}	Gly → Asp	+	
β^{87}	Thr → Lys	+	
	Lys → Glu	+	
β^{95}	Lys → Asn	+	

Source: Compiled primarily from data in RL Nagel, L Johnson, RM Bookchin, et al., β-chain contact sites in hemoglobin S polymer, *Nature* 283 (1980): 832.

lecular approach of mapping the intermolecular contact regions to a wide variety of other β-chain variants and have identified many intermolecular contact points involving the β-chain. The basic philosophy of this experimental approach is that if the mutation site of the molecular variant used in the polymerization assay is indeed forming an intermolecular contact region of the polymer, the molecular variant studies will result in an increased solubility of deoxy Hb S. The absence of the stabilization energy provided by this particular intermolecular contact region of mutant Hb S allows the mutant deoxy Hb S to remain in solution even at a protein concentration at which the parent Hb S is not soluble. If the particular mutation site under investigation is not involved in the contact region, it will not influence the polymerization process (i.e., it will not influence the solubility of Hb S).

Bookchin, Nagel, and colleagues have used the above experimental strategy with a wide variety of β-chain variants of Hb and have delineated the inter-molecular contact residues of the β-chain (38, 50). Hb C$_{Harlem}$ (Glu-6[β]→ Val; Asp-73[β]→ Asn) gels less readily than Hb S (37), implicating the role of the Asp-73(β) in the polymerization reaction. Complementary, and also confirma-tory, to this information is the observation that Hb Korle-Bu (Asp-73[β] → Asn) participated less readily in the gelation of Hb S compared to that of Hb A (38). Thus, Asp-73(β) appears to have an active role in the polymerization process. On the other hand, β-chain variants with a mutation of Glu-121 (to Lysine in the Hb O$_{Arab}$ (51), and to Gln in Hb D$_{Los Angeles}$) (52) interact strongly with Hb S, (i.e., a mixture of Hb S and these mutant hemoglobins gels readily), com-parable to that of a mixture of Hb A and Hb S. The various β-chain contact residues are listed in Table 2.1.

Table 2.2
α-Chain Intermolecular Contact Regions of Deoxy Hb S

Position	Structure	Influence on Inhibits	Polymerization Potentiates
α^6	Asp → Ala		+
α^{11}	Lys → Glu	+	
α^{16}	Lys → Glu	+	
α^{20}	His → Glu	+	
α^{23}	Glu → Gln	+	
α^{47}	Asp → His	+	
α^{54}	Glu → Gln	+	
α^{68}	Ans → Lys	+	
α^{75}	Asp → Lys		+
α^{78}	Asn → Lys	+	
α^{116}	Glu → Lys	+	

Source: Compiled from data in RE Benesch, S Kwong, R Benesch, et al., Location and bond type of intermolecular contacts in the polymerization of hemoglobin S, *Nature* 269 (1976): 772; RE Benesch, S Yung, R Benesch, et al., α-chain contacts in the polymerization of sickle hemoglobin, *Nature* 260 (1976): 219; and RE Benesch, S Kwong, R Edalji et al., α-chain mutations with opposite effects on the gelation of hemoglobin S, *J Biol Chem* 254 (1979): 8169.

The contact residue regions of α-chain in the polymer have been identified by R. E. Benesch, R. Benesch, and colleagues (53–55). In their studies, β^S chains were hybridized with mutant α-chains to generate new molecular variants of Hb S. The gelation behavior of a number of these molecular variants of Hb S have lead to the identification of many of the α-chain contact residues, and these have been summarized in Table 2.2. Most of the intermolecular contact regions are indeed the contact residues implicated by x-ray diffraction and electron microscopic studies. Thus, this molecular engineering approach is complementary to the crystallographic and electron microscopic studies.

The gelation experiments with Hb S and non-S Hb may fail to provide some of the unique structural interpretations that one may wish to delineate from such experiments using the molecular variants. Simple mixing experiments certainly fail to establish whether the contact site that is being investigated is cis or trans to the Val-6(β) contact site (primary site). More definite information could, however, be obtained by refining these experimental protocols. A mixture of Hb S and non-S Hb will contain the hybrid tetramer of the type α2βsβx, besides the two parent molecules (48), thus making the interpretation of the results of the gelation experiments very difficult. However, if the two Hb samples are deoxygenated before mixing, the hybrid tetramers are not generated (42, 48). Asymmetric hybrids of the type α2βsβx could also be chemically cross-linked to prevent the dissociation and formation of symmetrical tetramers (56, 57). Such an approach is very useful to generate the information about the cis–Trans position of the contact residues with respect to Val-6(β). Using such refined protocol, it has been demonstrated that the Asp-73(β) contact region is trans to the Val-6(β) region. The preparation of molecular variants using genetic engineering approaches or semisynthetic approaches will have to be adopted to locate the contact sites cis to Val-6(β). In the years ahead, we should certainly see more of these approaches being used to delineate the energetics of the interactions of the contact regions.

CHEMICAL MODIFIERS OF Hb S INFLUENCING POLYMERIZATION

Chemical modification studies of Hb S have helped us to understand the role and the reactivity of a number of side chain functional groups of amino acid residues of the intermolecular contact region of the protein and are in some respects complementary to the studies with the molecular variants of Hb S. Many reagents have been shown to increase the solubility of deoxy Hb S as a consequence of the modification of one or more functional groups of the protein.

Broadly, the chemical modifiers of Hb S are of two types: covalent and noncovalent. Urea and guanidine hydrochloride are the noncovalent reagents that first showed the inhibition of the polymerization reaction. These increase the solubility by interfering with some of the noncovalent intermolecular interactions of deoxy Hb S in much the same way as the mutations in molecular variants of Hb S perturb the intermolecular interactions. The studies with covalent modifiers are complementary to the molecular engineering approach (the preparation of hybrid Hb S) and try to probe the chemical reactivity of one or more of the functional groups of the amino acid residues of contact regions.

NONCOVALENT MODIFIERS OF POLYMERIZATION

With the recognition of the major role of the hydrophobic interactions in the polymerization process (36), urea was introduced as an antisickling agent (58, 59). However, because of the high levels of urea needed to disrupt the polymerization reaction, it did not prove to be a very useful therapeutic agent. Nonetheless, it provided the momentum for investigators to look for other antisickling agents and has lead to the investigation of the chemically similar alkyl ureas which contain a urea-like head on an aliphatic side chain (60, 61). The chain length of the aliphatic side of the alkyl ureas appears to correlate directly with the propensity of these reagents to inhibit polymerization (61).

The search for noncovalent stereospecific inhibitors of polymerization that will prevent the gelation of Hb S by competing for the noncovalent interaction of one or more of the intermolecular contact sites of the polymer is an interesting approach that has been investigated by many researchers (62–65). The better understanding of the areas of the intermolecular contact region as a consequence of x-ray and, electron microscopic studies, as well as the solubility studies of new molecular variants of Hb S, have provided a new impetus in this direction. The hypothesis of a stereospecific inhibition was invoked for a proposed inhibition of oligopeptides (63) that might have a conformation in solution resembling the parts of the polypeptide chain of Hb S (66, 67) that form the contact regions between the Hb S tetramer. Based on the immunological cross-reactions, it was suggested by Schechter and his associates that peptides corresponding to the amino terminal sequence of the β^S-chain would have a small but a finite probability of adopting a native-like conformation (68). This probability of adopting the native-like conformation should also afford a propensity for these peptides to compete effectively for Hb S-polymer contact sites. The amino acid phenylalanine and some peptides containing phenylalanine as well as peptides corresponding to the α-amino terminal region of the β^S-chain have been shown to have the antigelation properties (69, 70, 71, 72). Mimicking the conformational restrictions of the native protein into these peptides in order to increase the probability of these peptides adopting the native-like conformation has also been an active area of biochemical research. Design and synthesis of stereospecific inhibitors with a conformation that is sufficiently rigid and complementary to the acceptor site has also been described recently (73). Cliofibrate and its second-generation compound represent another class of noncovalent stereospecific inhibitors that have shown a promising inhibition of polymerization (74).

With the demonstration that stable conformation elements, such as α-helix, could be designed even into shorter segments by appropriately positioned Glu-Lys side chain interactions (75) is expected to stimulate further investigation into the development of noncovalent stereospecific inhibitors of polymerization. We have recently designed these aspects into the peptides of the amino terminal region of the β^S-chain 13 residue segment to increase their helical propensity and are in the process of evaluating the influence of this design on the antigelation property of the parent peptide.

COVALENT MODIFIERS OF SICKLE CELL HEMOGLOBIN

Interest in the inhibition of polymerization of deoxy Hb S by urea has lead to the study of the reaction of cyanate with Hb S by Cerami and Manning (76). Sodium cyanate became the first reported covalent modifier of Hb S with an antigelation influence, and this discovery has laid the foundation for investigations of other covalent modifiers. Under the physiological conditions of pH 7.4 and 37°C, cyanate predominantly reacted at the amino terminal Val-1(α) of Hb S (77). The carbamoylation of this α-amino group of Hb S increased the oxygen affinity of the protein, thereby decreasing the propensity of the carbamoylated Hb S to be converted to the deoxy conformation at a given oxygen tension. This is the primary molecular event that affords the antisickling propensity for the reaction of Hb S with cyanate (78). Besides the dominant reaction at Val-1(α), cyanate was also found to react at the α-amino group of β-chain to a lesser degree compared to that at Val-1(α). This latter derivatization on Val-1(β) has a direct influence on the solubility, in other words, it interfered with the integration of one or more of the intermolecular contact regions of the deoxy protein to form the polymer (74).

Amino groups of proteins represent one of the readily amenable functional groups for derivatization. The inhibition of erythrocyte sickling with cyanate (76) and the increased understanding and appreciation of the role of the interactions of intermolecular contact regions in the polymerization reaction have stimulated a host of other chemical modification studies of Hb S and sickle cell erythrocytes in an attempt to identify and/or establish the role of other side chain functional groups in the polymerization reaction on one hand and as the development of a chemical manipulative procedure to inhibit sickling *in vitro* and/or *in vivo,* on the other hand. Structures of some of the covalent modifiers of Hb S that increase the solubility of the protein are shown in Figure 2.6. Modification of the α-amino group of the α-chain of Hb S with pyridoxal sulfate has been shown to inhibit the polymerization reaction (79, 80). Thus, the influence of derivization by pyridoxal sulfate is distinct from carbamoylation of Val-1(α). The Schiff base adducts of pyridoxal and its derivative with the amino groups of Hb S have significantly higher stability compared to those of the simple aliphatic aldehydes. Aspirin was also found to have an antisickling influence as a consequence of acetylation of the amino groups, predominantly the α-amino group of Val-1(β) (81, 82). Several other aliphatic and aromatic aldehydes have also been tested as potential antipolymerizing as well as antisickling agents (83).

Glyceraldehyde, an aldotriose (2,3-dihydroxypropionaldehyde), is another aliphatic aldehyde that exhibits selectivity for amino groups of Hb S (84, 85). In addition, it has shown a very good antisickling, as well as antipolymerizing influence (80). The chemistry of this reaction also turns out to be interesting (86). The reaction of this α-hydroxyaldehyde is analogous to the nonenzymatic glycosylation reaction of proteins with glucose (Figure 2.7). The initial reversible Schiff base adducts of the aldotriose (glyceraldehyde) with the amino group of proteins undergoes an intramolecular rearrangement reaction, known as the Amadori rearrangement (87–89). The resulting product, a 2-oxo, 3 hydroxypropyl derivative of the amino group (i.e., the ketoamine adduct of Hb S) has a higher stability compared to its parent Schiff base adduct (90). The formation of the ketoamine adduct shows a high selectivity; in other words, there is a degree of site selectivity in this reaction (91). Not all the amino groups of Hb S that show the propensity to form aldimine exhibit the same potential for the formation of ketoamine adducts. Thus, the mechanistic aspects of ketoamine formation are distinct from aldimine formation, the latter being predominantly dictated by the pKa of the amino groups. Though the propensity of Val-1(α) and Val-1(β) to form aldimine is nearly the same, the propensity of the aldimine at Val-1(α) to rearrange to ketoamine adduct is nearly an order of magnitude slower than that of Val-1(β) (92). Thus, the sites of Hb S that form the ketoamine adducts with glyceraldehyde have a microenvironment that could catalyze the intramolecular rearrangement of the Schiff base adducts of glyceraldehyde to the ketoamine

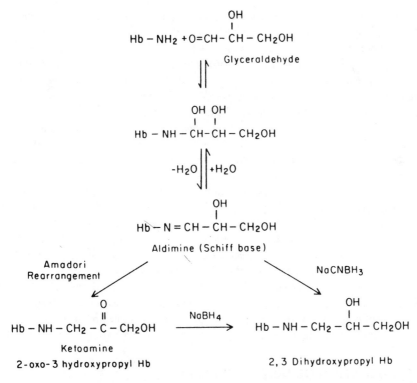

Figure 2.7. Schematic representation of the covalent modification of Hb S with glyceraldehyde.

reaction, a dihydroxypropyl group is placed on Lys-16(α) and the positive charge of the original amino group is retained. Nonetheless, both types of perturbations increase the solubility of Hb S.

Thus, the reaction of glyceraldehyde with Hb S suggests that some, if not all, of the side chain functional groups of the intermolecular amino acid residues of contact regions may dictate some unusual reactivity. It also raises the possibility of whether the stereochemistry around Lys-16(α) that is responsible for the facile Amadori reagent could play some role in providing the complementary surface for the noncovalent interactions that are present at this intermolecular contact region of deoxy Hb S fiber.

In addition to Lys-16(α), Val-1(β) of Hb S is also modified by a glyceraldehyde to a considerable degree during the nonreductive modification of the protein (87). The alkyl chains can be readily introduced onto the α-amino groups of both the α- and β-chains through reductive alkylation (modification of the protein with an aldehyde in the presence of sodium cyanoborohydride) using a limiting concentration of aliphatic aldehydes (94). Ethyl, hydroxyethyl, carboxymethel, dihydroxypropyl, and dihydroxyisopropyl groups have been introduced on the Val-1(β) and/or Val-1(α) of Hb S through this reductive alkylation procedure (95).

These substitutions have shown that the presence of alkyl chains on the amino terminals of either chain increases the solubility of deoxy Hb S. The presence of a ketoamine adduct of glucose on Val-1(β) of Hb S has also been shown to have an antipolymerizing influence (96). Thus, the antisickling potential of glyceraldehyde is apparently a consequence of the perturbation of two contact regions, namely Val-1(β) and Lys-16(α). The potential therapeutic value of an antisickling agent should be higher if the test antisickling reagent is targeted to two or more intermolecular contact sites and the antipolymerizing influence of derivatization at each site is at least additive, if not synergetic. (See also the section on additivity/synergy in the antipolymerization influence of the perturbation of intermolecular contact regions.)

The other amino group reagents that have been tried as covalent modifiers of Hb S to increase the solubility of deoxy Hb S include the imidates (97–100) and diaspirins (101–103). Methylacetyl phosphate has been recently introduced as an acetylating agent of the amino group of the anion-binding sites of Hb S (104). Various analogues of double-headed aspirins have also been used, which introduce specific intramolecular (interchain, intratetramer) covalent cross-links (97–99). The cross-links introduced by these diaspirins increased the solubility of deoxy Hb S. The high specificity with which these cross-links could be generated has also provided a new methodology for the formation of heterodimers to dissect out cis–trans positions of various intermolecular contact regions.

MODIFICATION OF HISTIDINE RESIDUES

The reaction of nitrogen mustard with Hb S has been shown to increase the solubility of deoxy Hb S. The reaction of nitrogen mustard shows a good selectivity to His-2(β) (105–107). Under suitable conditions, this compound could also cross the erythrocyte membrane and react with Hb S in a reasonably specific fashion. The modification of the sulfhydryl groups of Hb S through a thiol sulfide exchange reaction has also shown a good antipolymerizing influence (108).

AMIDATION OF CARBOXYL GROUPS

A number of side chain carboxyl groups of Hb S have also been implicated as part of the intermolecular contact regions (11,12). However, the carboxylates of proteins are more difficult targets for chemical modification compared to the amino groups, and generally require conditions of pH 4.0 for modification by amidation. Even more acidic conditions, as well as anhydrous conditions, are needed to carry out the esterification reactions. However, in view of the unusual reactivity of Lys-16(α), an intramolecular contact residue for nonreductive modification with glyceraldehyde, it is conceivable that some of the carboxylates of contact regions may have a higher pKa and may be accessible for amidation around neutral pH. Indeed, some of the carboxyl groups of Hb S were found to be accessible for carbodiimide-mediated amidation around pH 6.0 and at room

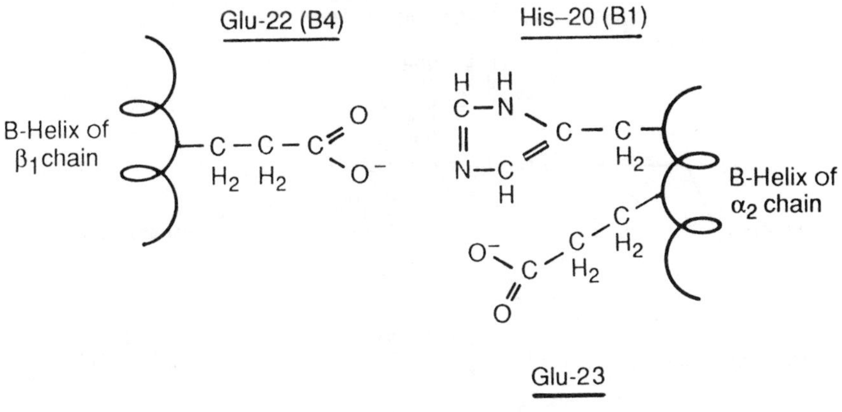

Figure 2.8. Schematic representation of the carboxylate–imidazole interaction of the intermolecular contact region of deoxy Hb S.

temperature (109). A very high degree of site selectivity was observed in the amidation reaction, and the amine used for amidation also dictated the site selectivity of the reaction considerably. With glycine ester, Glu-43(β) was the most predominant site of amidation, whereas with glucosamine and galactosamine, the gamma-carboxylates of both Glu-22(β) and Glu-43(β) are derivatized to nearly the same degree (110). Both these residues have been implicated as the intermolecular contact region by x-ray crystallography (12). Consistent with this finding, amidation of these sites increased the solubility of deoxy Hb S (111).

The high reactivity and the selectivity of the gamma-carboxylates of these two glutamic acid residues (112) of Hb S which are also the amino acid residues of intermolecular contact regions, making these reactive carboxylates ideal candidates to pursue the changes in the reactivity of these residues as the protein undergoes deoxygenation or the deoxyprotein undergoes the polymerization reaction. The Glu-22(β)/His-20(α) interaction is an intrastrand contact region (Figure 2.8), and Glu-43(β) is an interfiber contact region implicated by studies of Padlan and Love (12). Thus, a comparative study of the chemical reactivity of these two carboxylates (i.e., pKa) during the progress curve of polymerization could yield information when the reactivity of intrastrand contact site changes before that of an interfiber contact site. To further facilitate the amidation studies, the selectivity of the reaction has been increased by using N-hydroxysulfosuccinimide (NHS) as the "rescuer" of the activated carboxyl groups in order to get a quantitative amidation of activated carboxylates (Figure 2.9). In the presence of NHS, the amidation of carboxylate appears to correspond to their pKa. It is conceivable that as the concentration of Hb S increases, the pKa of these carboxylates may change. In fact, we have recently seen that in the pregelation stage of deoxy Hb S, the overall reactivity of the carboxylates for amidation is increased by about 20% (113). Further studies should help to

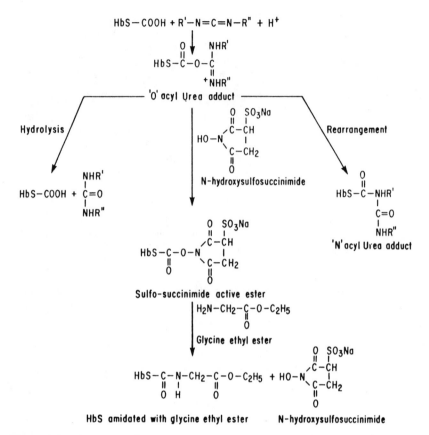

Figure 2.9. Chemistry of the amidation of carboxylates of Hb S.

determine whether the increase in the reactivity is a structural element that facilitates these sites to take part (i.e., to interact with the complementary site) in the nucleation or growth or alignment phases of the polymerization.

ADDITIVITY AND/OR SYNERGY IN THE ANTIPOLYMERIZATION INFLUENCE OF THE PERTURBATION OF THE INTERMOLECULAR CONTACT REGION

A number of amino acid residues of α- and β^s-chains of Hb S have been implicated by x-ray crystallographic and electron microscopic studies. The stabilizing influence of these intertetrameric contact regions have been demonstrated by studying the functional consequences of the mutations of the contact region by preparing new molecular variants and/or derivatives of Hb S. Except in the case of the Asp-47(α) mutation, the concentration of the protein in the gel is nearly the same as that of the gel of unmodified Hb S. This suggests that the structure of the gel of most variants is comparable to that of Hb S. Of considerable interest is the observation that the perturbations of none of the regions, either by mutations or by chemical modification studies of intermolecular contact residue so far, could completely neutralize the polymerizing influence of mutation at the sixth position of the β-chain. Thus, none of the mutation studies so far are capable of restoring the solubility of Hb S to a level comparable to that of Hb A. This can be considered as a clear reflection of the strong stabilizing interaction provided to the polymerization reaction by the interaction of the Val-6(β) region with the acceptor pocket. Therefore, as the next level of structural analysis of interactions of the intertetrameric interactions by deoxy Hb S, it seems reasonable to engineer mutations or chemical perturbations or two or more intertetrameric contact regions of Hb S and determine the additivity and/or possible synergy of two or more perturbations on the solubility of deoxy Hb S. However, the unavailability of α-chains with two or more mutations, as well as β^s-chains with additional mutations in it, is the rate-limiting factor for undertaking these studies. The preparation of molecular variants by genetic engineering or the semisynthesis of chains are the avenues that are available to pursue these aspects of the polymerization process.

In the meanwhile, approaches to chemical modification have been sought for generating information about these aspects of the polymerization reaction. Simply, this involves the use of two or more chemical modification approaches, each of which has been previously shown to have a high selectivity for a particular functional group of a residue implicated to be part of the intertetrameric contact region. As discussed earlier, amidation with glycine ethyl ester is highly selective to the gamma-carboxylate of Glu-43(β), and this modification increases the solubility of deoxy Hb S. Similarly, hydroxyethylation of Val-1(α) and Val-1(β) also increases the solubility of Hb S. Amidated Hb S has been now subjected to reductive hydroxyethylation to see the cumulative effect of hydroxyethylation and amidation of Hb S on the solubility (114). The results of these studies have clearly shown the additivity of the solubilizing influence of amidation and hydroxyethylation of Hb S. On the other hand, the influence of reductive alkylation of Val-1(α) and Val-1(β) with galacturonic acid on the solubility of Hb S are not additive (115). Reductive alkylation of either Val-1(α) or Val-1(β) increased the solubility of Hb S by about 20 percent; however, the solubility of Hb S with both of these modifications did not exhibit the additivity. Thus, from the results of these derivatives of Hb S with two modifications, it is clear that an interaction linkage map of the intermolecular contact regions will be essential to understand the mechanistic and energetic aspects of this macromolecular assembly process. This macromolecular assembly process could be considered as the higher order of protein folding/assembly reaction (i.e., the generation of quinary structure). Protein engineering studies of intermolecular contact regions of Hb S should help us to generate such an interaction linkage map, and the results of these studies would also complement with the current electron microscopic studies delineating the various intermolecular contact regions.

MUTATIONS OF Hb S POTENTIATING THE POLYMERIZATION

Just as the additivity and/or synergy of the antipolymerizing influence of the mutations/chemical modification of amino acid residues of intermolecular contact regions of deoxy Hb S seen in the chemical modification studies, it is also conceivable that mutations at some sites of Hb S could have a polymerization potentiating influence; namely, these facilitate the polymerization reaction. This would imply that such sites, if they exist, show additivity and/or synergy with the polymerizing influence of Val-6(β). Two such sites of the α-chain have been identified by Benesch et al., (55) and the result suggests that this macromolecular assembly (generation of the quinary structure of deoxy Hb S) represents a dynamic event of competing noncovalent interactions. One set of interactions facilitates the polymerization and the other destabilizes the polymerization reaction.

The two contact sites, the mutations of which facilitate the polymerization, are Ala-6(α) and Tyr-74(α) (55). Similarly, in the β-chain the influence of Lys-66(β)$\rightarrow$ Glu mutation has been shown to have a potentiating influence. The polymerizing influence of the mutations identified by Benesch et al. (55) is latent in the absence of the Val-6(β) mutation. The additivity/synergy of the polymerizing influence of these secondary potentiating sites could also be investigated by preparing double mutants using genetic engineering or semisynthetic methods. β_{23} and β_{121} are the two polymerizations potentiating contact sites of the β-chain.

GENERAL CONCLUSIONS

The brief discussion of the molecular aspects of the polymerization of deoxy Hb S presented in this chapter clearly demonstrates that the polymerization reaction is a stereospecific macromolecular assembly process and should be considered as the higher order protein folding/assembly reaction. The assembly reaction represents a dynamic event of a number of intermolecular (intertetrameric) interactions, some potentiating the polymerization, and some presumably destabilizing intermediates of the polymerization reaction. Given the fact that Hb A contains all the intermolecular contact regions of deoxy Hb S except the Val-6(β), it is certainly intriguing to see that the presence of Glu-6(β) is very critical to keep this oxygen-carrying protein in a soluble (unpolymerized) state under the physiological conditions, though the mutation is silent with respect to the function of the protein (i.e., the binding of oxygen). Thus, Glu-6(β) of Hb S has a very crucial structural role. In this era of protein engineering studies of structure and function relationships of proteins, we should caution ourselves that the mere absence of a detectable influence of a mutation on the enzymic activity or the receptor binding *in vitro* should not be construed as the lack of a structural or physiological role for a particular mutation *in vivo*. If nature had not presented us with this interesting molecular variant of Hb A, namely Hb S, one wonders whether hemoglobinologists would have attempted to study the possible structural and physiological roles of Glu-6(β) through mutational analysis, simply based on the structural information derived from the x-ray crystallographic analysis of Hb A. This only reflects the fact that we still have a long way to go to decode all the "structural memory" (such as the quinary structural memory) that is coded within the given amino acid sequence of a segment of a protein and in identifying the parts played by other segments of the protein in facilitating the translation of that structural memory of a particular segment *in vivo*.

ACKNOWLEDGMENTS

The results of the author's laboratory research presented in this article are supported by NIH Grants HL-27183, DK-35869, HL-38665, and a grant-in-aid from the American Heart Association, New York City Affiliate. The author is also indebted to Drs. G. Sahni and R. P. Roy for their helpful comments on the manuscript. The assistance of Ms. Sara Ruiz in the preparation of the manuscript is gratefully acknowledged.

REFERENCES

1. Pauling L, Itano HA, Singer SJ, et al.: Sickle cell anemia: A molecular disease. *Science* 110 (1949): 543–548.
2. Dean J, and Schechter AN: Sickle cell anemia: Molecular and cellular bases of therapeutic approaches. *N Engl J Med* 299 (1978): 752–763; 804–811; 863–870.
3. Bunn HF, and Forget BG: *Hemoglobin: Molecular and genetic aspects*. Philadelphia: W. B. Saunders, 1986.
4. Noguchi CT, and Schechter AN: Sickle cell hemoglobin polymerization in solution and in cells. *Ann Rev Biophys Chem* 14 (1983): 239–263.
5. Schechter AN, Noguchi CT, and Rogers GP: Sickle cell disease. In G Stamatoyannopoulos, AW Neinhus, P Leder, et al. eds.; *Molecular basis of blood diseases*, pp. 179–218. Philadelphia: W. B. Saunders, 1987.
6. Marotta CA, Wilson JT, Forget BG, et al.: Human β-globin messenger RNA. *J Biol Chem* 252 (1977): 5040–5053.
7. Embury S: The clinical pathophysiology of sickle cell disease. *Ann Rev Med* 37 (1986): 361.
8. Benesch RE, Edalji R, Kwang S, et al.: Oxygen affinity as an index of hemoglobin S polymerization: A new micromethod. *Analytical Biochem* 89 (1978): 162–173.
9. Ho C, Fund LW, and Lin KC: Recent high resolution proton nuclear magnetic resonance studies of sickle cell hemoglobin. In JI Hercules, GL Cottam, MR Waterman, et al., eds.: *Proceedings of the symposium on molecular and cellular aspects of sickle cell disease*, pp. 65–86 (DHEW Publication 76–1007), 1976.
10. Fronticielli C: Effect of the $\beta6$ Glu $\rightarrow$ Val mutation on the optical activity of hemoglobin S and β subunits. *J Biol Chem* 253 (1978): 2288–2291.

11. Wishner WC, Ward KB, Lattman EE, et al.: Crystal structure of sickle cell deoxy hemoglobin at 5 A° resolution. *J Mol Biol* 98 (1975): 179.

12. Padlan EA, and Love WE: Refined crystal structure of deoxyhemoglobin S. *J Biol Chem* 260 (1985): 8280.

13. Rosen LS, and Magdoff-Fairchild G: X-ray diffraction studies of 14 filament models of deoxygenated hemoglobin S fibers. I: Models based on electron micrograph reconstruction. *J Mol Biol* 183 (1985): 565.

14. Edelstein SJ: Molecular topology in crystals and fibers of hemoglobin S. *J Mol Biol* 150 (1981): 557.

15. Potel MJ, Williams TC, Vassar RJ, et al.: Macrofiber structure and the dynamics of sickle cell hemoglobin crystallization. *J Mol Biol* 177 (1984): 819.

16. Watowich SJ, Gross LJ, and Josephs R: Intermolecular contacts within sickle hemoglobin fibers. *J Mol Biol* 209 (1989): 821–828.

17. Moffat K, and Gibson H: The rate of polymerization and depolymerization of sickle cell hemoglobin. *Biochem Biophys Res Commun* 61 (1974): 237.

18. Hofrichter J, Ross PD, and Eaton WA: Kinetics and mechanism of deoxy HbS gelation: A new approach to understanding sickle cell disease. *Proc Natl Acad Sci USA* 71 (1974): 4864.

19. Malfa R, and Steinhardt J: A temperature dependent latent period in the aggregation of sickle cell hemoglobin. *Biochem Biophys Res Commun* 59 (1974): 887.

20. Harris JW, and Bensusan HB: The kinetics of the sol gel transformation of deoxy hemoglobin S by continuous monitoring of viscosity. *J Lab Clin Med* 86 (1975): 564.

21. Eaton WA, Hofrichter J, Ross PD, et al.: Comparison of sickle cell hemoglobin gelation kinetics by NMR and optical methods. *Biochem Biophys Res Commun* 69 (1976): 538.

22. Waterman MR, and Cottam GL: Kinetics of the polymerization of hemoglobin S. Studies below normal erythrocyte hemoglobin concentration. *Biochem Biophys Res Commun* 73 (1976): 639.

23. Shibata K, Waterman MR, and Cottam, GL: Alteration in the rate of deoxy HbS polymerization. Effect of pH and percentage of oxygenation. *J Biol Chem* 252 (1977): 7468.

24. Ferrone FA, Hofrichter J, Sunshine HR, et al.: Kinetic studies on photolysis induced gelation of sickle cell hemoglobin suggest a new mechanism. *Biophys J* 32 (1980): 361.

25. Ferrone FA, Hofrichter J, and Eaton WA: Kinetics of sickle hemoglobin polymerization. I: Studies using temperature jump and laser photolysis techniques. *J Mol Biol* 183 (1985): 591.

26. Ferrone FA, Hofrichter J, and Eaton WA: Kinetics of sickle hemoglobin polymerization. II: A dual nucleation mechanism. *J Mol Biol* 183 (1985): 611.

27. Wilson WW, Luzzana MR, Penniston JT, et al.: Pregelation aggregation of sickle cell hemoglobin. *Proc Natl Acad Sci USA* 71 (1974): 1260.

28. Elbaum D, and Nagel RL: Aggregation of deoxy hemoglobin S at low concentration. *J Biol Chem* 251 (1976): 7657.

29. Danish EH, and Harris JW: Viscosity studies of deoxyhemoglobin S: Evidence for formation of microaggregates during lag phase. *J Lab Clin Med* 101 (1983): 515.

30. Russu IM, and Ho CH: Proton longitudinal relaxation investigations of histidyl residues of normal human adult and sickle deoxyhemoglobin: Evidence for existence

of pregelation aggregations in sickle deoxyhemoglobin solutions. *Proc Natl Acad Sci USA* 77 (1980): 6577.

31. Hu CC, and Johnson ME: Spin label detection of aggregation of deoxygenated sickle cell hemoglobin under nongelling conditions. *FEBS Lett* 125 (1981): 231.

32. Briehl RW: Solid like behavior of unsheared sickle hemoglobin gels and the effects of shear. *Nature* 288 (1980): 622.

33. Briehl RW: The effects of shear on the delay time for the gelation of deoxy hemoglobin S. *Blood Cells* 8 (1982): 201.

34. Magdoff-Fairchild B, and Chiu EE: X-ray diffraction studies of fibers and crystals of deoxygenated sickle cell hemoglobin. *Proc Natl Acad Sci USA* 76 (1979): 223.

35. Allison AC: Properties of sickle cell hemoglobin. *Biochem J* 65 (1957): 212.

36. Murayama M: Molecular mechanism of red cell "sickling." *Science* 153 (1966): 145.

37. Bookchin RM, and Nagel RL: Molecular interactions of sickling hemoglobins. In H Abraham, JF Bertle and DL Wethers, eds.: *Sickle cell disease*, p. 140. St. Louis: C. V. Mosby, 1974.

38. Bookchin RM, Nagel RL, and Ranney HM: Structure and properties of Hb C-Harlem, a human hemoglobin variant with amino acid substitutions at two residues of the β-polypeptide chain. *J Biol Chem* 242 (1967): 248.

39. Bookchin RM, Nagel RL, and Ranney HM: The effect of $\beta^{73\ Asn}$ on the interaction of sickling hemoglobin S. *Biochim Biophys Acta* 221 (1970): 373.

40. Behe MJ, and Englander SW: Mixed gelation theory: Kinetics, equilibrium and gel incorporation in sickle hemoglobin mixtures. *J Mol Biol* 133 (1979): 137.

41. Ross PD, and Minton AP: Analysis of non-ideal behavior in concentrated hemoglobin solutions. *J Mol Biol* 112 (1977): 437.

42. Goldberg MA, Husson MA, and Bunn HF: Participation of hemoglobins A and F in polymerization of sickle hemoglobin. *J Biol Chem* 252 (1977): 3414–3421.

43. Sunshine HR, Hofrichter J, and Eaton WA: Gelation of sickle cell hemoglobin in mixtures with normal adult and fetal hemoglobins. *J Mol Biol* 133 (1979): 435–467.

44. Waterman MR, Cottam GL, and Shibata K: Inhibitory effect of deoxyhemoglobin A_2 on the rate of deoxyhemoglobin S polymerization. *J Mol Biol* 128 (1979): 337.

45. Cheetam RC, Huenhs ER, and Rosemeyer MA: Participation of hemoglobins A, F, A_2 and C in the polymerization of hemoglobin S. *J Mol Biol* 129 (1979): 45.

46. Benesch RE, Edalji R, Benesch R, et al.: Solubilization of hemoglobin S by other hemoglobins. *Proc Natl Acad Sci USA* 77 (1980): 5130.

47. Bunn HF, Noguchi CT, Hofrichter HJ, et al.: Molecular and cellular pathogenesis of hemoglobin S disease. *Proc Natl Acad Sci USA* 79 (1982): 7527.

48. Bookchin RM, Nagel RL, and Balazs T: Role of hybrid tetramer formation in gelation of hemoglobin S. *Nature* 265 (1975): 667.

49. Singer K, and Singer L: The gelling phenomenon of sickle cell hemoglobin: Its biological and diagnostic significance. *Blood* 8 (1953): 1008.

50. Nagel RL, Johnson L, Bookchin RM, et al.: β-chain contact sites in hemoglobin S polymer. *Nature* 283 (1980): 832.

51. Milner PF, Miller C, Grey R, et al.: Hemoglobin O-Arab in four Negro families and its interaction with hemoglobin S and hemoglobin C. *N Engl J Med* 283 (1970): 1417.

52. McCurdy PR: Clinical and physiological studies in a Negro with sickle cell hemoglobin D disease. *N Engl J Med* 262 (1960): 961.
53. Benesch RE, Kwong S, Benesch R, et al.: Location and bond type of intermolecular contacts in the polymerization of hemoglobin S. *Nature* 269 (1976): 772.
54. Benesch RE, Yung S, Benesch R, et al.: α-chain contacts in the polymerization of sickle hemoglobin. *Nature* 260 (1976): 219.
55. Benesch RE, Kwong S, Edalji R, et al.: α-chain mutations with opposite effects on the gelation of hemoglobin S. *J Biol Chem* 254 (1979): 8169.
56. Bookchin RM, Balazs T, Nagel RL, et al.: Polymerization of hemoglobin SA hybrid tetramers. *Nature* 269 (1977): 526.
57. Benesch RE, Kwong S, and Benesch R: The effect of α-chain mutations cis and trans to the β-6 mutation on the polymerization of sickle cell hemoglobin. *Nature* 299 (1982): 231.
58. Nalbandian RM, Henry RL, and Barnhart MI: Sickle cell disease: Clinical advances by Murayama molecular hypothesis. *Melit Med* 137 (1972): 215–220.
59. Nalbandian RM, Schultz G, and Lusher JM: Sickle cell crisis terminated by intravenous urea in sugar solutions: A preliminary report. *Am J Med Sci* 261 (1971): 309–324.
60. Elbaum D, Nagel RL, and Bookchin RM: Effect of alkylureas on the polymerization of hemoglobin S. *Proc Natl Acad Sci USA* 71 (1974): 4718–4722.
61. Elbaum D, Roth EF Jr., Neuman G, et al.: Molecular and cellular effects of antisickling concentration of alkylureas. *Blood* 48 (1976): 273–282.
62. Yang JT: Intermolecular contacts of deoxy hemoglobin S, a hypothesis and search for antisickling agents. *Biochem Biophys Res Commun* 63 (1975): 232–238.
63. Kobota S, and Yang JT: Oligopeptides as potential antiaggregation agents for deoxy hemoglobin S. *Proc Natl Acad Sci USA* 74 (1977): 5431–5434.
64. Schechter AN: Synthetic β^s oligopeptides. II: Use as potential stereospecific inhibitors of hemoglobin S gelation. In JS Hercules, GL Cottam, and MR Waterman, eds.: *Proceedings of the Symposium on Molecular and Cellular Aspects of Sickle Cell Disease,* pp. 317–326 (CDHEW Publication), 1976.
65. Poillon WN: Noncovalent inhibition of sickle hemoglobin gelation: Effect of alphatic alcohols, amides and ureas. *Biochemistry* 19 (1980): 3194–3199.
66. Sachs DH, Schechter AN, Eastlake A, et al.: An immunologic approach to the conformational equilibria of polypeptides. *Proc Natl Acad Sci USA* 69 (1972): 3790–3994.
67. Furie B, Schechter AN, Sachs DH, et al.: An immunological approach to the conformational equilibrium of staphylococcal nuclease. *J Mol Biol* 92 (1975): 497–506.
68. Young NS, Eastlake A, and Schechter AN: The NH_2-terminal region of sickle hemoglobin β-chain. II: Characterization of monospecific antibodies. *J Biol Chem* 251 (1976): 6431–6438.
69. Noguchi CT, and Schechter AN: Effect of amino acids on gelation. Kinetics and solubility of sickle hemoglobin. *Biochem Biophys Res Commun* 74 (1977): 637–642.
70. Noguchi CT, and Schechter AN: The inhibition of sickle hemoglobin gelation by amino acids and related compounds. *Biochemistry* 17 (1978): 5455.
71. Gorecki M, Acquaye CTA, Wilchek M, et al.: Antisickling activity of amino acid benzyl esters. *Proc Natl Acad Sci USA* 77 (1980): 181.

72. Altman J, Gorecki M, Wilchek M, et al.: Synthesis of pyridine derivatives of L-pheynylalanine as antisickling agents. *J Med Chem* 27 (1984): 967.
73. Sheh L, Mokotoff M, and Abraham DJ: Design, synthesis and testing of potential antisickling agents: 9 cyclic tetrapeptides homologs as mimics of the mutation site of hemoglobin S. *Int J Peptide Prot Res* 29 (1987): 509–520.
74. Abraham DJ, Perutz MF, and Phillips SE: Physiological and x-ray studies of potential antisickling agents. *Proc Natl Acad Sci USA* 80 (1983): 824.
75. Margusee S, and Baldwin RL: Helix stabilization by Glu^--Lys^+ salt bridges in short peptides of denovo design. *Proc Natl Acad Sci USA* 84 (1987): 8898–8902.
76. Cerami A, and Manning JM: Potassium cyanate as an inhibitor of sickling of erythrocytes *in vitro*. *Proc Natl Acad Sci USA* 68 (1970): 1180–1183.
77. Njikam N, Jones WM, Nigen AM, et al.: Carbamylations of the chains of hemoglobin S by cyanate *in vitro* and *in vivo*. *J Biol Chem* 248 (1973): 8052.
78. Nigen AM, Njikam N, Lee CK, et al.: Studies on the mechanism of action of cyanate in sickle cell disease: Oxygen affinity and gelling properties of hemoglobin S carbamylated on specific chains. *J Biol Chem* 249 (1974): 6611.
79. Benesch RE, Yung S, Suzuki T, et al.: Pyridoxal compounds as specific reagents for the α and the β N termini of hemoglobin. *Proc Natl Acad Sci USA* 70 (1973): 2595.
80. Benesch R, Benesch RE, and Yung S: Chemical modifications that inhibit gelation of sickle hemoglobin. *Proc Natl Acad Sci USA* 71 (1974): 1504.
81. Klotz JM, and Tam JWO: Acetylation of sickle cell hemoglobin by aspirin. *Proc Natl Acad Sci USA* 70 (1973): 1313–1315.
82. Walder JA, Zuagg RH, Iwaoka RS, et al.: Alternative aspirins as antisickling agents: Acetyl 3:5 dibromosalicylic acid. *Proc Natl Acad Sci USA* 70 (1973): 3707–3710.
83. Klotz IM, Haney DN, and King LC: Rational approaches to chemotherapy: Antisickling agents. *Science* 213 (1981): 724.
84. Nigen AM, and Manning JM: Inhibition of erythrocyte sickling *in vitro* by DL-glyceraldehyde. *Proc Natl Acad Sci USA* 74 (1977): 367–371.
85. Nigen AM, and Manning JM: Effects of glyceraldehyde on the structural and functional properties of sickle erythrocytes. *J Clin Invest* 61 (1978): 11–19.
86. Acharya AS, and Manning JM: Amadori rearrangement of glyceraldehyde-hemoglobin Schiff base adducts. *J Biol Chem* 255 (1980): 7218–7224.
87. Koenig RJ, and Cerami A: Synthesis of hemoglobin A_{1c} in normal and diabetic mice: Potential model for basement membrane thickening. *Proc Natl Acad Sci USA* 72 (1975): 3687.
88. Bunn HF, Haney DN, Gabbay KH, et al.: Further identification of the nature and linkage of the carbohydrate in HbA^{1c}. *Biochem Biophys Res Commun* 67 (1975): 103.
89. Higgins PJ, and Bunn HF: Kinetic analysis of the nonenzymic glycosylation of hemoglobin. *J Biol Chem* 256 (1981): 5204–5208.
90. Acharya AS, and Sussman LG: The reversibility of the ketoamine linkages of aldoses with proteins. *J Biol Chem* 259 (1984): 4372–4378.
91. Acharya AS, and Manning JM: Reactivity of the amino groups of carbonmonoxy-hemoglobin S with glyceraldehyde. *J Biol Chem* 255 (1980): 1406.
92. Acharya AS, Sussman LG, and Manning JM: Schiff base adducts of glyceraldehyde with hemoglobin: Differences in the Amadori rearrangement at the α-amino groups. *J Biol Chem* 258 (1983): 2296–2302.

 93. Acharya AS, Sussman LG, Jones WM, et al.: Inhibition of deoxy hemoglobin S polymerization by glyceraldehyde. *Analytical Biochem* 136 (1984): 101–109.
 94. Acharya AS, and Sussman LG: Reductive hydroxyethylation of hemoglobin A. *J Biol Chem* 258 (1983): 13761–13767.
 95. Acharya AS, Sussman LG, and Manning JM: Selectivity in the modification of the α-amino groups of hemoglobin on reductive alkylation with aliphatic carbonyl compounds. *J Biol Chem* 260 (1983): 6039–6046.
 96. Abraham EC, and Elseweidy E: Nonenzymic glycosylation influences HbS polymerization. *Hemoglobin* 10 (1986): 173–183.
 97. Pennathur-Das R, Heath RH, Mentzer WC, et al.: Modification of hemoglobin S with dimethyl adipimidate. Contribution of intertetrameric cross-linking to changes in properties. *Biochim Biophys Acta* 706 (1982): 80.
 98. Chao TL, and Berenfeld MR: Prevention of the immune agglutination of methylacetimidate reacted sickle erythrocytes by prior reaction with pyridoxal 5-phosphate. *J Biol Chem* 256 (1971): 5324.
 99. Guis MS, Lande WM, Mohandas N, et al.: Prolongation of sickle cell survival by dimethyl adipimidation compromised by immune sensitization. *Blood* 64 (1984): 161.
100. Chao TL, Berenfeld MR, and Gabuzda TG: Inhibition of sickling by methyl acetimidate. *FEBS Lett* 62 (1976): 57.
101. Walder JA, Zaugg RH, Walder RY, et al.: Diaspirins that cross-link β-chains of hemoglobin: Bis(3,5-dibromosalicyl) succinate and Bis(3,5-dibromosalicyl) fumarate. *Biochemistry* 18 (1979): 4265.
102. Walder JA, Walder RY, and Arnone A: Development of antisickling compounds that chemically modify hemoglobin S with 2:3 diphosphoglycerate binding site. *J Mol Biol* 141 (1980): 195.
103. Chatterjee Y, Walder RY, Arnone A, et al.: Mechanism for the increase in the solubility of deoxyhemoglobin S due to cross-linking of β-chains between Lys 82β_1 and Lys 82β_2. *Biochemistry* 21 (1982): 5901.
104. Ueno H, Bai Y, and Manning JM: Covalent chemical modifiers of sickle cell hemoglobin. *Ann NY Acad Sci* 565 (1989): 239–246.
105. Roth EF, Nagel RL, Bookchin RM, et al.: Nitrogen mustard: An *in vivo* inhibitor of erythrocyte sickling. *Biochem Biophys Res Commun* 48 (1972): 612.
106. Fung LWM, Ho C, Roth EF, et al.: The alkylation of hemoglobin S by nitrogen mustard. *J Biol Chem* 250 (1975): 4786.
107. Roth EF, Nagel RL, and Bookchin RM: Mechanisms of the inhibitory effect of nitrogen mustard on sickling of hemoglobin S containing red cells. *Clin Res* 21 (1973): 565.
108. Hassan W, Beuzard Y, and Rosa J: Inhibition of erythrocyte sickling by cystamine: A thiol reagent. *Proc Natl Acad Sci USA* 73 (1976): 3288.
109. Seetharam R, Manning JM, and Acharya AS: Specific modification of the carboxyl groups of Hemoglobin S. *J Biol Chem* 258 (1983): 14810–14815.
110. Acharya AS, and Seetharam R: Reactivity of Glu-22(β) of hemoglobin S for admidation with glucosamine. *Biochemistry* 24 (1985): 4885–4890.
111. Kandke LS, and Acharya AS: Influence of amidation of Glu-43(β) on the polymerization of deoxy hemoglobin S. *Ann NY Acad Sci* 565 (1989): 416.
112. Kandke LS, and Acharya AS: Selective amidation of carboxyl groups of the inter-

molecular contact regions of hemoglobin S structural aspects. *J Prot Chem* 8 (1989): 231–237.

113. Rao MJ, and Acharya AS: [unpublished data].
114. Acharya AS, Sussman LG, and Seetharam R: Reductive hydroxyethylation of the α-amino groups of amidated hemoglobin S. *J Prot Chem* 4 (1985): 215–225.
115. Acharya AS: [unpublished data].

3

Pathophysiology of the Sickle Cell

R. Blaine Moore

As described in the previous chapters, the molecular change responsible for sickle cell anemia has been identified as a single nucleotide change in the gene that codes for the β-chain of hemoglobin. More precisely, the triplet nucleotide sequence codes for a valine residue rather than a glutamate residue at position number six of the beta chain. The presence of this valine residue appears to alter the shape of the hemoglobin molecule, particularly in the deoxygenated state, allowing several molecules to associate with one another to form long crystalline rods which can then align to form fibrils. These fibrils may be capable of changing some physical properties of the cell, such as deformability and shape. Upon reoxygenation, the hemoglobin molecules dissociate and dissolve back into the cytoplasm, allowing the cell to regain its original normal state (or apparently so).

The sickle-shaped cells observed through a microscope are often considered to be the hallmark of sickle cell anemia and other sickling disorders, yet these cells possess little or no polymerized hemoglobin. They do not become more strikingly sickled upon *in vitro* deoxygenation, nor do they resume a normal biconcave shape when gassed with pure oxygen. These *irreversibly sickled cells,* as they are termed, have quite different properties than those with normal morphology. Most probably, they contribute to changes in vascular flow, to the way in which other cells in the vascular system interact, and, eventually, to the dysfunction of tissues and organs that are observed clinically. Unfortunately, the mechanism by which hemoglobin polymerization leads to irreversible sickling remains obscure. This chapter will attempt to address some of the effects that hemoglobin polymerization and/or sickling have on cellular metabolism, membrane structure, and cellular membrane physiology.

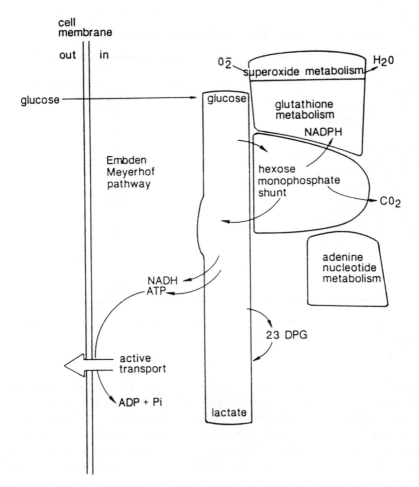

Figure 3.1.   Red cell metabolism.

ERYTHROCYTE METABOLISM

The mature erythrocyte, which lacks a nucleus, mitochondria, endoplasmic reticula, and other organelles, has a more limited metabolic system than other cells (1–3). (See Figure 3.1.) The cytoplasm of erythrocytes contains enzymes that convert glucose to lactate through the Embden-Meyerhof pathway (anaerobic glycolysis). The hexose monophosphate shunt represents a second pathway which arises from glucose-6-phosphate in the Embden-Meyerhof pathway and then, through a number of reactions, returns to this same pathway in the forms of fructose-6-phosphate and glyceraldehyde-3-phosphate. This pathway can be described as one of oxidative glycolysis because of its importance in generating reduced nicotinamide adenine dinucleotide phosphate (NADPH). Shorter path-

Table 3.1
Concentrations of Human Erythrocytle Glycolytic Intermediates

Intermediate	μM
Glucose	5,000
Glucose-6-phosphate	83
Fructose-6-phosphate	14
Fructose-6-phosphate	31
Dihydroxyacetone phosphate	138
Glyceraldehyde-3-phosphate	19
1,2-diphosphoglycerate	1
2,3-diphosphoglycerate	4,000
3-phosphoglycerate	118
2-phosphoglycerate	30
Phosphoenol pyruvate	23
Pyruvate	51
Lactate	2,900
ATP	1,850
ADP	138
Pi	1,000

Source: S Minikami and H Yoshikawa, Thermodynamic considerations on erythrocyte glycolysis, *Biochem Biophys Res Commun* 19 (1965): 347.

ways also exist for the purpose of synthesizing reduced glutathione, converting superoxide to water, and metabolizing adenosine to either adenosine-5'-monophosphate (AMP) (phosphorylation) or inosine (deamination), synthesizing adenosine-5'-triphoshate (ATP) from adenine, synthesizing NAD from nicotinic acid, and so forth. Table 3.1 shows a list of metabolites and their normal concentrations. These pathways are all linked at specific points and serve two major functions: (1) to generate metabolic energy through the formation of high energy phosphates and (2) to generate reducing energy through the formation of metabolites that defend against transient oxidative stress.

The Embden-Meyerhof pathway of glycolysis consists of 11 enzymes whose major purpose is to synthesize reduced nicotinamide adenine dinucleotide (NADH), ATP, and 2,3-diphosphoglycerate (DPG) (Figure 3.2). NADH is needed in the enzymic restoration of ferric methemoglobin to normal ferrous hemoglobin (4). ATP is a high-energy metabolite required in pumping cations such as sodium, potassium, and calcium across the cell membrane and for synthesizing glutathione, an important metabolite used in the removal of hydrogen peroxide (see Figure 3.2). The erythrocyte also contains two unique enzymes, namely diphosphoglyceromutase and diphosphoglycerate phosphatase, which synthesize and dephosphorylate, respectively, 2,3-diphosphoglycerate, an important regulator of hemoglobin oxygen affinity. This side reaction of the glycolytic pathway determines whether the energy stored in 1,3-diphosphoglycerate

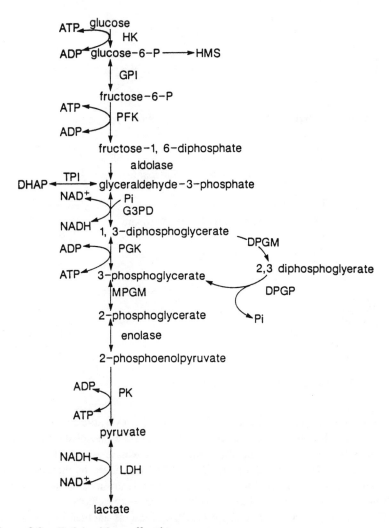

Figure 3.2.   Embden-Meyeroff pathway.

will be used to generate ATP via phosphoglycerate kinase or to synthesize 2,3-diphosphoglycerate via diphosphogyceromutase. The direction of metabolism from 1,3-diphosphoglycerate depends on several factors, including the concentrations of 2,3-DPG and hydrogen ions, which inhibit diphosphoglycerate mutase (DPGM) and the concentration of adenosine-5'-diphosphate (ADP), which activates phosphoglycerate kinase (PGK) and, thereby, the synthesis of ATP. The 3 most important of the 10 or so enzymes in this pathway are hexokinase, phosphofructokinase, and pyruvate kinase, because their reactions are essentially irreversible and they are regulated by the levels of glycolytic products. Both phosphofructokinase and pyruvate kinase are inhibited by ATP, while hexokinase

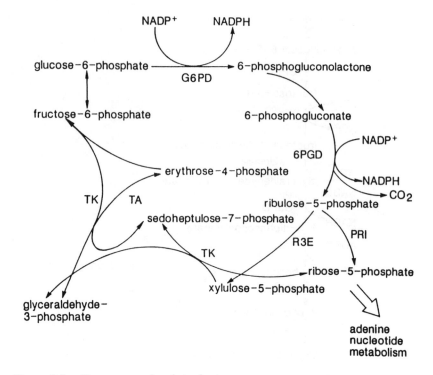

Figure 3.3.   Hexose monophosphate shunt.

is inhibited by its product, glucose-6-phosphate. However, the net effect of ATP inhibition of phosphofructokinase is to cause fructose-6-phosphate and glucose-6-phosphate to accumulate, thereby inhibiting hexokinase as well. The feedback inhibition by ATP of phosphofructokinase (PFK) is relieved by increased levels of AMP. Thus, phosphofructokinase and glycolysis are most active when the cell needs energy as signaled by a low adenylate energy charge.

The hexose monophosphate shunt (HMS) represents another very important side chain of the Embden-Meyerhof pathway. This shunt is comprised of seven enzymes which convert glucose-6-phosphate to glyceraldehyde-3-phosphate and fructose-6-phosphate (refer to Figure 3.3). The major purpose of the HMS is to produce NADPH, an essential molecule which contains reducing equivalents needed for the replenishment of reduced glutathione. NADPH is generated from NADP and glucose-6-phosphate by glucose-6-phosphate dehydrogenase (G6PD). The phosphorylated sugar is converted to 6-phosphogluconolactone, which spontaneously hydrolyzes to 6-phosphogluconate. Alternatively, the gluconolactone may be converted enzymatically by lactomase. The G6PD reaction lies far to the right and is readily inhibited by the product NADPH, thus exhibiting negative feedback on the shunt. The next reaction involves the conversion of 6-phosphogluconate to ribulose-5-phosphate and carbon dioxide. The CO_2 is derived from the first carbon position of glucose. This reaction is catalyzed by 6-phosphogluconate dehydrogenase and, like G6PD, converts NADP to NADPH.

Aside from the formation of NADPH, this reaction is important for the formation of pentoses used for the salvage of nucleotides. Ribulose-5-phosphate is converted to either xylulose-5-phosphate by an epimerase or to ribose-5-phosphate by an isomerase. The latter two pentose phosphates (i.e., ribose-5-phosphate and xylulose-5-phosphate) can be converted to fructose-6-phosphate (of the glycolytic pathway) by transketolase and transaldolase reactions via sedoheptulose-7-phosphate. Alternatively, the hexose monophosphate can be produced from xylulose-5-phosphate and erythrose-4-phosphate (a byproduct of the transaldolase reaction). It is now possible for the fructose-6-phosphate to be converted to glucose-6-phosphate and to be recycled through the hexose monophoshate shunt or for it to proceed normally through the glycolytic pathway to pyruvic acid. The first carbon of the original glucose-6-phosphate is lost during one cycle of the HMS, and the second carbon of this sugar now becomes the first carbon of fructose-6-phosphate following the transketolase reaction. Thus, glucose channeled through the HMS for the first cycle can be assessed by using $^{14}C_1$-glucose and measuring the amount of radioactive CO_2 produced, and glucose-6-phosphate recycled through the HMS can be assessed by using $^{14}C_2$-glucose and measuring the amount of radioactive CO_2.

The formation of pentose phosphates is important because ribose-5-phosphate is directly linked with the metabolism of adenosine and inosine. Two enzymes, namely adenosine kinase and adenosine deaminase, play critical roles in regulating the metabolism of adenosine. The former enzyme phosphorylates adenosine to AMP, which then can form ADP in the presence of adenylate kinase using ATP as a cosubstrate. Adenosine deaminase removes an ammonium group from adenosine to form inosine. In the presence of inorganic phosphate, inosine is split to form ribose-1-phosphate and hypoxanthine. Through phosphoribomutase, ribose-1-phosphate is converted to ribose-5-phosphate, the high-energy phosphate intermediate associated with the HMS. In the presence of ATP, ribose-5-phosphate can be pyrophosphorylated to 5-phosphoribosyl-1-pyrophosphate, which can then be used by phosphoribosyltransferase to convert hypoxanthine to inosine monophosphate or adenine to AMP. High concentrations of adenosine (i.e., about 40 μM) result in deamination of the purine nucleoside, whereas low concentrations of adenosine tend to be preferrentially phosphorylated.

In addition to the metabolism of adenosine, the HMS plays an important role in the removal of hydrogen peroxide through the turnover of glutathione (Figure 3.4). The dissociation of oxygen from hemoglobin is not always homogeneous, and occasionally a heterogeneous split occurs, resulting in the formation of methemoglobin (the ferric form of hemoglobin) and superoxide (a highly reactive species of oxygen). Methemoglobin is converted back to its normal ferrous state by an NADH cytochrome b_5 reductase (referred to in earlier research as methemoglobin reductase). In this regard, the maintenance of normal ferrous hemoglobin depends greatly on the Embden-Meyerhof pathway rather than the hexose

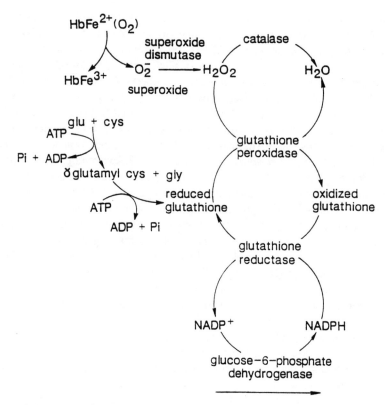

Figure 3.4. Superoxide and glutathione metabolism.

monophosphate shunt. Superoxide anion is made less reactive by its conversion
to hydrogen peroxide. The enzyme responsible for this conversion is superoxide
dismutase. In the human red blood cell, this enzyme is a zinc metalloenzyme.
This may be important in sickle cell anemia since nutritional zinc deficiency is
quite common among people with this disease (this will be discussed in more detail
later). Hydrogen peroxide is not as potent an oxidant as its precursor, superoxide, but
it has a longer half-life and may be converted chemically in the presence of iron to an
extremely potent oxidant, namely, the hydroxyl radical. Fortunately, the red cell contains two enzymes that can rapidly catalyze hydrogen peroxide to water. These enzymes are catalase and glutathione peroxidase. The latter enzyme uses the sulfhydryl
electrons of reduced glutathione to convert hydrogen peroxide to water. In this process, oxidized glutathione (the disulfide form of glutathione) is formed.

The presence of micromolar quantities of this metabolite activates the enzyme
glutathione reductase, whose primary function is to replenish the reduced form
of glutathione needed in the removal of hydrogen peroxide, as mentioned above.
Glutathione reductase uses NADPH, which is produced from glucose-6-
phosphate dehydrogenase and 6-phosphogluconate dehydrogenase, to supply

electrons in the reduction process of glutathione. This reductase is an interesting enzyme in that it requires flavin adenine dinucleotide (FAD) as a cofactor and is therefore dependent on the nutritional status of riboflavin, a vitamin that may also be deficient in persons with sickle cell anemia. The concentration of reduced glutathione in the cytoplasm of normal erythrocytes is very high, about 2 mM (only hemoglobin and 2,3-diphosphoglycerate exceed this value), while that of oxidized glutathione is very low, usually in the micromolar range. This ratio is maintained by the different K_ms that glutathione peroxidase and glutathione reductase have for their respective glutathione substrates, the former having a high K_m of 650 μM and the latter having a low K_m of 25–40 μM. When oxidized glutathione accumulates, during an acute episode of oxidative stress, for example, the metabolite can be removed by transport out of the cell. This is not true for reduced glutathione, however, which does not have a transport pathway through the cell membrane. Reduced glutathione levels are also maintained by a two-step process that links the amino acids glycine, cysteine, and glutamic acid together. This is accomplished by two enzymes, namely, γ-glutamyl cysteine synthetase and glutathione synthetase. The synthesis of glutathione is an energy-requiring process, and both enzymes use ATP for their energy source. In summary, reactive oxygen species such as superoxide anion and hydrogen peroxide are removed by superoxide dismutase and a cyclic glutathione pathway.

In conclusion, the metabolism of glucose through the Embden-Meyerhof pathway serves the purpose of (a) producing ATP which is needed in the pumping of ions such as sodium, potassium, and calcium across the cell membrane and in the synthesis of reduced glutathione; (b) forming NADH for the reduction of methemoglobin back to its normal ferrous state; and (c) synthesizing 2,3-diphosphoglycerate which is needed in the regulation of the oxygen dissociation curve. The hexose monophosphate shunt serves the purpose of (a) producing the NADPH used by the glutathione pathway to reduce oxidized glutathione and glutathione mixed disulfides which are formed through oxidative reactions, and (b) synthesizing pentose sugars which are needed as substrates in the production of nucleotides.

ERYTHROCYTE METABOLISM IN SICKLE CELL ANEMIA

To determine that persons with sickle cell anemia have an altered erythrocyte metabolism is very difficult. Clearly, the major parameters to measure are metabolites and enzyme activities. The caution that must be taken whenever one assesses the concentrations of metabolites or the specific activities of enzymes is in the denominator. The most frequent units for the denominator include hemoglobin in gm, volume of packed red blood cells in ml, and number of red blood cells—usually 10^{10}. Depending on the denominator used, some variation in the results can be obtained. This arises because some persons with sickle cell anemia have a high proportion (>40%) of cells that have become dehydrated and, consequently, have lower mean cell volumes. For example, if the level of

Table 3.2
Enzymophies Resulting in Nonspherocytic Hemolytic Anemia

Enzyme Deficiency	Degree of Hemolysis	Sensitivity to Oxidative Stress
Glucose-6-P-dehydrogenase	mild-severe	+ +
6-phosphogluconate dehydrogense	very mild	+
Glutathione reductase	moderate	+
Glutathione synthetase	moderate	+
Glutathione peroxidase	mild	+
Hexokinase	mild-moderate	
Glucose phosphate isomerase	moderate	
Phosphofructokinase	mild	
Triose phosphate isomerase	moderate	
Glyceraldehyde-3-P-dehydrogense	mild	
Phosphoglycerate kinase	moderate	
2,3-diphosphoglycerate mutase	mild-severe	
Pyruvate kinase	mild-severe	
Adenylate kinase	mild	
Adenosine deaminase (increased activity)	very mild	

a metabolite is expressed in units/10^{10} RBC or units/ml-packed RBC, there may be some discrepancy compared to normal cells for one expression but not the other. Also, the measurement of individual enzyme activities may be affected by the age of the cell (5), and most erythrocytes in persons with sickle cell anemia are very young. As a result, other hemolytic anemias with reticulocytosis are often used for comparison. Even when it is determined that an individual enzyme activity is decreased or increased, it is difficult to know whether the change is significant enough to alter the entire metabolic pathway. This evaluation becomes even more complicated when several enzyme activities are changed, with some being increased and some decreased. Fortunately, there are two other avenues of investigation that have been helpful in assessing enzyme changes and their overall effects on metabolic pathways. The first is the study of persons with enzymopathies, namely, deficiencies or excesses of individual enzyme activities (6–9). A list of these enzymopathies and their degree of nonspherocytic hemolytic anemia is presented in Table 3.2. The second is the *in vitro* evaluation of products from a metabolic pathway such as CO_2 production in the Hexose Monophosphate Shunt. I will begin the evaluation of erythrocyte metabolism in sickle cell anemia with studies concerning the Embden-Meyerhof pathway.

Embden-Meyerhof Pathway

As mentioned above, the Embden-Meyerhof pathway includes approximately 10 enzymes, the most important of which are hexokinase, phosphofructokinase, and pyruvate kinase. The activities of these enzymes derived from erythrocytes of persons with sickle cell anemia have been studied by several investigators (10–18) the most comprehensive study being that of Lachant, Davidson; and Tanaka (16). They found that all enzymes of this pathway, with the exception of glucose phosphate isomerase, phosphoglycerate kinase, and enolase, were elevated relative to normal controls. However, the activities of the enzymes were also increased in hemolytic anemia controls with reticulocytosis, indicating that the elevated activities may be due to the presence of reticulocytes. Studies of these enzymes in normal cells over the life span of the cell show that the activities decline (5). The enzymes that suffer the greatest losses in activity are pyruvate kinase, aldolase and hexokinase with half-lives of 29, 77, and 33 days, respectively. Effectively, this means that the elevated enzyme activities observed by Lachant et al. (16) and other investigators may be due in large part to the presence of much younger cells in persons with sickle cell anemia compared to normals. Specific deficiencies in individual glycolytic enzymes have been noted, and most of these result in a nonspherocytic hemolytic anemia (Table 3.2). The enzyme whose deficiency causes the most commonly seen clinical manifestations is pyruvate kinase (other than glucose-6-phosphate dehydrogenase of the Hexose Monophosphate Shunt). Since most of the enzymes have elevated activities, their direct influence on anemia is of little concern. What effect do these elevated activities have on the metabolic products of interest, namely, ATP; 2,3-diphosphoglycerate; and NADH? The levels of these three metabolites are altered. ATP is elevated, but only marginally (4.9 μmoles/gm Hb in sickle cell disease; 4.8 μmoles/gm Hb is the upper limit of the normal range). The consequences of this higher ATP level are not only a slowdown of the glycolytic pathway but also inhibition of glucose-6-phosphate dehydrogenase, an important enzyme in the hexose monophosphate shunt. Lachant et al. (16) found that the increased level of ATP was strongly correlated with the reticulocyte count, indicating that this elevation may be due largely to the presence of reticulocytes and very young red cells. The level of 2,3-DPG was not correlated with the reticulocyte count, however, and its increase must be attributed to other effects. In this case, it is most probably related to the enhanced activity of the glycolytic pathway. The effects of high 2,3-DPG levels on the hemoglobin-oxygen dissociation curve must also be considered. The redox potential of the red blood cell is assessed by the ratios of NADH/(NADH + NAD$^+$) and NADPH/(NADPH + NADP$^+$). Zerez, Lachant, Lee, et al. (18) found that the total levels of pyridine nucleotides were increased, even above hemolytic anemia controls, and the ratio of NADH/NAD$_{total}$ was decreased in sickle cell erythrocytes. The authors speculated that the increased level of NAD$^+$ may be responsible for the increased consumption of glucose through the Embden-Meyerhof pathway since this metabolite is the rate-limiting factor for glyceraldehyde-3-phosphate dehydogenase activity. The decreased level of NADH may be the result of oxidant stress brought about by the elevated levels of reactive oxygen species in the presence of an unstable hemoglobin molecule, in this case hemoglobin S.

In summary, the Embden-Meyerhoff pathway in erythrocytes from persons with sickle cell anemia has an increased activity due in large part to the presence of a very young cell population which is rich in reticulocytes. Most of the enzyme activities are high and the major metabolites, ATP, 2,3-DPG, and total pyridine nucleotides are normal or elevated. Also, it is probable that this pathway could easily cope if stimulated by increased concentrations of glucose or inorganic phosphate. Due to the increased oxidative stress placed on Hb SS erythrocytes it is likely that the major changes in metabolism may occur in the hexose monophosphate shunt and glutathione pathway since these represent the primary channels of antioxidant defense.

Hexose Monophosphate Shunt

In vitro analyses of glucose-6-phosphate dehydrogenase (G6PD), 6-phosphogluconate dehydrogenase, transketolase, and transaldolase show that the first three enzymes have elevated activities compared to normal (only G6PD has significantly higher levels relative to hemolytic anemia controls with reticulocytosis); the latter enzyme had normal activity (16). Considerable attention has been focused on glucose-6-phosphate dehydrogenase in sickle cell anemia (19–26) not only because of its importance in generating NADPH for the glutathione pathway but because there is an incidence of G6PD deficiency that crosses over with sickle cell anemia. The most comprehensive of these studies was reported by Steinberg, West, Gallagher, et al. (26) in collaboration with the Cooperative Study of Sickle Cell Disease group. After examining 801 male patients (G6PD deficiency is X-linked recessive), they found that 10.4 percent had decreased G6PD activities (3.8 vs. 19.0 IU/gHb) with the genotype GdA$^-$. Another 18.4 percent of these males were identified to be of the GdA$^+$ genotype and had activities similar to those of sickle cell males with the normal G6PD genotype (16.6 vs 19.0 IU/gHb). Surprisingly, the impact of G6PD deficiency on the hematologic parameters and clinical symptoms of sickle cell disease was insignificant.

Assessment of the hexose monophosphate shunt can be made by examining the production of CO_2 from radiolabelled $^{14}C_1$-glucose. Carbon dioxide is produced by 6-phosphogluconate dehydrogenase in the conversion of 6-phosphogluconate to ribulose-5-phosphate. The advantages of studying CO_2 production are (1) the ability to study the effects of several enzymes working together in a pathway (in this case, hexokinase, glucose-6-phosphate dehydrogenase, and 6-phosphogluconate dehydrogenase), and (2) the ability to study the effects of inhibitors or stimulants on a pathway (in this case ATP or 2,3-DPG as inhibitors and new methylene blue or phenazine methosulfate as stimulants). The results of Lachant et al. (16) showed that the production of $^{14}CO_2$ from $^{14}C_1$-glucose without stimulants in subjects with sickle cell anemia was not significantly different from that in hemolytic anemia controls with reticulocytosis, which, in turn was not significantly different from that in normal controls. However, stimulation of the hexose monophosphate shunt with 1 μM methylene blue caused a significant increase in the production of CO_2 in subjects with sickle cell anemia compared to hemolytic anemia or normal controls ($3.61 \pm 0.95 > 2.83 \pm 1.09 > 2.15 \pm 0.55$ μmoles glucose oxidized/ml RBC/hr, respectively). Despite the ability to demonstrate the presence of high enzyme activities and an active shunt (i.e., $^{14}CO_2$ production) *in vitro*, Lachant et al. proposed that this pathway may be depressed *in vivo*. This proposal originates from the facts that (1) hexokinase may be the rate-limiting enzyme for the pathway, and (2) the high levels of ATP and 2,3-DPG would be expected to inhibit glucose-6-phosphate dehydrogenase, an important initial enzyme in the pathway. It would appear, however, that while the basal shunt rate may be depressed *in vivo*, the shunt is more than capable of increasing its rate in the presence of oxidative stress. This is of particular importance in sickle cell anemia because of the high levels of reactive oxygen species that are formed.

Glutathione Metabolic Pathway

One of the major functions of the hexose monophosphate shunt is to provide NADPH to the cyclic glutathione metabolic pathway for the removal of hydrogen peroxide. The important enzymes of this pathway are glutathione reductase and glutathione peroxidase, which recycle glutathione between its reduced and oxidized states to transfer electrons from NADPH to H_2O_2, producing water. In sickle cell anemia it has been shown that the activity of glutathione peroxidase is high (16, 27) and that of gluthathione reductase is low (16, 28). Also, the levels of reduced glutathione (GSH) appear to be significantly lower in many subjects with sickle cell anemia compared to black or white controls (29). Finally, the levels of $NADP^+$ and NADPH are also higher in subjects with sickle cell anemia (18). What does this all mean? First, the reasons for the low levels of reduced glutathione are not clear, although one might speculate that they are due to the decreased activity of glutathione reductase which is unable to keep up with the stimulated activity of glutathione peroxidase in the presence of increased levels of hydrogen peroxide. One might consider that the decreased level of GSH would be corrected by the presence of the GSH synthetic pathway which is composed of γ-glutamylcysteine synthetase and glutathione synthetase. Both these enzymes require ATP, and a decrease in this metabolite might explain the reduction in GSH. However, ATP would appear not to be deficient in subjects with sickle cell anemia (30). Although it has not been reported, it is probable that the precursor amino acids, glutamate, cysteine, and glycine, are also not deficient. As mentioned above, the only mechanism for reducing the GSH/GSSG level is by transporting GSSG out of the cell. Possibly, GSH is oxidized faster than it can be synthesized and the excess GSSG, which accumulates in the face of decreased glutathione reductase activity, diffuses from the cell. The end result would be a decrease in the GSH level. The reason for the decreased activity of glutathione reductase would appear to be a decrease in the cofactor flavin adenine dinucleotide (FAD). FAD is an important nutritional cofactor since the electron from NADPH is not transferred directly to the disulfide bond of oxidized glutathione directly. Rather, the electron of NADPH is transferred to the FAD molecule first and then to the oxidized glutathione molecule. The levels of erythrocyte FAD have not been measured directly in subjects with sickle cell anemia, but indirect measurements involving an *in vitro* assay of glutathione reductase in the absence and presence of exogenously added FAD indicate that the FAD level is decreased. The levels of FAD are decreased in black controls relative to white controls. However, the GSH levels of controls may not be decreased because of the absence of oxidative stress.

As described in the section on erythrocyte metabolism, the dissociation of oxyhemoglobin occasionally results in the formation of methemoglobin and superoxide anion. This reactive oxygen species is removed by first converting it to hydrogen peroxide by the enzyme superoxide dismutase (SOD) and then to water by either catalase and/or glutathione peroxidase. In addition, the presence of iron or iron-containing compounds may transform the less toxic hydrogen peroxide into the very toxic hydroxyl radical. Hb SS (31) and Hb AS (32) erythrocytes produce significantly higher levels of all three of these reactive oxygen species. The activity of superoxide dismutase has been reported both to be higher (33) and to be slightly lower (34) in Hb SS erythrocytes compared to erythrocytes of controls. In any event, SOD levels do not appear to be severely depressed. The cause of the increased oxygen radical formation is not known but it is speculated (35) that Hb S may be more prone to heterogeneous dissociation resulting in higher levels of superoxide and methemoglobin, with the latter degrading to hemichromes. Increased levels of iron-containing compounds associated with the sickle cell membrane (see the section on the interaction of hemoglobin S with the membrane) create an environment conducive to the formation of other reactive oxygen species such as hydroxyl and alkoxyl radicals. Compounding the increased formation of reactive oxygen species is the reduced ability of the sickle cell to defend itself against this oxidative stress. Subjects with sickle cell disease have decreased levels of zinc (36) (needed for superoxide dismutase activity), decreased levels of riboflavin (28) (needed for glutathione reductase activity), and decreased levels of vitamins E (37, 38) and C (39). Evidence for the increased oxidative stress has been found with increased levels of thiobarbituric acid–reactive products (40, 41) (byproducts of lipid peroxidation), decreased levels of free sulfhydryl groups (42) (an indicator of protein sulfhydryl group oxidation), and the presence of methionine sulfones (43). It has been proposed that this increased oxidative stress in sickle cells may be responsible for their increased hemolytic rate (44) as well as their protection from parasitic infection due to malaria (45).

To summarize, the Hb SS erythrocyte is, on the average, a young cell with typically high enzyme activities. Glycolysis appears to be normal, producing adequate levels of ATP, NADH, and 2,3-DPG. However, the cell is overly burdened with reactive oxygen species which create an environment of oxidative stress. Depressed levels of reduced glutathione and deficiencies of the essential vitamins and nutrients that are needed for oxidant defense exacerbate the existing oxidative state. The oxidative injury to the cell, particularly the cell membrane, has important ramifications for the pathophysiology of irreversibly sickled cell formation. To more fully understand the relevance of hemoglobin polymerization and altered metabolism to the pathophysiology of the sickle cell, a discussion of normal and sickle cell membrane structure and function follows.

INTRODUCTION TO CELL MEMBRANES

The membrane of a cell has many functions, the simplest of which is to provide a barrier that defines the inside from the outside of the cell. This is important because it allows the cell to maintain an internal environment that is quite different from the external environment. More than this, the membrane permits the two environments to interact somewhat so that the cell can adapt to changes in either the internal or external environment. The membrane must provide structural support for the cell to ensure that it survives the physical stresses to which it is constantly subjected. Often, this structural support confers a unique shape to the cell that may be necessary for its function or its interaction with other cells. Although the composition and distribution of the cell membrane components differ from cell to cell, there are some common features about cell membranes that should be discussed. Principally, all membranes are composed of lipids, proteins, and sugars.

The actual lipids that are present in membranes vary widely, but they all provide a hydrophobic barrier that separates the two hydrophilic environments inside and outside the cell. Lipids are described as *amphipathic*, which means that they have both a hydrophobic component (i.e., a portion that is immiscible, or not very soluble with water) and a hydrophilic component, usually consisting of a polar or charged headgroup which can interact with water. The bulk of the membrane is composed of a bilayer of lipids in which the hydrophobic portions of each lipid monolayer meet in the middle while the hydrophilic portions interact with the aqueous environments inside and outside the cell. This hydrophobic lipid bilayer by itself would be quite impermeable to most molecules, allowing only those that are small and somewhat hydrophobic, like glycerol, to pass through the membrane, and then only to a limited degree. Moreover, a membrane the size of a normal cell that was composed just of lipids would be structurally very fragile, fragmenting under the smallest stress. This is overcome by the presence of proteins. As with lipids, there are many different kinds of proteins associated with cell membranes, and they provide different functions. For simplicity's sake I will divide the proteins into the structural and the functional, although there is some overlap between these groups. Structural proteins form a cytoskeletal framework, usually at the inner surface of the membrane, which can interact with membrane lipids and integral membrane proteins (i.e., those proteins that have a strong interaction with the hydrophobic lipid environment). Indeed, some of these integral proteins are known to transcend the lipid bilayer, with portions being exposed to the extracellular and intracellular environments.

The cytoskeletal framework appears like a lattice attached to posts inserted into the lipid environment. In this way the lattice offers strength to the lipid bilayer, and shape as well. Shape is created by the conformation of the cytoskeletal proteins and by their distribution or arrangement within the cytoskeleton. Most, if not all, of the sugar component of the membrane is located on its external surface of the membrane and is attached to either lipids or proteins. Sugars, linked linearly or in short branches, act as antigens or, in some cases, receptors for antibodies or other proteins. Excellent articles (46, 47) reviewing the structure and function of cell membranes can provide further information. In order to understand the changes to erythrocyte membrane structure in sickle cell anemia, it is worth studying the normal erythrocyte membrane in detail first.

ERYTHROCYTE MEMBRANE STRUCTURE

Lipids and Membrane Asymmetry

The normal human erythrocyte membrane is composed of lipids, proteins, and carbohydrate moieties. The lipid portion of the membrane can be divided into three major groups: (1) neutral lipids, (2) glycolipids, and (3) phospholipids. For an excellent review of this subject, the reader is encouraged to read the chapter by van Deenan and De Gier in *The Red Blood Cell,* edited by Bishop and Surgenor (48). Table 3.3 shows the approximate percentages of these lipids, including their subclasses. The bulk of the neutral lipids is represented by cholesterol and its esters (principally stearoyl, palmitoyl, and oleoyl) (49). Using the procedure of filipin binding to cholesterol, Blau and Bittman (50) demonstrated that this neutral lipid was divided evenly between the inner and outer bilayers of the membrane. Glycolipids of the erythrocyte membrane are made from sphingosine, a fatty acid, and one or more hexoses. Glucosamine and galactosamine may also be included in the carbohydrate portion. In addition, some glycolipids contain the negatively charged sugar n-acetylneuraminic acid. Glycolipids containing this sugar are referred to as gangliosides. By labelling galactose residues with tritium (galactose oxidase followed by tritiated sodium borohydride), Steck and Dawson (51) determined that lipids and proteins containing this group were allocated to the outer bilayer exclusively. It is believed that glycolipids, as well as glycoproteins, contain many, if not all, the antigens that form the "blood groups" of the red cell on its external surface. Phospholipids—that is, those lipids containing one or more molecules of phosphorus—constitute nearly 60 percent of the total lipid of the membrane. The major phospholipids of the human erythrocyte membrane are sphingomyelin, phosphatidylcholine, phosphatidylethanolamine, and phosphatidylserine. The former two are choline-containing lipids and the latter two are often referred to as cephalins because they were first isolated from the brain. Other minor phospholipids include phosphatidic acid, phosphatidylinositol, phosphatidylinositol-4-phosphate, and phosphatidylinositol-4,5-bisphosphate. The latter three phospho-

Table 3.3
Lipid Subclasses within Human Erythrocyte Membranes

Lipid Classes	% Within Subclass	% of Total Lipid	Total % of Each Subclass
Neutral Lipids			29
Cholesterol	79	23	
Cholesterol esters	4	1	
Free fatty acids		5	
Di- & tri-glycerides	17		
Glycolipids			13
Cerebrosides			
Gangliosides			
Phospholipids			58.0
Sphingomyelin	23.8	13.8	
Phosphatidyl Choline	31.6	18.3	
Phosphatidyl ethanolamine	22.6	13.1	
Phosphatidyl serine	13.5	7.8	
Phosphatidyl acid	1.4	0.8	
Phosphoinosides	4.5	2.6	
Tysophospholipids	2.4	1.4	
Other phospholipids	0.2	0.2	

lipids are often grouped together as phosphoinositides. A number of different studies have been performed to determine the topographic distribution of these phospholipids in membranes (52–59). These reports showed that the choline-containing phospholipids, phosphatidylcholine and sphingomyelin, were located predominantly in the outer bilayer, while phosphatidylethanolamine was located predominantly in the inner bilayer (see Figure 3.5). Of greatest significance was the finding that phosphatidylserine (PS) was present exclusively in the inner bilayer. This appears to be important in the normal function of the human erythrocyte, since changes in the distribution of phospatidylseine (PS) across the membrane may be associated with the pathophysiology of sickle cell anemia (refer to the section on changes in lipid composition and bilayer asymmetry). The phosphoinositides and phosphatidic acid are linked metabolically on the inner bilayer of the membrane. A portion of phosphatidylinositol which cannot be metabolized is known to be located on the outer surface of the membrane, forming a covalent anchor for the enzyme acetylcholinesterase (60) and perhaps other enzymes. The phosphoinositide pathway is very sensitive to hydrolysis by a membrane-bound phosphodiesterase in the presence of low calcium concentrations. The pathway may act as a monitor for the presence of elevated intracellular calcium concentrations since there will be an irreversible depletion of phosphoinositides with a concomitant increase in phosphatidic acid (61, 62). I

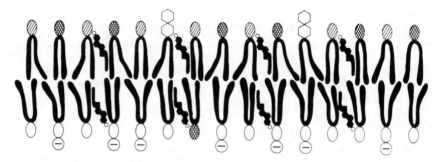

Figure 3.5. Erythrocyte membrane lipid bilayer asymmetry.

mention this minor pathway because of its potential importance to sickle cell formation (see the section on changes in lipid composition).

Cytoskeletal Proteins

Erythrocyte membrane proteins have been classified in a number of different ways (e.g., solubility or nonsolubility in nonionic detergent, location in the membrane, function, ability to interact and form protein complexes, etc). For the purpose of this discussion, I will divide them into three major groups: (1) cytoskeletal proteins, (2) transport proteins, and (3) enzymes. Not all these proteins or enzymes have been isolated and characterized, but what current knowledge has been gained and its relevance to sickle cell anemia will be discussed.

The cytoskeletal proteins have been described best because of their direct influence on membrane shape, deformability, and membrane integrity (63–66). They also have the most importance to the formation of irreversibly sickled cells (refer to the section on protein and cytoskeletal changes). The major cytoskeletal proteins are defined by numbers according to their monomer molecular weights as observed on sodium-dodecyl sulfate polyacrylamide gels. In some instances, the proteins have been given names. A typical protein separation by SDS-polyacrylamide gel electrophoresis (PAGE) showing these bands and their nomenclatures is shown in Figure 3.6. The major cytoskeletal proteins include bands 1, 2, 2.1, 4.1, 4.9, and 5. Bands 1 and 2 are often referred to as α- and β-spectrin, respectively. They are both long, thin flexible proteins (100 nm in length) which together form a heterodimer by aligning themselves in an antiparallel configuration with respect to their amino and carboxyl terminals. Under native conditions on the inner surface of the membrane, spectrin is believed to be a tetramer; that is, two heterodimers linked end to end where the β-spectrin of one heterodimer binds to the α-spectrin of the opposing heterodimer, and vice versa (67–69). As expected, the tetramer is about 200 nm in length. A smaller portion of isolated spectrin is found in larger oligomers which take on a spider-like appearance by electron microscopy (EM) (70). The spectrin tetramer or

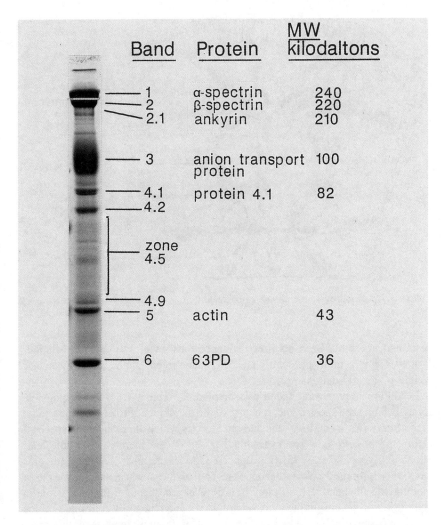

Figure 3.6. Erythrocyte membrane proteins: separation by SDS polyacrylamide gel electrophoresis.

oligomer clearly forms the building block for the lateral framework that forms the cytoskeleton at the inner surface of the membrane. However, other proteins are needed to cross-link these tetramers and to attach the framework to integral membrane proteins. Two important proteins involved in cross-linking are actin and protein 4.1. Although spectrin dimers and tetramers can bind F-actin (and not G-actin), only the spectrin tetramer–F-actin interaction results in cross-linking (71). The formation of spectrin–actin gels is promoted by the presence of protein 4.1 and stabilizes this complex. While direct binding of spectrin to protein 4.1 (K_D = 200 nM) has been demonstrated and spectrin binding to actin has been

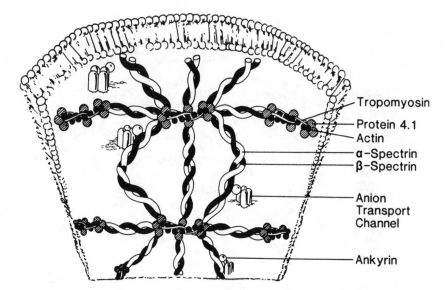

Tropomyosin

Protein 4.1
Actin
α-Spectrin
β-Spectrin

Anion
Transport
Channel

Ankyrin

Figure 3.7.   Erythrocyte membrane cytoskeleton.

described, there has been no direct evidence for protein 4.1–actin association. Protein 4.1 is a multi-phosphorylated globular protein which has a molecular weight of 80,000 daltons (72).

In addition to promoting spectrin–actin binding, protein 4.1 is also responsible for associating the spectrin–actin matrix to the membrane. Protein 4.1 binds with high affinity (K_D = 40 nM) to inside-out vesicles which are deficient in spectrin, actin, and protein 4.1. The exact binding site on the membrane is not clear, although glycophorin A (73), glycophorin C (74), and phosphatidylserine (75) have been proposed. Near the opposite end of the spectrin heterodimer is a binding site for band 2.1, or ankyrin (76). Ankyrin plays an important role in connecting or anchoring the cytoskeleton to the membrane by forming a bridge between β-spectrin and band 3 protein, an integral membrane protein that functions as the anion transporter. A pictorial sketch of the cytoskeletal framework described above is shown in Figure 3.7. An understanding of the functional role of these proteins in maintaining cell shape and integrity has come from the examination of patients with hemolytic anemias that are expressed through changes in red cell shape. The most studied of these anemias are hereditary spherocytosis, hereditary elliptocytosis, and hereditary pyropoikilocytosis. The review by Platt (77) has addressed the role of cytoskeletal protein defects in the membrane changes associated with these anemias.

A hypothesis has been put forward to help understand how defective cytoskeletal proteins cause the observed membrane lesions (78). The hypothesis proposes two major types of cytoskeletal proteins: those that interact laterally

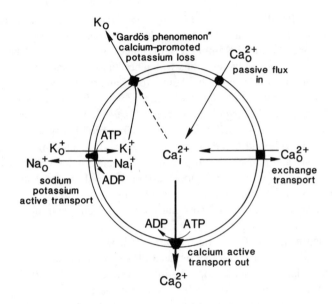

Figure 3.8.   Method of cation transport in human erythrocytes.

or parallel to the membrane surface and those that interact vertically or perpendicular to the membrane surface. Lateral changes in the interactions of spectrin heterodimers, actin, and protein 4.1 prevent reversible deformability resulting in permanent elliptocytosis or fragmentation, as is seen in pyropoikilocytosis. Vertical changes in the interactions of spectrin–ankyrin or ankyrin–protein 3 tend to render the membrane less stable, resulting in loss of membrane material and spherocytosis. I only raise this information to help explain the membrane lesion in irreversibly sickled cells which will be discussed later. Other membrane proteins of major interest in the cell include transport proteins and enzymes.

Transport Proteins

The mature erythrocyte is known to carry out several forms of transport. These include: (1) passive anion transport, (2) facilitated glucose transport, (3) nucleoside transport, (4) active sodium and potassium transport, (5) active calcium transport and (6) calcium-dependent potassium transport (the Gardös phenomenon; see Figure 3.8). Of these transport pathways, only the anion transporter, glucose transporter, nucleoside transporter, and the two active cation transport proteins have been elucidated biochemically.

The anion transport protein (79, 80) has been identified as band 3 with an average molecular weight of 95,000 daltons (the band appears diffuse on SDS-polyacrylamide gels). In many ways it is an unusual membrane protein which provides several functions. It associates as a dimer or tetramer, with each monomer transcending the lipid bilayer of the membrane several times. In contrast to most membrane proteins, the carboxyl terminal faces the cytoplasmic surface of the membrane while the amino terminal faces extracellularly. The extended carboxy-terminus not only functions to anchor the cytoskeleton by binding to band 2.1 (ankyrin) but also to bind hemoglobin and other cytoplasmic enzymes such as glyceraldehyde-3-phosphate dehydrogenase. The amino-terminus is glycosylated but lacks the negatively charged N-acetylneuraminic acid, which is characteristic of some red cell glycoproteins. The anion transport protein allows the flux of chloride and bicarbonate anions as well as other multivalentanions such as sulfate and phosphate. Of greatest importance is the understanding that the rate of passive anion flux is about a thousandfold higher than the passive cation flux under normal steady-state conditions. This allows the cell to compensate for changes in cation fluxes and maintain electroneutrality (i.e., no net charge across the membrane).

The glucose transporter of the red blood cell is a 43,000 MW glycoprotein (monomer) which is believed to exist as a dimer in the membrane (81–84). On SDS-polyacrylamide gels, it appears diffusely over a 45,000 to 72,000 MW range with an average MW of 55,000 (i.e., zone 4.5) (81). This diffuse range of molecular weights probably results from the glycosylation of this protein which is known to affect the way in which proteins run on SDS-gels. The transporter facilitates the passive diffusion of glucose and other monosaccharides through the membrane for the purpose of glycolysis. The transporter has now been purified and reconstituted into liposomes (82).

The transport of adenosine and other nucleosides also occurs through a protein with the same MW range as the glucose transporter (85). Indeed, the glucose transporter copurifies with the nucleoside transporter (86), and the nucleoside transporter is identified as a component of zone 4.5 (87). Like the glucose transporter, the nucleoside transporter has been purified and functionally reconstituted into liposomes (88). The nucleoside transporter plays an important role in erythrocytes in maintaining cellular levels of ATP.

In contrast to simple or facilitated diffusion where molecules move in the direction of their concentration or electrochemical gradients, some molecules, especially cations, are pumped against their concentration gradients, in other words; from a low concentration to a high concentration. For example, the concentration of potassium inside the cell is usually 10 to 15 times higher than that outside the cell. Sodium, on the other hand, is the reverse, with a higher concentration outside the cell compared to inside it. These differences in concentrations are maintained by a sodium-potassium pump (89). Because these monovalent cations are "pumped" against their electrochemical gradients, energy is required, usually in the form of ATP. It is now known that the pumping of potassium into the cell and sodium out of the cell are linked in a ratio of $2K^+$ to $3Na^+$ (i.e., three sodium ions are pumped out of the cell for every two potassium ions that are pumped in). Although this stoichiometry is not equivalent, it compensates for the unequal rates of passive diffusion for these cations which is about the same ratio ($3Na^+$ vs. $2K^+$).

The enzyme, which catalyzes the hydrolysis of ATP to ADP and inorganic phosphate and is associated with the pump protein, is called the ($Na^+ + K^+$)-ATPase. Both the enzyme activity and the Na^+-K^+ pump are inhibited by ouabain, a cardiac glycoside. The structure of the ($Na^+ + K^+$)-ATPase has been determined (90–92) and is believed to be composed of three subunits: a large transmembrane component that contains the catalytic site for ATP hydrolysis (alpha subunit with MW = 100,000), a smaller glycoprotein (beta-subunit with M.W. = 55,000), and a polypeptide of molecular weight 10,000 known as the gamma subunit. When the complex of these subunits is reconstituted into liposomes, a functional ($Na^+ + K^+$) pump can be demonstrated (93).

The divalent cation, calcium, represents another example whereby a transmembrane protein containing an ATPase maintains a very low concentration inside the cell compared to the outside. In contrast to the sodium-potassium pump, the calcium pump produces a concentration gradient that is about 100,000-fold higher outside the cell (i.e., 10^{-8} M inside vs. 10^{-3} M outside). The Ca^{2+}-ATPase has been purified and found to have a molecular weight of 140,000 (94–96). Reconstitution of the enzyme into liposomes results in calcium pump activity (97), and both are stimulated by anionic phospholipids or polyunsaturated fatty acids (96, 98). Calcium pumping and Ca^{2+}-ATPase activity are enhanced significantly by a cytoplasmic protein known as calmodulin (99–101). Micromolar concentrations of calcium cause conformational changes in the protein that allow it to associate with the calcium transport protein in the membrane to enhance the pumping activity. It appears that the stimulation of the enzyme by calmodulin in a reconstituted system is also regulated by certain phospholipids.

Enzymes

There are a number of enzymes associated with the membrane that have not been numbered on an SDS-gel and are not associated with a transport function. These enzymes include acetylcholinesterase, adenylate cyclase, phosphoinositide monoesterases, phosphoinositide phosphatases, polyphosphoinositide phosphodiesterase, diglyceride kinase, the protein and phospholipid methyltransferases, protein kinase C, spectrin kinase, and transglutaminase.

Acetylcholinesterase in an enzyme located on the external surface of the erythrocyte membrane that specifically hydrolyzes acetylcholine into choline and acetate. Its presence on the membrane would seem superfluous since there are excessive levels of pseudo-cholinesterase in the plasma which can carry out the same function. The membrane acetylcholinesterase has a monomer MW of 80,000 on SDS-polyacrylamide gels but it probably exists as a dimer (102, 103). Most important, the protein portion of the enzyme appears to be entirely at the surface of the membrane linked to the hydrophobic domain by an ethanolamine-glycosyl-phosphatidylinositol anchor (60, 104). Further evidence indicates that acetylcholinesterase is a disulfide-linked dimer in its native state (105). Although its direct contact with the lipid bilayer would seem minimal, it copurifies, and is influenced by, anionic phospholipids such as phosphatidylserine (102, 106). In addition, the enzyme activity can be inhibited by nonionic detergents including Triton X-100 (107). Reconstitution of the enzyme activity following incorporation into liposomes has been achieved (108), although most of the activity can be demonstrated in a soluble form following Triton X-100 extraction or treatment with papain (103, 109, 110).

The regulation of cell function by many hormones and biochemicals often involves the stimulation or inhibition of adenylate cyclase, an enzyme that converts ATP to cyclic AMP within the cell. The regulation of adenylate cyclase involves a transmembrane signal composed of (1) binding of a ligand to its receptor on the outer surface of the membrane, (2) interaction of the receptor with a guanine nucleotide-binding protein in the membrane, and (3) stimulation or inhibition of the adenylate cyclase by the guanine nucleotide-binding proteins. Stimulation of adenylate cyclase produces cyclic AMP which is important in the activation of protein kinases. These phosphorylate a variety of proteins, including membrane proteins. Changes in the phosphorylation state of many proteins appear to confer changes in enzyme activities and protein interactions. Human erythrocyte membranes contain very few β-adrenergic receptors and very little adenylate cyclase activity; however, they do contain normal levels of the guanine nucleotide-binding protein. This binding protein confers Gpp(NH)p, fluoride, and GTP stimulation of the adenylate cyclase; cholera toxin labels the protein with NAD. Purification of the guanine nucleotide-binding protein has been accomplished and the end product has a molecular weight of 39,000 to 42,000 on SDS-polyacrylamide gels (111, 112). Because of its excess over the adrenergic receptor and the catalytic enzyme, the GTP-binding protein of human erythrocytes has been used in reconstitution studies involving mixed membranes (112) or liposomes (113) in order to probe the mechanisms of signal transduction. Although the human erythrocyte lacks adrenergic receptors on its surface, it does contain receptors for the prostaglandins PGE_1, PGE_2 thromboxane, and prostacyclin (114–117), and for leukotriene C_4 (118). Apparently, PGE_1 and PGE_2 do not produce significant levels of cyclic AMP, and it is yet to be established whether any of these agents elicit their effects on human erythrocytes by activating the adenylate cyclase to produce cyclic AMP (cAMP).

Many cells contain another mechanism of membrane signal transduction involving hormone- or ligand-induced turnover of the phoshoinositide phospholipids (119, 120). The breakdown of these lipids results in the formation of 1,2-diacylglycerol (i.e., the fatty acid–glycerol backbone of the lipid) and inositol-1,4,5-trisphosphate (the polar headgroup of the lipid). The former component binds a cytoplasmic protein kinase, protein kinase C, which forms a tight bond with the membrane in the presence of phosphatidylserine (121). The formation of this complex activates the kinase to phosphorylate a variety of proteins, many of which are different from those proteins phosphorylated by cAMP-stimulated protein kinases. The inositol-1,4,5-trisphosphate interacts with intracellular reticulum membranes to initiate the release of calcium ions, which then bring about a number of different reactions. In most cells the turnover of phosphoinositides is

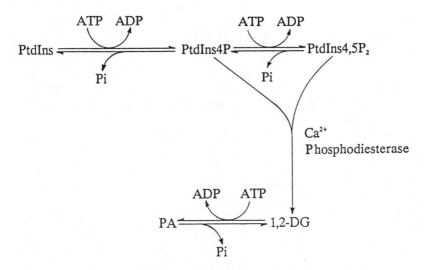

Figure 3.9. Phosphoinositide metabolism in human erythrocytes.

cyclic; that is, the products of the phosphoinositide breakdown are used to resynthesize phosphatidylinositol. Human erythrocyte membranes contain the three phosphoinositide lipids, diacylglycerol, and phosphatidic acid, as well as some of the enzymes
required for this metabolic pathway (see Figure 3.9). However, human erythrocytes
lack the enzymes needed to resynthesize phosphatidylinositol from phosphatidic acid.
Moreover, the polyphosphoinositide phosphodiesterase, which degrades PtdIns4P
and PtdIns4,5P$_2$, is irreversible and calcium-dependent (62).

Normal human erythrocytes are capable of maintaining a very low intracellular
calcium concentration throughout their life span, thereby preventing the inevi-
table depletion of the phosphoinositides and the accumulation of phosphatidic
acid. However, under pathophysiologic conditions such as sickle cell disease,
it has been speculated that the calcium concentration may rise, even transiently
within the cell. This being the case, one might predict lower levels of the
polyphosphoinositides and higher levels of inositol-1,4,5-trisphosphate and phosphatidic acid, and perhaps higher levels of membrane-bound protein kinase C.
Studies on polyphosphoinositides and their metabolism have been made in sickle
cell disease and will be discussed in the next section. In summary, the normal
erythocyte maintains steady state levels of the three phosphoinositide lipids,
phosphatidylinositol, phosphatidylinositol-4-phosphate and phosphatidylinositol-
4,5-bisphosphate, through a balance of the PI kinases (which are Mg^{2+}- and
ATP-dependent) and PI phosphomonoesterases (122). This may be important
also because of the possible importance of these lipids in maintaining the cytoskeleton (123) and activation of the $(Ca^{2+} + Mg^{2+})$-ATPase required for
pumping calcium out of the cell (124).

Erythrocytes and many other cell types contain a protein kinase C in their
cytoplasms which becomes associated with the inner surface of the membrane

upon the formation of 1,2-diacylglycerol (125). This protein kinase has a molecular weight of 80,000 on SDS-polyacrylamide gels and can be purified by anion exchange and hydroxyapatite chromatography. In erythrocytes, protein kinase C can become associated with the membrane by introducing calcium to the cytoplasm by means of A23187 (a calcium-selective ionophore) or by adding a nonmetabolizable analogue of 1,2-diacylglycerol. Two of these analogues include 12-O-tetra-decanoyl phorbol 13-acetate (TPA) and phorbol dibutyrate. Once attracted to the inner surface of the membrane by 1,2-diacylglycerol or TPA, the protein kinase C forms a complex with phosphatidylserine and calcium (Ca^{2+} < 10μM) which cannot be easily removed (126). Once the complex is formed, the enzyme is capable of phosphorylating a number of membrane-bound proteins. These proteins include protein 4.1, protein 4.9 (126–129), two minor peripheral proteins named alpha and beta adducin (130), and the glucose transporter (131). These two adducin proteins have molecular weights of 120,000 and 110,000 and may form a heterodimer in their native states (130). Of particular interest is the finding that adducin can form a complex with spectrin and actin and, after being formed, can further recruit other spectrin molecules (132). This would indicate that the protein kinase C of human erythrocytes may have an important role in the arrangement of spectrin–actin complexes and in the phosphorylation of the two other cytoskeletal proteins, bands 4.1 and 4.9. One report indicates that the phosphorylation of protein 4.1 reduces its association for spectrin, a condition that might destabilize the cytoskeletal network (133). As described above, a physiological role for protein kinase C in the normal mature erythrocyte may be insignificant since this cell is capable of maintaining a very low intracellular calcium concentration; calcium inside the cell is the initiator of events leading to the activation of the protein kinase C. However, pathophysiological conditions that would invite transiently higher calcium concentrations than normal (i.e., above 1 μM) could precipitate the cascade of events described above.

Another important group of enzymes located in both the cytoplasm and the membrane portions of the erythrocyte are the methyltransferases (134). These enzymes function to transfer a methyl group from S-adenosyl methionine to some acceptor molecule; the type of acceptor molecule is used to classify the methyltransferase specifically. The major methyltransferases of the human erythrocyte include (1) phospholipid methyltransferases (135, 136), (2) catechol O-methyltransferase (137), (3) histamine N-methyltransferase (138), (4) thiolmethyltransferase (139, 140), and (5) carboxyl methyltransferase (141, 142). The methyltransferases are generally inhibited by S-adenosyl homocysteine (143). Of these enzymes, the catechol-, histamine-, and thiolmethyltransferases are involved in the methylation of small biological molecules or drugs and will not be discussed in detail here. The phospholipid methyltransferases of the membrane and the carboxyl methyltransferases of the cytoplasm have the most importance in the possible modification of the erythrocyte membrane. The phospholipid methyltransferases of the membrane catalyze the methylation of phosphatidyle-thanolamine to monomethyl-phosphatidylethanolamine, monomethyl-phosphatidy lethanolamine to dimethyl-phosphatidylethanolamine, and, finally, dimethyl-phosphatidylethanolamine to phosphatidylcholine. In simple terms, the enzyme sequentially adds three methyl groups to the amine group on the polar head of phosphatidylethanolamine (PE). Evidence shows that as the PE is being methylated it becomes transported from the inner leaflet of the bilayer to the outer leaflet of the bilayer. As might be expected, this process has a disturbing effect on the membrane, and an increase in membrane fluidity attributed to the methylation has been reported (144). The carboxyl methyltransferases, unlike the phospholipid methyltransferases, are located in the cytoplasm of the erythrocyte and catalyze the methylation of proteins both in the cytoplasm (145, 146) and associated with the membrane (147, 148). The reaction of this enzyme functions to neutralize the carboxyl groups of acidic amino acid residues of proteins thereby potentially altering the protein's structure and function. In addition, the carboxymethyl esterification of proteins is reversible under physiological conditions and may represent a mechanism of regulation for certain proteins. The proteins of the erythrocyte membrane most affected by carboxyl methylation are bands 2.1 (ankyrin), 3, 4.1, and 4.5 (147, 148). The enzymatic methylation of band 3 has been further studied, and the results show that this protein modification does not appear to affect its anion transport function (149, 150). Aged erythrocytes exhibit increased methyl esterification with preference for the cytoskeletal proteins ankyrin and protein 4.1 (151). Of potential interest to sickle cell anemia is the recent finding that membrane-associated hemoglobin is more actively methylated compared to that found in the cytosol (152) and that the presence of intracellular calcium at micromolar concentrations decreases carboxyl methylation of the membrane proteins (153). Clearly, the phospholipid and protein methyltransferases could potentially play a role in the pathophysiology of sickle cell membrane changes.

The cytoplasm of erythrocytes also contains a transglutaminase, which, in the presence of intracellular calcium, can induce the cross-linking of membrane proteins (154, 155). This cross-linking is created by the catalytic formation of γ-glutamyl-ε-lysine bridges between membrane proteins (156, 157). This covalent bridging is irreversible and would have the effect of fixing the cytoskeletal network. However, the concentration of intracellular calcium required to catalyze this reaction is above 50 μM, and this rarely occurs in erythrocytes, even under pathophysiologic conditions. Nonetheless, the possibility that transglutaminase cross-linking of membrane proteins may explain the fixed shape and decreased deformability of the irreversibly sickled cell has been entertained. A search for cross-linked proteins in sickle cells, including fractions which were poor or rich in irreversible sickled cells, was found to be negative, indicating that the transglutaminase reactions do not play a role in sickle cell membrane pathophysiology (158).

ERYTHROCYTE MEMBRANE STRUCTURE AND ENZYME
FUNCTION IN SICKLE CELL ANEMIA

As mentioned above and in previous chapters of this book, the molecular change responsible for sickle cell anemia occurs in the β-chain of hemoglobin. The self-association of deoxyhemoglobin S into polymers and the effect of these rod-like fibers on erythrocyte sickling have been studied extensively (see Chapter 2). However, the deformed cells, including sickle-shaped cells, which are observed under the microscope in an oxygen-rich atmosphere do not contain large amounts of the polymerized hemoglobin S fibers, which would explain the distorted shape. Indeed, treatment of these cells with high concentrations of oxygen or carbon monoxide, which ensure the depolymerization of any existing hemoglobin fibers, do not revert these cells to normal biconcave discs. Because of the irreversibility in their morphological shape and physical properties, these cell types have been defined as *irreversibly sickled cells* (ISCs). Cells that are sickled in the presence of deoxygenated conditions but that appear to resume their normal shape upon reoxygenation are defined as *reversibly sickled cells* (RSCs).

Two major approaches have been taken to understand the changes that take place in SS cells, namely, (1) to demonstrate metabolic, compositional, structural, and enzymatic differences between SS cells and controls (usually age-, sex-, and race-matched control subjects or those with a nonsickling, reticulocyte-rich hemolytic anemia such as hereditary spherocytosis, etc.); and (2) to demonstrate these differences between ISCs and non-ISCs. The latter have been studied either statically or dynamically. That is, studies have been done that isolate fractions of blood cells that are rich in ISCs and fractions that are deficient in ISCs and that compare their differences: This is the *static* model. Alternatively, studies have been performed to make ISCs *in vitro* from an ISC-poor fraction of cells in order to evaluate the changes that take place over time: This is the *dynamic* model. It is important to understand the limitations of each of these models. First, the static model provides clear and real differences between normal cells, nonirreversibly sickled cells, and ISCs but does not reveal how these changes took place and, more particularly, in what order, since many of these changes could be very indirect consequences of the primary cause of ISC formation. Second, the dynamic model may yield useful information about how ISCs are formed in the laboratory; however, it presumes that the environmental conditions used *in vitro* mimic those conditions *in vivo* that are responsible for ISC formation. Theoretically, the information gained from the dynamic model should corroborate that obtained by the static model; however, this is not always the case. Regardless of these difficulties, studies continue to shed light on the mechanism(s) of ISC formation and the way in which hemoglobin S polymerization brings about changes in erythrocyte metabolism, membrane composition, membrane shape, and membrane physiology.

Interaction of Hemoglobin S with the Membrane

In the early 1970s when the polymerization of hemoglobin S was proposed as the molecular basis of sickling (159–161), investigators soon began to explore the mechanism by which polymerized or denatured hemoglobin S might alter or damage the red cell membrane. Studies showed that purified hemoglobin S bound to a greater extent to the purified erythrocyte membrane than did hemoglobin A (162, 163). In addition, the levels of hemoglobin S associated with the membrane were higher in a dense fraction of cells (i.e., the fraction that is rich in irreversibly sickled cells) and in ISCs as observed by freezed fracture electron microscopy (164). The binding was independent of temperature and little affected by sulfhydryl reagents. However, the binding was very sensitive to pH, being inhibited above 7.0, and could be disrupted at high ionic strength. In addition, the experiments were performed with very low hemoglobin/membrane ratios. Because the conditions of binding were so different from those found in the normal red cell, it was difficult to predict whether there was increased association of hemoglobin S with the membrane under physiological conditions and whether such association, if it existed, resulted in changes to the membrane. More recent work by Eisinger, Flores, and Bookchin (165) has clarified this question somewhat. Incorporating fluorescent-labelled stearic acid (a free fatty acid) probes into the outer lipid bilayer of the membrane, these researchers could measure the close proximity of hemoglobin, in this case Hb S, to the inner surface of the membrane bilayer using resonant energy transfer. Their results showed that the concentration of hemoglobin S at the membrane surface of oxygenated Hb SS cells increased with cell density to almost twice the level measured for hemogobin A to oxygenated Hb AA cells. In contrast membrane ghosts obtained from these different fractions of dense cells did not show the increased association of hemoglobin S near the membrane. Deoxygenation of Hb SS cells caused the elevated concentrations of hemoglobin S at the membrane surface to fall (reversibly) for all density fractions tested. The researchers proposed that the withdrawl of hemoglobin S from the membrane surface upon deoxygenation was consistent with an increased net negative charge on deoxygenated Hb S and/or the possibility that the cytoskeleton presents a barrier to polymeric Hb S but not to the monomeric form of the protein. While membrane-associated hemoglobin S is believed to play an unimportant role in Hb S polymerization (166, 167), its presence near the cytoplasmic surface of the membrane may affect the properties of the cytoskeleton and perhaps other membrane proteins through electrostatic or, less likely, hydrophobic interactions.

Through the use of instruments that measure various physical properties of Hb SS cells and their membranes, it has become quite clear that hemoglobin polymers and cellular distention arising from these polymers cause significant changes to the properties of the membrane. One of the most commonly used techniques to measure cell membrane viscoelasticity and membrane rigidity is micropipette aspiration. Upon suctioning a cell partially into the end of a micropipette, the ability of the cell to deform can be ascertained. When the cell is pushed out of the pipette there is a tendency for it to resume its original state. The rate at which the cell recovers this shape, if at all, is a reflection of membrane elasticity and of the dissipation of viscosity in the membrane and the cytoplasm. Studies using Hb SS cells showed that those cells that had higher hemoglobin concentrations (i.e., those richer in ISCs) had increased viscoelastic behavior and increased membrane elasticity (168). This has been measured as a function of PO_2 and concentration (169). As the PO_2 level decreased there was a corresponding increase in membrane rigidity. However, some SS cells did not sickle even at low PO_2 levels, and these cells maintained normal membrane elasticity and normal membrane viscosity. That cytoplasmic hemoglobin S contributes to the membrane shear modulus (i.e., static rigidity) was demonstrated by crossover experiments in which purified normal or sickle cell membranes (i.e., membranes from red blood cells of a subject with sickle cell anemia and not the membranes from irreversibly sickled cells per se) were reconstituted with different concentrations of Hb A or Hb S (170). The results showed that normal membranes reconstituted with Hb SS expressed the high static rigidity typical of oxygenated sickle cells while sickle cell membranes reconstituted with Hb A exhibited relatively normal static rigidity. The degree of membrane distention by hemoglobin polymers appears also to affect the rate of net potassium loss and cellular dehydration (171, 172). Slow deoxygenation of cells causes greater elongation of cells than does rapid deoxygenation, which results in star-shaped cells. The observations support the concept that sickling formed upon slow deoxygenation leads to an increase in membrane permeability related to mechanical stress that is imposed on the membrane by bundles of hemoglobin S polymers. The increased permeability consequently leads to cellular dehydration and an increased probability of ISC formation (172). Although the reasons for increased membrane rigidity in dense ISCs is not known, there is evidence that indicates that the formation of a spectrin–hemoglobin complex may be responsible (173). In addition, hemoglobin-catalyzed oxidative changes in the cytoskeleton may lead to changes in the morphology and physical properties of the membrane.

In addition to its ability to polymerize, hemoglobin S is known to be unstable to mechanical shaking resulting in precipitation (174). This helped to explain the presence of inclusion bodies (presumably due to precipitated hemoglobin) which are sometimes seen in Hb SS cells (175). Further research demonstrated the presence of hemichromes bound to the membranes of Hb SS cells (176, 177). Hemichromes represent hemoglobin molecules altered upon hemoglobin denaturation or oxidation. Using specrophotometric measurements it was demonstrated that the membranes from Hb SS cells had significantly higher levels of hemichromes than did Hb AA cells. The increased levels of membrane associated hemichromes was not found to the same degree in other anemias with reticulocytosis, namely, hereditary spherocytosis and autoimmune hemolytic anemia. Separation of Hb SS cells into various density fractions by stractan density gradient centrifugation did not show any differences in the levels of hemichromes bound to the membranes (177). This may be due in part to the ability of plasma albumin to extract hemin from the membrane (178). Indeed, it has been proposed that excess hemin, formed upon hemoglobin denaturation, may be removed by drainage through the membrane and adsorption to plasma albumin. Increased levels of hemin in Hb SS cell membranes appear to be associated with both the lipid-soluble portion and the cytoskeletal protein portion (178, 179). The extraction of heme-containing compounds (i.e., hemoglobin, hemichromes, or free heme) from inside-out membranes prepared from Hb SS cell membranes was achieved partially by spectrin elution, proteolysis of band 3, and treatment with dithiothreitol. Sequential treatment with all these procedures still allowed about 40 percent of the heme-containing compounds to be associated with inside-out membranes, and at least part of this could be attributed to free heme without globin (179). A recent report (180) confirmed that the denaturation of hemoglobin S by mechanical shaking results in the release of significantly higher levels of hemin to the cytoplasm compared to hemoglobin A in normal cells. Following the formation of hemin and its association with the membrane, the further release of iron (i.e., nonheme iron), may also occur. Kuross and Hebbel (181) found that inside-out membranes from SS cells contained not only higher levels of heme-containing iron but also nonheme iron. Although some of the nonheme iron may be in the form of ferritin, a portion is associated with another chelate. This portion can be removed by phospholipase D, indicating that it is iron-bound to amino phosopholipids, particularly the negatively charged phosphatidylserine. In summary, the presence of hemoglobin, hemichromes, hemin, or chelated iron in the membrane has significant ramifications regarding iron-catalyzed oxidative damage to both proteins and lipids of the membrane, which could result in structural and functional changes.

In addition to the formation of heme-containing compounds, the presence of free globin chains (i.e., without heme) has been considered. An early report (182) indicated that the levels of free alpha- and beta-globin chains in hemolysates (i.e., the protein portion of hemoglobin without the heme) were not significantly higher than those observed in normal cell hemolysates. More recent studies (183, 184) demonstrated that membranes prepared from normal erythrocytes contained alpha- and beta-chains and that sickle cell membranes, particularly those derived from the most dense fraction, possessed more globin than normal membranes. Some of this protein was without heme. This raises the possibility that more free-globin S and denatured-globin S associated or bound to the membranes of sickle erythrocytes might influence the status of the membrane.

Changes in Lipid Composition and Bilayer Asymmetry

The contents or concentrations of neutral lipids and phospholipids in subjects of sickle cell anemia have been examined without significant changes in the major classes (185, 186). Some differences in plasma cholesterol levels (186, 187), plasma cholesterol esterifying activity (188) and plasma–erythrocyte membrane cholesterol exchange (188) have been reported. The levels of the major phospholipid classes (i.e., phosphatidylcholine, sphingomyelin, phosphatidylethanolamine, and phosphatidylserine) in sickle cells are roughly normal, although their transbilayer distribution appears to be altered (see discussion to follow). Regarding the minor phospholipids, increased levels of phosphatidic acid in ISCs have been reported (189). Since the formation of phosphatidic acid (PA) in erythrocytes is dependent on the level of 1;2-diacylglycerol, which, in turn, is produced from phospholipase action on phospholipids (primarily the phosphoinositides), one would expect the levels of the phosphoinositides in sickle cells and specifically ISCs to be decreased. This would be in keeping with the activation of the polyphosphoinositide phosphodiesterase (a phospholipase C-type enzyme) by possible transient increases in calcium concentration during sickling episodes. It is somewhat surprising, however, that the levels of phosphatidylinositol and its phosphorylated products, phosphatidylinositol-4-phosphate and phosphatidylinositol-4,5-bisphosphate, have been determined to be within normal limits for sickle cells and ISCs (190).

Changes in the distribution of phospholipids across the membrane have been reported also. As previously described, the external surface of the normal erythrocyte membrane contains primarily phosphatidylcholine (PC) and shingomyelin with small amounts of phosphatidylethanolamine (PE), while the inner surface is comprised of PE and phosphatidylserine (PS). For this reason only small amounts of PE and no PS should be detected on the external surface of the membrane by nonpenetrating chemical probes or enzymes. However, the addition of trinitrobenzene sulfonate (TNBS), a nonpenetrating probe that can react with the amino groups of PS and PE, to irreversibly sickled cells showed an increased labelling reaction with PE and a 4 percent labelling of PS (191, 192). Normal cells, cells from subjects with sickle cell trait, and reversibly sickled cells exposed to room air failed to show PS on the outer surface. Deoxygenating sickle-trait cells, reversibly sickled cells, and irreversibly sickled cells also increased the levels of PE labelling with TNBS (17 to 22%; 11% for normal cells) and exposed the presence of 6 to 9 percent of the PS on the external surface. The lack of reactivity of this chemical probe with the amino groups of hemoglobin under all these conditions indicated that the increased reactivity of the TNBS was due to the increased levels of PE and PS on the external surface and not due to the increased permeability of the membrane to the probe. Despite one report (287) that claimed that there was no change in the phospholipid asymmetry of sickled cells, the results found with TNBS have been corroborated with studies utilizing phospholipase A_2 (an enzyme that cleaves the fatty acyl group from the second position of the glycerol backbone of PC, PE, and PS) and sphingomyelinase (192, 193) along with spin-labelled analogues of PE, PC, and PS (194). These experiments demonstrated that deoxygenated reversibly sickled cells and oxygenated irreversibly sickled cells contained increased levels of PE and PS on the outer surface of the membrane, compensated by increased levels of PC on the inner surface of the membrane. Sphingomeylinase results indicated that sphingomyelin levels remained constant for these cells under all conditions.

Of particular interest was the observation that the increase in the PS level in reversibly sickled cells upon deoxygenation returned to normal (i.e., no PS on the outer surface) upon reoxygenation of the cells. The overall results were interpreted to mean that during polymer formation and sickling there is a disruption in the membrane that allows the movement of some PS and PE from the inner to the outer surface of the membrane. This increase in phospholipid content is compensated for by a movement of PC from the outer surface to the inner surface of the membrane. This altered distribution of the lipids supposedly corrects itself during conditions of oxygenation when the hemoglobin polymer dissociates and sickling is reversed. At some point, however, when the reversibly sickled cell is transformed to an irreversibly sickled cell, the altered distribution of PE and especially PS becomes permanent. This proposal is supported by evidence that at least one acidic phospholipid, PIP_2, is involved in the linkage of the cytoskeleton to the membrane (123) and that destabilization of the membrane results in the increased flip-flop of phospholipids across the bilayer (195–197).

It appears that the exposure of small amounts (4–6%) of PS on the external surface of the membrane causes serious physiological complications related to blood coagulation. The involvement of lipids in accelerating blood coagulation leading to clot formation has been known for many years. The procoagulant activity is normally derived from activated platelets, and normal erythrocytes do not appear to play a role. However, irreversibly sickled cells and deoxygenated reversibly sickled cells do shorten the blood clotting time as measured by the Russell's viper venom assay (191, 198). To test the relevence of membrane phospholipids to this assay, liposomes of known composition were prepared with purified erythrocyte phospholipids. Only those liposomes containing phosphatidylserine exhibited the shortened blood clotting effect seen with ISCs and deoxygenated RSCs. In addition to changes in blood coagulation, the presence of PS in the outer membranes of sickle cells appears to be associated with their recognition by macrophages and consequent rosette formation (199). While the exact pathophysiologic consequences of these two observations are yet to be determined, it is probable that the exposure of PS on the outer surface of sickle cell membranes leads to vascular complications *in vivo*.

Deoxygenated Hb SS erythrocytes are more susceptible to lipid peroxidation when treated with hydrogen peroxide than are oxygenated sickle cells or normal cells under either condition, as evidenced by the formation of thiobarbituric reactive products such as malondialdehyde (181, 192, 200). In the case of malondialdehyde (MDA) the presence of two aldehyde groups on the molecule allows the possible formation of two Schiff bases with compounds containing amino groups. The identification of a novel phospholipid–MDA adduct (201–203) strongly indicates that increased membrane oxidation occurs in sickle cells.

Protein and Cytoskeletal Changes

Since their first discovery, irreversibly sickled cells have stimulated much interest among investigators. This interest was enhanced when it was learned that the molecular alteration responsible for the disease was located in the hemoglobin molecule rather than in a membrane component. How could a single amino acid substitution in the hemoglobin molecule cause significant changes in the morphology of the cell? Furthermore, why did the cell maintain this morphology under oxygenating conditions when most of the hemoglobin was in its soluble rather than its polymerized state? Questions regarding the causes of ISC formation continue to baffle scientists, although research is beginning to elucidate this process.

Sickle or crescent-shaped cells were first described in animals (i.e., pigs and deer) as early as 1840. It was not until 1910 that Herrick first published his finding of sickle-shaped cells in humans (204). An excellent article reviewing sickle cell shape and structure was published by Bessis and Delpech (205) and is recommended for further reading on this subject. The presence of ISCs took on greater importance when it was realized that there was a direct correlation between the ISC count and red cell survival (206). At the same time, further characterization of sickle cells was completed (207–209) which helped to distinguish between reversibly sickled cells and irreversibly sickled cells and to identify the presence of endocytic vesicles in ISCs. The mid-1970s witnessed a growing realization that spectrin and other structural proteins formed a matrix or cytoskeleton and that these proteins were responsible for erythrocyte shape and deformability (64, 65, 210, 211). An initial examination of the major membrane proteins by SDS-polyacrylamide gel electrophoresis failed to reveal any differences between normal and sickle cell membranes (212, 213). A more careful scrutiny of these proteins and glycoproteins did, however, reveal some minor differences including increased binding of bands 4.5a (nomenclature of Riggs and Ingram), 6, 7, and 8 (214, 215). The staining of glycoproteins with periodic acid Schiff (PAS) reagent in sickle cell membranes was decreased relative to controls. However, normal levels of N-acetylglucosamine and N-acetylgalactosamine were found, indicating that the decrease was due to the absence of N-acetylneuraminic acid (the sugar that stains with PAS) and that the glycoprotein levels were probably normal (214). Of particular interest is the increase in band 8 that has been observed (214, 215). Ballas and Burka (213) acknowledged that this protein and others were higher in sickle cell membranes that were prepared in a manner comparable to normal membranes, but they reported that more vigorous washing of the membranes could remove these proteins. Indeed, it has been demonstrated that band 8 is a cytoplasmic protein that has the ability to associate with the erythrocyte membrane under particular conditions. This may be important since the association of cytoplasmic proteins with the membrane may be associated with a change in membrane deformability.

Not only proteins but also polyamines such as putrescine, spermidine, and spermine appear to be higher in the blood of sickle cell subjects compared to controls (216), and the increased levels are associated with membrane proteins (217). This takes on greater relevance since the association of polyamines with erythrocyte membranes has been found to decrease the deformability (218). Further research (219) has shown that the incorporation of ^{14}C-histamine and ^{3}H-spermine into sickle erythrocyte membranes following incubation of these amines with intact erythrocytes in the presence of calcium and the ionophore A23187 is decreased relative to control cells. This was true despite the fact that sickle cells were more permeable to these amines than normal cells. It was proposed that the γ-glutamyl sites of membrane proteins in sickle erythrocytes are less accessible to cross-linking by calcium-activated transglutamination of histamine and polyamines due to prior *in vivo* activation of this enzyme and/or shielding secondary to the changed membrane topography. While the concentrations of polyamines in erythrocyte membranes may not reach levels sufficient to dramatically alter deformability, it has been proposed that these compounds may at least contribute to the decreased deformability.

Because of the very minor changes in the quantities of the membrane proteins, investigators looked for qualitative changes. These have included (1) self- or intermembrane protein association, that is, polymerization, (2) redistribution of membrane proteins within the membrane, and (3) altered binding of proteins that normally associate with one another, that is, cytoskeletal proteins.

In the mid-1970s it became apparent that the introduction of calcium into normal erythrocytes caused them to be more rigid and less deformable. This was often associated with the formation of protein polymerization catalyzed by the enzyme transglutaminase. Since irreversibly sickled cells were known to have higher calcium contents than normal cells or non-ISCs, studies (220–224) were initiated to investigate the possibility that ATP depletion increased calcium and activated transglutaminase polymerization of proteins, which could represent a pathophysiological event in ISC formation. Palek, Liu, and Liu (221) investigated protein polymerization in ISCs using a two-dimensional SDS-polyacrylamide gel system in which proteins were separated in the absence of the sulfhydryl reducing agent dithiothreitol (DTT) in the first dimension and then again in the presence of DTT in the second dimension. This procedure allowed the identification of protein polymers that were artificially formed by either $CuSO_4$ + O-phenanthroline oxidation, glutaraldehyde fixation (i.e., cross-linking of protein amino groups), or by ATP depletion in the presence of calcium, or by calcium loading with the ionophore A23187. The latter two methods, at calcium concentrations below 100 μM, produced spectrin aggregates that could be reduced by DTT. In contrast, when calcium concentrations above 500 μM were used, irreversible protein polymers were formed that could not be reduced by DTT. The high calcium protein polymers included not only spectrin but also band 3, another major membrane protein. When a dense cell fraction containing >80 percent ISCs was examined, no high-molecular-weight protein polymers could be detected. The authors concluded that ''neither a Ca^{2+} dependent irreversible crosslinking of membrane proteins nor a spectrin rearrangement characteristically seen in ATP depleted cells is responsible for a permanent fixation of ISCs in a sickled shape'' (221: p. 85). These results were attributed to the facts that the ATP concentration is only moderately decreased in ISCs, if at all; the increased calcium content in ISCs did not exceed 80 micromoles/10^{13} cells (assuming a mean cell volume of about 70 fl for dense cells, this would be a calcium concentration of less than 114 μM). Indeed, the possibility of transglutaminase activation by calcium as well as calcium-induced spectrin aggregation appears remote since it has been recently shown that most of the increased calcium in ISCs is sequestered in endocytic vesicles and that the cytoplasmic ionic calcium is maintained at a very low concentration during steady state periods (see discussion below). This does not preclude the possibility, however, that transient rises in calcium concentrations during sickling episodes might lead to distributional or associative changes among membrane proteins.

Evidence for changes in the distribution of proteins across the surfaces of the membrane are derived somewhat indirectly from studies investigating the adherence of normal and sickle erythrocytes to endothelial cells (for a more indepth discussion of this topic, see Chapter 4). Initial studies showed that erythrocytes from sickle cell subjects adhered to a monolayer of endothelial cells in culture to a much greater extent than did normal erythrocytes (225, 226). It became clear from crossover experiments that this increased adherence was due to factors present in the plasma and in the erythrocyte membranes of sickle cell subjects (227). Recent data attribute the plasma component responsible for this adherence to high-molecular-weight polymers of von Willebrand factor. The membrane component has been more elusive to understand. Although all sickle erythrocytes exhibited abnormal adherence to endothelial cells, there was a positive correlation with the density of the cells (228). Aberrant shape did not appear to be a major factor since deoxygenation of sickle cells reduced the adherence. Also, the depletion of N-acetylneuraminic acid, the sugar that provides the net negative charge on the external surface, likewise reduced the adherence significantly.

Manipulation of normal red blood cells to mimic the sickle cell adherence effect was attempted with the result that low-dose loading of calcium (10 micromolar) caused an increase in the number of cells bound to the endothelial cell layer. This concentration of calcium did not result in a change in morphology but probably caused the cells to undergo a loss of potassium and intracellular water, leading to an increase in density of the cells. Depletion of N-acetylneuraminic acid from these cells prior to calcium loading prevented the increased adherence. These results suggest that sickle cells undergo a topographical distribution of proteins such as glycophorin, the major transmembrane protein which contains the majority of N-acetynueuraminic acid, on the surface of the membrane and that this rearrangement, which is perhaps just a reduction in the distance between these proteins, results in a greater propensity of these cells to associate with endothelial cells in the presence of plasma factors. It should be mentioned that an independent study by Clark, Chan, Powars, et al. (229) using colloidal iron hydroxide labelling followed by glutaraldehyde fixation and electron microscopy did not support the findings by Hebbel, Yamada, Moldow, et al. (228) that the negative charge distribution on the surface of sickle erythrocytes was altered relative to controls. Further research will be required to resolve this difference. Regardless, the evidence indicates that changes in the topographical distribution of surface components occurs, and possibly results from, transmembrane associations with the cytoskeleton since previous evidence has indicated that antibodies to spectrin cause an aggregation of negative charges (glycophorin) at the membrane surface (230). Studies such as these have spurred the interest in changes in the cytoskeleton of sickle cells.

The role of the cytoskeletal network in the morphological change of ISCs was strengthened by the finding that not only the membranes derived from these cells, but also the Triton shells (i.e., the cytoskeletal protein framework, which remains after treatment with Triton X-100 and removal of the solubilized proteins), maintained the sickled shape (231, 232). Reversibly sickled cells do not yield the abnormal Triton shells and membrane skeletons derived from hereditary elliptocytes and hereditary pyropoikilocytes also maintain similar shape alterations, indicating that the shape change in sickle cells may be attributed to the cytoskeletal matrix. A more recent study by Platt, Falcone, and Lux (233) demonstrated that the binding of spectrin dimers (derived from normal cells) to inside-out vesicles (IOVs) derived from sickle cell membranes was significantly decreased. This decrease was most pronounced when IOVs were prepared from irreversibly sickled cells. In contrast, spectrin dimers extracted from either normal erythrocyte membranes or sickle cell membranes exhibited the same binding to IOVs derived from normal cells. Finally, the binding of purified ankyrin from control and SS cells to purified spectrin from normal cells was the same. The authors speculated that the decreased binding of spectrin to sickle cell IOVs may be due to an altered topography of ankyrin molecules on the cytoplasmic surface of the membrane. Possibly, the repetitive process of sickling and unsickling brings about such a topographical change in ankyrin as well as in other proteins.

Finally, the sickling process is associated with a loss of membrane material in the form of spicules (223, 234). The formation of these spicules can be demonstrated during *in vitro* sickling and can be isolated from the fresh blood of sickle cell subjects. As opposed to spectrin-depleted vesicles, which are formed during the ATP depletion of normal cells, spicules derived from sickle cell membranes appear to possess all the major membrane components (223).

Clearly, the process of irreversible sickling results in subtle changes in the sickle erythrocyte membrane, including cytoplasmic protein adherence to the inner surface, the possible alteration in membrane topography, the decreased binding of spectrin to the cytoplasmic membrane surface, and the homogeneous loss of membrane material. Further studies are underway to investigate the oxidation of membrane proteins and lipids and to elucidate the possible role that this might have in ISC formation. In addition to membrane structure, changes in enzyme activities have been a focus of attention for many investigators who are interested in the sickling phenomenon.

Changes in Ion Transport That Lead to Cellular Dehydration

The isolation of cell fractions that are rich in irreversibly sickled cells is most often accomplished by density gradient centrifugation. Although there is not a perfect correlation, it is apparent that most ISCs are more dense than normal. It should be kept in mind that some dense cells are not ISCs. Regardless, it appears that the process of sickling is accompanied by or preceded by cellular dehydration, (i.e., a loss of intracellular water), which causes the cells to become more dense. An excellent and concise evaluation of the current theories regarding the changes in ion fluxes that may cause cellular dehydration in HbSS cells has been reported by Bookchin, Ortiz, and Lew (235), and I recommend it highly.

It is generally agreed that the loss of water from sickle cells is caused by a net loss of monovalent cations, principally potassium. This efflux of potassium is not compensated for by an equivalent influx of sodium, although the intracellular sodium concentration does rise considerably (236–238). Rather, the cell loses chloride anions in order to maintain electroneutrality. The combined loss of potassium and chloride causes the inside of the cell to become hypo-osmotic relative to the outside, and to compensate for this difference, the cell loses water. The proteins inside the cell become more concentrated due to the dehydration and the cell becomes more dense. The controversy over the years has concerned the possible causes for the net loss of potassium.

Throughout the 1970s there were several reports of a calcium abnormality in HbSS cells. Fractions that were rich in irreversibly sickled cells formed *in vivo* or *in vitro* had higher levels of calcium than normal (239–241). Deoxygenated sickle cells took up 2.6 times more calcium than normal cells or control cells during a 2-hour incubation (242, 243). Calcium exchange across the sickle cell membrane was reported to be both high (244) and low (245). The ability of sickle cells to extrude preloaded calcium was abnormal (243, 245), leaving a residual level of calcium within the cell which could only be removed by the ionophore A23187. In addition, most of the calcium in normal red cells was not extracted when the cells were permeabilized to calcium by ionophore in the presence of EGTA, and therefore was tightly bound, whereas nearly all the excess calcium in HbSS cells was easily extracted. From 1979 to 1981, reports were published demonstrating decreased activity of basal and/or calmodulin-stimulated $(Ca^{2+} + Mg^{2+})$-ATPase, the enzyme responsible for providing the energy to pump calcium out of the cell (246–248). Purification of the enzyme from sickle cell membranes demonstrated that the change could be attributed to a decrease in the specific activity rather than the number of enzyme molecules (249). A recent paper (250) proposed that the decreased enzyme activity may be due to increased oxidative stress, and there is evidence (251–253) that could support this theory. The overwhelming evidence indicated that sickle cells were more leaky to calcium, particularly under deoxygenation conditions; that the calcium pump was unable to remove all the intracellular calcium; and that the enzyme responsible for supplying energy for the calcium pump was depressed. This might explain the increased intracellular calcium and also the loss of potassium via the calcium-dependent potassium transport pathway described by Gardös (254) in the late 1950s.

More recent studies (255, 256) have shown that most, if not all, of the increased intracellular calcium is sequestered within endocytic vesicles and is not cytoplasmic. Indeed, when the cytoplasmic ionic calcium concentration in sickle erythrocytes was measured using an NMR probe (257), it was found to be within the normal range (10–30 nM). The possibility still remains, however, that ionic calcium concentrations rise transiently during sickling, after which the calcium is pumped out of the cell or into the endocytic vesicles. It is possible that repetitive transient rises in intracellular ionic calcium may lead to a net potassium loss and cellular dehydration, and a case for this hypothesis has recently been put forward (235). Our own results have recently identified a cytoplasmic protein that is involved in calcium-dependent potassium transport in human erythrocytes. Levels of this cytoplasmic protein bound to the membrane are higher in dense sickle cells (i.e., those cells that have undergone dehydration) than normal cells or light sickle cells, and the levels increase with the formation of dense cells *in vitro*. Further studies are needed to verify conclusively that this protein is involved in the cellular dehydration of sickle cells, but these results support the argument for the hypothesis involving calcium-dependent potassium transport. Because of the controversy regarding the actual cytoplasmic calcium concentrations, other models have been explored to explain the net potassium loss.

One theory suggests that a net potassium loss might take place because of the inequivalent stoichiometry of the sodium-potassium pump. Normal cells have very slow passive flux rates to potassium and sodium, and the concentrations of these monovalent cations are regulated principally by active transport (i.e., the pump). The pump normally transports two potassium ions into the cell for every three sodium ions pumped out of the cell. During reversible sickling (i.e., a short period of deoxygenation), however, Hb SS cells express an increased rate of passive leak to sodium and potassium ions in an equivalent manner (one Na^+ in for one K^+ out) (258, 259). Following such a leak, the sodium-potassium pump within the cell membrane would restore two potassium ions for every three sodium ions removed, resulting in a net loss of the former cation. Theoretically, this would result in cellular dehydration and an increase in the formation of dense cells. When tested, Clark, Guatelli, White, et al. (260) found that the response of the pump to an equivalent loss of sodium and potassium did indeed cause dehydration and could potentially account for at least some of the dehydration observed in Hb SS cells. Joiner, Platt, and Lux (261) found that incubation of Hb SS cells *in vitro* for 18 hours under deoxygenating conditions caused a loss of cations and that this loss could be prevented by the addition of ouabain, an inhibitor of the sodium-potassium pump. The authors proposed that the net cation loss observed in irreversibly sickled cells or during irreversible sickling *in vitro* could be contributed by the 3:2 stoichiometry of the pump. This mechanism, however, cannot fully account for the significant loss of potassium which occurs in dense Hb SS cells with an only moderate sodium gain (235). In addition, our own research using the repetitive deoxygenation/reoxygenation procedure for forming dense Hb SS cells showed highly variable effects with ouabain (many sickle subjects showed no prevention of dense cell formation in the presence of this inhibitor). Quinine, a selective inhibitor of calcium-dependent potassium transport, was found to be a more reliable inhibitor of dense cell formation (see also Ohnishi, Horiuchi, and Horiuchi [262]). Regardless, the mechanism of net cation loss due to the inequivalent transport of the sodium and potassium through the pump has the potential of contributing to dense cell formation in Hb SS cells.

Another mechanism for net cation loss and cellular dehydration in human erythrocytes is chloride- and volume-dependent potassium efflux (263). It was found that cells that were artificially swollen underwent a volume-regulated decrease in size through a net loss of potassium. This loss of potassium ions was dependent on chloride but not ATP and was insensitive to both ouabain and bumetanide, an inhibitor of Na-K-Cl transport. Canessa and colleagues (264, 265) have demonstrated that this process can take place in Hb SS cells and that the transport is elevated in young red cells (266). It has been shown that erythrocytes swell under conditions of low pH, an environment that is known to exist in some organs, particularly the kidney. Possibly, young Hb SS cells may undergo pH-dependent swelling as they traverse acidified sections of the circulation and then undergo a volume-regulated decrease through net K-Cl efflux. The contribution of this transport pathway to dense cell formation is probably limited due to the finding that it is inhibited under conditions of deoxygenation (265). A review of this subject may be gained by reading Nagel, Fabry, Kaul et al. (267). An N-ethylmaleimide–stimulated potassium transport that leads to a net loss of intracellular cations has also been described (268) in Hb AA and Hb SS cells. This transport process is ATP-dependent (M. Canessa, personal communation, 1989) and, therefore, may be distinct from the volume-dependent potassium transport pathway. Because N-ethylmaleimide acts by alkylating sulfhydryl groups and because sulfhydryl groups are also very sensitive to oxidation, an alternative hypothesis for net cation loss may be proposed: namely, the excessive formation of reactive oxygen species decreases the presence of free sulfhydryl groups (particularly those associated with NEM-stimulated K^+ transport) and elicits an increase in the net efflux of potassium and chloride ions. Of course, further research will be necessary to support such a hypothesis.

Altered Enzyme Activities

In addition to membrane structure, changes in enzyme activities have been a focus of attention for many investigators interested in the sickling phenomenon.

Table 3.4
Human Erythrocyte Protein Kinases

	cAMP-Dependent	c-AMP-Independent
<u>Endogenous</u> <u>Acceptors</u>	bands 2.1, 4.5, (3 weak)	bands 2 and 3* several minor proteins
Properties	inhibited by 130 mM Na$^+$ or K$^+$ 1 mM Ca^{2+}	inhibited by low calcium concentrations
		stimulated by 0.1 mM Mg^{2+} 1 mM Ca^{2+} 50 mM Na$^+$ or K$^+$
<u>Exogenous</u> <u>Acceptors</u>	histones or protamine	casein or phosvitin
Properties	inhibited by 130 mM Na$^+$ or K$^+$	requires Mg^{2+}
	stimulated by cAMP	stimulated by 130 mM Na$^+$ or K$^+$
	70% membrane bound	26% membrane bound

*Band 3 includes proteins 2.9, 3, and PAS-1.

The enzymes that have received the most attention include the protein kinases, the enzymes of the phosphoinositide cycle, the methyltransferases and adenylate cyclase. The subjects will be discussed in that order.

The protein kinases are enzymes that can phosphorylate other proteins. These enzymes may be located in the cytoplasm and/or the membrane and may phosphorylate proteins that are soluble in the cytoplasm or are membrane-bound. The erythrocyte protein kinases have been categorized (269) under the following criteria: (1a) cyclic AMP-dependent phosphorylating endogenous membrane proteins, (1b) cyclic AMP-dependent phosphorylating exogenous acceptor proteins (histones or protamine are preferred), (2a) cyclic AMP-independent phosphorylating endogenous membrane-bound proteins, and (2b) cyclic AMP-independent phosphorylating exogenous acceptor proteins (casein and phosvitin are preferred). Table 3.4 provides details regarding this classification. Note that although most of the membrane-associated protein kinase activity is of the cyclic AMP-dependent type, very little of this activity would be expressed under physiological conditions (i.e., monovalent cation concentrations approaching 130 mM). The cyclic AMP-independent protein kinases that are less associated with the membrane (only 26% bound) are active within the physiological environment. The major membrane proteins that are phosphorylated by these kinase(s) involve band 2 (beta-spectrin), band 3 (the anion transport channel), and glylcophorin (the major sialoglycoprotein). In addition, several other minor membrane proteins are phosphorylated (270). The properties of the membrane-bound casein kinase reflect those of spectrin kinase, which is cyclic AMP-independent, stimulated by salt concentrations above 50 mM, and extractable by treatment with 0.5 M NaCl. It would appear, however, that the spectrin kinase is not part of the spectrin molecule itself, since treatment of the erythrocyte membrane with low-ionic-strength solutions removes almost all of alpha- and beta-spectrin yet all the casein kinase activity remains with the unsolubilized membrane portion. It is also known that the addition of purified casein kinase to membranes results in the phosphorylation of many erythrocyte membrane proteins other than beta-spectrin. These results suggest that the spectrin kinase is a membrane-bound protein with casein kinase–like activity which is distinct from spectrin. Phosphorylation of spectrin occurs at the c-terminus of beta-spectrin.

Erythrocyte membrane protein phosphorylation has been studied in sickle cell disease by several investigators (270–277). Interpretation of the results must be made carefully since the rate of phosphorylation is often determined by the presence of the enzyme(s) that phosphorylate the various proteins, and phosphatases, the enzyme(s) that dephosphorylate proteins. Indeed, Beutler, Guinte, and Johnson (271) found that the rate of protein phosphorylation in isolated membranes was only linear for about 10 min after which it began to plateau, leveling off between 20 and 60 min. Consequently, the effects of membrane kinase activity were assessed after 5 min of incubation with ^{32}P-ATP and the effects contributed largely by membrane phosphatase activity were assessed after 60 min of incubation. The results showed that there was a significant decrease in the phosphorylation of spectrin but not band 3 after 5 min, indicating a reduced spectrin kinase activity. However, the degree of protein phosphate labelling after 60 min was severely depressed for both spectrin and band 3, indicating increased phosphatase activity.

These results have been repeated with other anemias and it is now known that decreased phosphorylation of spectrin occurs in hereditary spherocytosis and hereditary pyropoikilocytosis. Further work by Dzandu, Johnson, and Worth (274, 277) demonstrated that the decreased spectrin kinase activity in sickle cell disease could not be due to the relative cell age, the ATP levels within the cell, or the rate of ^{32}P labelling of the ATP pool. Moreover, calcium loading into normal cells using the ionophore A23187 initiated changes in ^{32}P labelling that reflected the changes normally seen in sickle cell disease, suggesting that potential transient increases in cytoplasmic calcium during sickling might cause the effects observed. Finally, it has been documented that there is increased phosphorylation of the sialoglycoproteins in sickle cell membranes relative to controls (278). The same study also contends that spectrin phosphorylation in sickle cells is normal and that the ratio of band 3/band 2 phosphorylation is increased.

Protein kinase C (discussed previously in the section on enzymes) has also been investigated in sickle cell disease (279). Briefly, protein kinase C becomes bound to the membrane following the formation of diglyceride, which is a consequence of increased cytoplasmic calcium. Upon binding to the membrane, this kinase becomes activated, phosphorylating predominantly bands 3, 4.1, and 4.9. The kinase can be artifically activated by the reagent phorbol-12,13-dibutyrate (PDBu), which acts as an analogue to diglyceride but is not metabolized. Sickle cells have abnormal protein kinase activity. First, sickle cell membranes showed a fourfold increase in ^{3}H-PDBu binding relative to control membranes. Second, phosphorylation of sickle cell membrane proteins was enhanced compared to that of controls. Third, induction of protein kinase C activity by calcium loading of cells resulted in elevated phosphorylation in both normal and sickle cells, but the elevation was greater in the latter. In summary, the phosphorylation of membrane proteins appears altered in sickle cell disease and this change apparently results from the pathophysiological changes that occur during the disease process.

In addition to the phosphorylation of proteins, membrane phospholipids, particularly the phosphoinositides, may also be phosphorylated. As with proteins, the phosphate groups are added by kinases, in this case phosphatidylinositol kinases, and the phosphate groups are removed by phosphatases (see Figure 3.9). An enzyme—a polyphosphoinositide phosphodiesterase—is responsible for hydrolyzing the molecule into two components, an inositol bis or tris phosphate and diglyceride. This enzyme is important because it depletes the membrane of phosphoinositides. The mature red cell does not resynthesize them and instead generates diglyceride, the molecule that initiates the association of protein kinase C to the membrane and contributes to its activation. The phosphodiesterase has received interest (189, 280, 281) in sickle cell disease because it is activated by cytoplasmic calcium within the micromolar concentration range. ^{32}P-labelling studies have shown less incorporation of phosphate into phosphatidylinositol 4,5-bisphosphate. Under deoxygenated conditions in the presence of calcium there is significantly less incorporation of the label into the polyphosphoinositides compared to the same conditions in the presence of ethylene-bis (oxylethyl-enenitrilo) tetra-acetic acid (EGTA) (280). The decreased label is presumed to be the consequence of phosphodiesterase activity (unpublished data from our own laboratory confirm these results). The fractionation of sickle erythrocytes on discontinuous isotonic stractan gradients revealed that dense cells that were rich in irreversibly sickled cells contained fewer polyphosphoinositides and more phosphatidic acid relative to the lighter fraction of sickle cells (189). In contrast to these results, Rhoda, Sulpice, Gascard, et al. (281) found little or no changes in the levels of polyphosphoinositides in light cells compared to dense cells and could not demonstrate any phosphoinositide change during *in vitro* incubation under deoxygenated conditions in the presence of calcium. This included the measurement of inositol-1,4,5-trisphosphate by ion-pair reverse-phase high-performance liquid chromatography. These conflicting results raise questions as to whether calcium concentrations rise significantly during sickling to initiate protein and lipid changes.

The methylation of erythrocyte membranes is altered in sickle cell anemia (282–285). Both phospholipid methylation and protein carboxyl methylation are decreased in Hb SS cells (282). The protein portion, which normally comprises about 70 percent of the methyl acceptors, was decreased in all fractions of SS cells separated by density gradient centrifugation (284). Furthermore, the decreased rate of methylation was similar for all methyl acceptor proteins (282), although Green et al. (283) claimed there were differences in the rates of demethylation, particularly in regard to proteins 2.1 and 4.1 (283). The decreased methylation has been attributed to differences in organizational structure of sickle erythrocyte membranes for the following reasons: (1) purified membranes treated with the same purified methylase II show the same 50 percent decrease for sickle cell samples, (2) the levels of methylase II and methyl acceptor proteins in the membrane are similar in Hb SS and Hb AA cells, and (3) the methylation of sickle cell glycophorin is decreased when the protein was located in the membrane but the methylation appeared normal after the protein was extracted from the membrane (diiodosalicylate) (285).

While the contribution of protein methylation to cellular function has been determined in bacteria, the exact role of membrane protein methylation in erythrocytes has yet to be elucidated. However, bands 2.1 and 4.1 are important cytoskeletal elements of the membrane. Consequently, changes in carboxyl methylation of these proteins may lead to serious alterations in the structure and shape of the membrane. A further understanding of membrane protein methylation is needed in order to better interpret the ramifications of the results heretofore reported.

Adenylate cyclase activities, although low in erythrocytes, have been examined in normal and sickle cells and have been found to be increased (286). Some, but not all, of the increased activity could be attributed to the increased presence of reticulocytes in the samples and perhaps the younger age of the cells. Both basal and sodium fluoride-stimulated activities were enhanced in sickle cells relative to normal. Unfortunately, there has been little subsequent documentation regarding the levels of the GTP regulatory proteins or their receptor proteins (e.g., PGE_1) and other prostaglandins. This subject is discussed more fully in the next chapter.

SPECULATION REGARDING THE FORMATION OF DENSE CELLS AND IRREVERSIBLY SICKLED CELLS

The correlation between dense cells and irreversibly sickled cells is not perfect, and the cellular changes that lead to their formations may be quite different. I am always reminded that dense cells are isolated and quantified from density gradients and probably result from changes in ion transport, while irreversibly sickled cells are characterized morphologically under the microscope and probably result from changes in the cytoskeletal architecture of the membrane. Granted, there may be some common causes to dense cell and ISC formation as well. Regardless, one fact is clear: The origin of these changes lies in the presence of the hemoglobin S molecule. A speculation as to some of the cellular changes that take place upon repeated Hb S polymerization and Hb S denaturation, which lead to the formation of dense cells and ISCs, is provided below and depicted in Figure 3.10. At present, it is difficult to assign any chronological order to these events other than Hb S polymerization, and, indeed, the sequence of these changes may be different from cell to cell and even between subjects with varying penetrance of the disease.

The polymerization of hemogolobin S into short rods causes an initial distortion of cell shape and probably some stretching of the membrane architecture. This might result in the elongation of spectrin tetramers and distortion of the normal cytoskeletal conformation. This distortion may then lead to local changes in the interphospholipid associations, thereby altering the normal function of enzymes and transport proteins. Increased passive fluxes of sodium, potassium, and possibly calcium change the ionic environment and activate enzymes such as phospholipid and protein kinases and, potentially, phospholipid and protein methyl transferases. Alterations in the phosphorylation and methylation states of these macromolecules may lead to further changes in structural orientation, enzyme activities, and transport kinetics. Longer periods of deoxygenation produce longer rods, which cause even greater stress on the membrane, even to the point of puncturing the cytoskeleton. This leads to the separation of the phospholipid bilayer and some integral membrane proteins, such as band 3, from the cytoskeletal matrix. This state of the cell worsens as the changes described above intensify and additional transformations take place. As expected, these alterations become less reversible. The asymmetry of the phospholipid bilayer changes as phosphatidylserine migrates from the inside to the outside of the membrane surface. The redistribution of surface proteins leads to local clustering, allowing for increased binding of antibodies. Puncturing the cytoskeleton leads to isolated areas of disruption which may be unable to be patched upon dissolution of the polymer. Elongated spicules on the cell, where significant portions of the membrane are detached from the cytoskeleton, are susceptible to removal due to rupture of the fragile lipid bilayer. This leads to the formation of small membrane vesicles and cells with decreased membrane surface area to volume.

Reexposure of the cell to normal oxygen pressures causes the hemoglobin S polymer to dissolve back into the cytoplasm. The removal of these polymers decreases the mechanical stress on the membrane and allows it to return to what appears to be the normal biconcave shape. The return of the cell to an apparently normal state has allowed these cells to be classified as "reversibly sickled cells." However, this is probably a misnomer since it implies that the cell has returned to its original state in all respects. Rather, the cell has undergone many biochemical and structural changes that are not detectable morphologically. Either repetitive sickling or extended periods of deoxygenation finally produce signicant

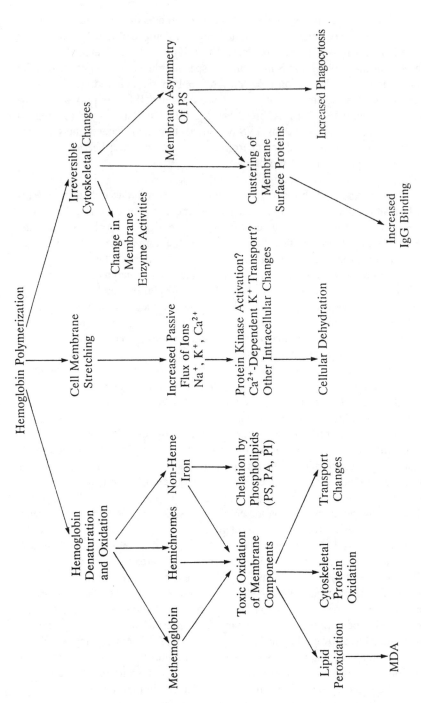

Figure 3.10. Sickle cell pathophysiology.

structural and functional changes to the cell that allow biochemical, physiological, and visual detection. At this stage, irreversibly sickled cells have sustained serious injury to the membrane.

In addition to the changes that result from hemoglobin polymerization, denaturation of the hemoglobin molecule to hemichromes and non-heme iron leads to increased formation of reactive oxygen species, such as superoxide anion, hydrogen peroxide, and hydroxyl radicals. This oxidative environment leads to lipid peroxidation and decomposition and to the oxidation of proteins that may be important for the maintenance of normal membrane structure and function. The non-heme iron forms complexes with the anionic phospholipids PS and PA, and with the phosphoinositides. These complexes potentially alter the normal associations of these phospholipids with membrane proteins, leading to changes in cytoskeletal attachment to the bilayer, the activities of many enzymes, and the transport of ions and other molecules.

Clearly, our understanding of the formation of dense cells and irreversibly sickled cells increases with the ongoing research that takes place. Nonetheless, there is still much that needs to be learned in the solution of this complex puzzle, and it will be interesting to see what future research will reveal.

REFERENCES

1. Hawkins CF, Kyd JM, and Bagnara AS: Adenosine metabolism in human erythrocytes: A study of some factors which affect the metabolic fate of adenosine in intact red cells *in vitro*. *Arch Biochem Biophys* 202 (1980): 380–387.
2. Beutler E: *Red cell metabolism: A manual of biochemical methods*, 3d ed. New York: Grune and Stratton, 1984.
3. Beutler E: *Hemolytic anemia in disorders of red cell metabolism*. New York: Plenum Medical, 1978.
4. Hultquist DE, Sannes LJ, and Schafer DA: The NADH/NADPH—Methemoglobin reduction system of erythrocytes. *Prog Clin Biol Res* 55 (1981): 291–305.
5. Seaman C, Wyss S, and Piomelli S: The decline in energetic metabolism with aging of the erythrocyte and its relationship to cell death. *Am J Hematol* 8 (1980): 31–42.
6. Brewer GJ: Inherited erythrocyte metabolic and membrane disorders. *Med Clin N Amer* 64 (1980): 579–596.
7. Jaffe ER, and Valentine WN: Human erythroenzymopathies of the anaerobic Embden-Meyerhof glycolytic and associated pathways. In RL Nagel, ed.: *Genetically abnormal red cells*, Vol. 1, pp. 106–136. Boca Raton, FL: CRC Press, 1988.
8. Miwa S, and Fujii H: Molecular aspects of erythroenzymopathies associated with hereditary hemolytic anemia. *Am J Hematol* 19 (1985): 293–305.
9. Mentzer WC, and Glader BE: Disorders of erythrocyte metabolism. In WC Mentzer and GM Wagner, eds.: *The hereditary hemolytic anemias*, pp. 267–318. New York: Churchill Livingstone, 1989.
10. Moll PP, Sing CF, and Brewer GJ: A path analysis of the causal relationships between red cell glycolytic intermediates, ADP and ATP in sickle cell anemia. *Biosystems* 9 (1977): 245–256.

11. Altay C, Alper C, and Nathan DG: Normal and variant isoenzymes of human blood cell hexokinase and isoenzyme patterns in hemolytic anemia. *Blood* 36 (1970): 219–227.

12. Charache S, Grisolia S, Fiedler AJ, et al.: Effect of 2,3-diphosphoglycerate on oxygen affinity of blood in sickle cell anemia. *J Clin Invest* 49 (1970): 806–812.

13. Huehns ER, and Bellingham AJ: Studies of oxygen dissociation in red cells with abnormal hemoglobins and some enzyme deficiencies. *Biochem Pharmacol* 20 (1971): 981–983.

14. Opalinski A, and Beutler E: Creatine, 2,3-diphosphoglycerate and anemia. *N Engl J Med* 285 (1971): 483–486.

15. Roth EF Jr, Rachmilewitz EH, Schifter A, et al.: Benign sickle cell anemias in Israeli-Arabs with high red cell 2,3-diphosphogycerate. *Acta Haematol* 59 (1978): 237–245.

16. Lachant NA, Davidson WD, and Tanaka KR: Impaired pentose phosphate shunt function in sickle cell disease: A potential mechanism for increased Heinz body formation and membrane lipid perioxidation. *Am J Hematol* 15 (1983): 1–13.

17. Lachant NA, and Tanaka KR: Antioxidants in sickle cell disease: The *in vitro* effects of ascorbic acid. *Am J Med Sci* 292 (1986): 3–10.

18. Zerez CR, Lachant NA, Lee SJ, et al.: Decreased erythrocyte nicotinamide adenine dinucleotide redox potential and abnormal pyridine nucleotide content in sickle cell disease. *Blood* 71 (1988): 512–515.

19. Lewis RA, Kay RW, and Hathorn M: Sickle cell disease and glucose-6-phosphate dehydrogenase. *Acta Haematol* 36 (1966): 399–411.

20. Piomelli S, Reindorf CA, Arzanian MT, et al.: Clinical and biochemical interactions of glucose-6-phosphate dehydrogenase deficiency and sickle cell anemia. *N Engl J Med* 287 (1972): 213–217.

21. Steinberg MH, and Dreiling BJ: Glucose-6-phosphate dehydrogenase deficiency in sickle cell anemia. *Ann Intern Med* 80 (1974): 217–220.

22. Beutler E, Johnson C, Powars D, et al.: Prevalence of glucose-6-phosphate dehydrogenase deficiency in sickle cell disease. *N Engl J Med* 290 (1974): 826–828.

23. Bienzle U, Sodeinde O, Effiong CE, et al.: Glucose-6-phosphate dehydrogenase deficiency and sickle cell anemia. Frequency and features of association in an African community. *Blood* 46 (1975): 591–597.

24. Gibbs WN, Wardle J, and Serjeant GR: Glucose-6-phosphate dehydrogenase deficiency and homozygous sickle disease in Jamaica. *Br J Haematol* 45 (1980): 73–80.

25. Samuel APW, Saha N, Acquaye JK, et al.: Association of red cell glucose-6-phosphate dehydrogenase with hemoglobinopathies. *Human Hered* 36 (1986): 107–112.

26. Steinberg MH, West MS, Gallagher D, et al.: Effects of glucose-6-phosphate dehydrogenase deficiency upon sickle cell anemia. *Blood* 71 (1988): 748–752.

27. Beretta L, Gerli GC, Farraresi R, et al.: Antioxidant system in sickle red cells. *Acta Haematol* 70 (1983): 194–197.

28. Varma RN, Mankad VN, Phelps DD, et al.: Depressed erythrocyte glutathione reductase activity in sickle cell disease. *Am J Clin Nutr* 38 (1983): 884–887.

29. Wetterstroem N, Brewer GJ, Warth JA, et al.: Relationship of glutathione levels and Heinz body formation to irreversibly sickled cells in sickle cell anemia. *J Lab Clin Med* 103 (1984): 589–596.

30. Clark MR, Unger RC, and Shohet SB: Monovalent cation composition and ATP and lipid content of irreversibly sickled cells. *Blood* 51 (1978): 1169–1178.
31. Hebbel RP, Eaton JW, Balasingam M, et al.: Spontaneous oxygen radical generation by sickle erythrocytes. *J Clin Invest* 70 (1982): 1253–1259.
32. Schacter LP: Generation of superoxide anion and hydrogen peroxide by erythrocytes from individuals with sickle trait or normal haemoglobin. *Eur J Clin Invest* 16 (1986): 204–210.
33. Das SK, and Rajagopalan CN: Superoxide dismutase, glutathione perioxidase, catalase and lipid peroxidation of normal and sickled erythrocytes. *Br J Haematol* 44 (1980): 87–92.
34. Schacter L, Warth JA, Gordon LM, et al.: Altered amount and activity of superoxide dismutase in sickle cell anemia. *FASEB J* 2 (1988): 237–243.
35. Hebbel RP: Auto-oxidation and a membrane-associated "Fenton Reagent": A possible explanation for development of membrane lesions in sickle erythrocytes. *Clin Haematol* 14 (1985): 129–140.
36. Fraker PJ, Gershwin ME, Good RA, et al.: Interrelationships between zinc and immune function. *Fed Proc* 45 (1986): 1474–1479.
37. Chiu D, and Lubin B: Abnormal vitamin E and glutathione peroxidase levels in sickle cell anemia: Evidence for increased susceptibility to lipid peroxidation *in vivo. J Lab Clin Med* 94 (1979): 542–548.
38. Natta C, and Machlin L: Plasma levels of tocopherol in sickle cell anemia subjects. *Am J Clin Nutr* 37 (1979): 1359–1362.
39. Jain SK, and Williams DM: Reduced levels of plasma ascorbic acid (vitamin C) in sickle cell disease patients: Its possible role in the oxidant damage to sickle cells *in vivo. Clin Chim Acta* 149 (1985): 257–261.
40. Hebbel RP, and Miller WJ: Phagocytosis of sickle erythrocytes: Immunologic and oxidative determinants of hemolytic anemia. *Blood* 64 (1984): 733–741.
41. Chiu D, Vichinsky E, Yee M, et al.: Peroxidation, vitamin E, and sickle cell anemia. *Ann NY Acad Sci* 393 (1982): 323–335.
42. Rank BH, Carlsson J, and Hebbel RP: Abnormal redox status of membrane-protein thiols in sickle erythrocytes. *J Clin Invest* 75 (1985): 1531–1537.
43. Schwartz RS, Rybicki AC, Heath RH, et al.: Protein 4.1 in sickle erythrocytes. Evidence for oxidative damage. *J Biol Chem* 262 (1987): 15666–15672.
44. Miller WJ, and Hebbel RP: Erythrophagocytosis as a determinant of hemolytic rate in sickle cell disease. *Prog Clin Biol Res* 165 (1984): 85–92.
45. Anastase J: Hemoglobin S-mediated membrane oxidant injury: Protection from malaria and pathology in sickle cell disease. *Med Hypotheses* 14 (1984): 311–320.
46. Alberts B, Bray D, Lewis J, et al.: *Molecular biology of the cell*, 2d ed., pp. 275–340. New York: Garland Publishing, 1989.
47. Bergelson LD, and Barsukov LI: Topological asymmetry and flip-flop of phospholipids in biological membranes. In G Benga, ed.: *Structure and properties of cell membranes*, Vol. 1, pp. 77–92. Boca Raton, FL: CRC Press, 1985.
48. Van Deenan LLM, and de Gier J: Chemical composition and metabolism of lipids in red cells of various animal species. In C Bishop and DM Surgenor, eds.: *The red blood cell*, pp. 243–307. New York: Academic Press, 1964.
49. Hanahan DJ, Watts RM, and Pappajohn D: Some chemical characteristics of the lipids of human and bovine erythrocytes and plasma. *J Lipid Res* 1 (1960): 412–432.

50. Blau L, and Bittman R: Cholesterol distribution between the two halves of the lipid bilayer of human erythrocyte ghost membranes. *J Biol Chem* 253 (1978): 8366–8368.

51. Steck TL, and Dawson G: Topographical distribution of complex carbohydrates in the erythrocyte membrane. *J Biol Chem* 249 (1974): 2135–2142.

52. Whiteley NM, and Berg HC: Amidination of the outer and inner surfaces of the human erythrocyte membrane. *J Mol Biol* 87 (1974): 541–561.

53. Gordesky SE, Marinetti GV, and Love R: The reaction of chemical probes with the erythrocyte membrane. *J Memb Biol* 20 (1975): 111–132.

54. Verkleij AJ, Zwaal RFA, Roelofsen B, et al.: The asymmetric distribution of phospholipids in the human red cell membrane. *BBA* 323 (1973): 178–193.

55. Kahlenberg A, Walker C, and Rohrlick R: Evidence for an asymmetric distribution of phospholipids in the human erythrocyte membrane. *Can J Biochem* 52 (1974): 803–806.

56. Demel RA, Geurts Van Kessel WSM, Zwaal RFA, et al.: Relation between various phospholipase actions on human red cell membranes and the interfacial phospholipid pressure in monolayers. *Biochim Biophys Acta* 406 (1975): 97–107.

57. Bloj B, and Zilversmit DB: Asymmetry and transposition rates of phosphatidylcholine in rat erythrocyte ghosts. *Biochem* 15 (1976): 1277–1283.

58. Rencoji W, VanGolde LMG, Zwaal RFA, et al.: Topological asymmetry of phospholipid metabolism in rat erythrocyte membranes. *Eur J Biochem* 61 (1976): 53–58.

59. Low MG, and Finean JB: Modification of erythrocyte membranes by a purified phosphatidylinositol specific phospholipase C (staphylococcus aureus). *Biochem J* 162 (1977): 235–240.

60. Roberts WL, Kim BH, and Rosenberry TL: Differences in the glycolipid membrane anchors of bovine and human erythrocyte acetylcholinesterase. *Proc Natl Acad Sci USA* 84 (1987): 7817–7821.

61. Downes P, and Michell RH: Phosphatidylinositol 4-phosphate and phosphatidylinositol 4,5-bisphosphate: Lipids in search of a function. *Cell Calcium* 3 (1982): 467–502.

62. Moore RB, and Appel SH: Calcium-dependent hydrolyses of polyphosphoinositides in human erythrocyte membranes. *Can J Biochem Cell Biol* 62 (1984): 363–368.

63. Tyler JM, and Branton D: Molecular interactions governing red cell membrane structure. *Prog Clin Biol Res* 56L (1981): 79–93.

64. Palek J, and Liu SC: Altered red cell cytoskeletal protein associations leading to membrane instability. *Prog Clin Biol Res* 55 (1981): 385–402.

65. Shohet SB, Card RT, Clark M, et al.: The erythrocyte cytoskeleton and its apparent role in cellular functions. *Prog Clin Biol Res* 51 (1980): 35–58.

66. Gardner K, and Bennett GV: Recently identified erythrocyte membrane skeletal proteins and interactions: Implications for structure and function. In P Agre and JC Parker, ed.: *Red blood cell membranes*, pp. 1–29. New York: Marcel Dekker, 1989.

67. Speicher DW: Structural and functional features of the alpha-1 domain from human erythrocyte spectin. *Prog Clin Biol Res* 165 (1984): 441–456.

68. Goodman SR, Krebs KE, Whitfield CF, et al.: Spectrin and related molecules. *Crit Rev Biochem* 23 (1988): 171–234.

69. Palek J, Liu SC, Lawler J, et al.: Molecular defects of α-spectrin in hereditary

elliptocytosis and pyropoikilocytosis. In V Bennett, CM Cohen, SE Lux, and J Palek ed.: *Membrane skeletons and cytoskeletal-membrane associations*, pp. 357–369. New York: A. R. Liss, 1986.

70. Shen BW: Ultrastructure and function of membrane skeleton. In P Agre and JC Parker, ed.: *Red blood cell membranes*, pp. 261–297. New York: Marcel Dekker, 1989.

71. Brenner SL, and Korn ED: Spectrin-actin interaction. Phosphorylated and dephosphorylated spectrin tetramer cross-link F-actin. *J Biol Chem* 254 (1979): 8620–8627.

72. Goodman SR, Shiffer K, Coleman DB, et al.: Erythrocyte membrane skeletal protein spectrin band 4.1: A brief review. *Prog Clin Biol Res* 165 (1984): 415–439.

73. Anderson RA, and Louvrien R: Glycophorin is linked by band 4.1 protein to the human erythrocyte cytoskeleton. *Nature* 307 (1984): 655–658.

74. Mueller TJ, and Morrison M: Glycoconnectin (PAS 2), a membrane attachment site for the human erythrocyte cytoskeleton. *Prog Clin Biol Res* 56 (1981): 95–116.

75. Sato SB, and Ohnishi S: Interaction of a peripheral protein of the erythrocyte membrane, band 4.1, with phosphatidylserine-containing liposomes and erythrocyte inside-out vesicles. *Eur J Biochem* 130 (1983): 19–25.

76. Bennett GV: The membrane skeleton of human erythrocytes and its implication for more complex cells. *Ann Rev Biochem* 54 (1985): 273–304.

77. Platt OS: Inherited disorders of red cell membrane proteins. In R Nagel, ed.: *Genetically abnormal red cells*, Vol. 2, pp. 149–160. Boca Raton FL: CRC Press, 1988.

78. Palek J: Disorders of red cell membrane skeleton: An overview. *Prog Clin Biol Res* 159 (1984): 177–189.

79. Jennings ML, Anderson MP, and McCormick SJ: Functional roles of carboxyl groups in human red blood cell anion exchange. In RB Gunn and JC Parker, eds.: *Cell physiology of blood*, pp. 163–180. New York: Rockefeller University Press, 1987.

80. Salhany JM, ed.: *Erythrocyte band 3 protein*. Boca Raton, FL: CRC Press, 1989.

81. Baldwin SA, and Lienhard GE: Immunological identification of the human erythrocyte monosaccharide transporter. *Biochem Biophys Res Commun* 94 (1980): 1401–1408.

82. Rampal AL, Jung EKY, Chin JJ, et al.: Further characterization and chemical purity assessment of the human erythrocyte glucose transporter preparation. *Biochim Biophys Acta* 135 (1986): 135–142.

83. Jung CY: Radiation target size measurement of glucose transport function in animal cells. In JC Venter and CY Jung, eds: *Target size analysis of membrane proteins*, pp. 137–151. New York: A. R. Liss, 1987.

84. Mueckler MM: Structure and function of the glucose transporter. In P Agre and JC Parker, eds.: *Red blood cell membranes*, pp. 41–45. New York: Marcel Dekker, 1989.

85. Gati WP, and Paterson AR: Nucleoside transport. In P Agre and JC Parker, eds.: *Red blood cell membranes*, pp. 635–661. New York: Marcel Dekker, 1989.

86. Jarvis SM, and Young JD: Extraction and partial purification of the nucleoside-transport system from human erythrocytes based on the assay of nitrobenzylthioinosine binding activity. *Biochem* 194 (1981): 331–339.

87. Wu JSR, Kwong FYP, Jarvis SM, et al.: Identification of the erythrocyte nucleoside

transporter as band 4.5 polypeptide. Photoaffinity labelling studies using nitro ben-zylthioinoside. *J Biol Chem* 258 (1983): 13745–13751.

88. Tse CM, Belt JA, Jarvis SM, et al.: Reconstitution of the human erythrocyte nucleoside transporter. *J Biol Chem* 260 (1985): 3506–3511.

89. Sarkadi B, and Tosteson DC: Active cation transport in human red cells. In G Giebisch, DC Tosteson, and HH Ussing, eds.: *Membrane transport in biology.* Volume 2: *Transport across single biological membranes,* pp. 117–160. New York: Springer Verlag, 1979.

90. Cantley LC: Structure and mechanisms of the (Na, K) ATPase. *Curr Topics Bio-energet* 11 (1983): 201–237.

91. Shull GE, Schwartz A, and Lingrel JB: Amino acid sequence of the catalytic subunit of the (Na^+-K^+) ATPase deduced from a complimentary DNA. *Nature* 316 (1985): 691–695.

92. Mercer RW, Schneider JW, and Benz EJ: Na, K-ATPase structure. In P Agre and JC Parker, eds.: *Red blood cell membranes,* pp. 135–165. New York: Marcel Dekker, 1989.

93. Sweadner KJ, and Goldin SM: Active transport of sodium and potassium ions: mechanism function and regulation. *N Engl J Med* 302 (1980): 777–783.

94. Niggli V, Penniston JT, and Carafoli E: Purification of the $(Ca^{2+} + Mg^{2+})$-ATPase from human erythrocyte membranes using a calmodulin affinity column. *J Biol Chem* 254 (1979): 9955–9958.

95. Minocherhomjee AM, Beauregard G, Portier M, et al.: The molecular weight of the calcium-transport-ATPase of the human red blood cell determined by radiation inactivation. *Biochem Biophys Res Commun* 116 (1983): 895–900.

96. Steiger J, and Luterbacher S: Some properties of the purified $Ca^{2+} + Mg^{2+}$ ATPase from human red cell membranes. *Biochim Biophys Acta* 641 (1981): 270–275.

97. Niggli V, Adunya ES, Penniston JT, et al.: Purified $Ca^{2+} + Mg^{2+}$ -ATPase of the erythrocyte membrane. Reconstitution and effect of calmodulin and phospholipids. *J Biol Chem* 256 (1981): 395–401.

98. Ronner P, Gazzotti P, and Carafoli E: A lipid requirement for the $Ca^{2+} + Mg^{2+}$ -activated ATPase of erythrocyte membranes. *Arch Biochem Biophys* 179 (1977): 578–583.

99. Carafoli E: Calmodulin-sensitive calcium pumping ATPase of plasma membranes: Isolation, reconstitution and regulation. *Fed Proc* 43 (1984): 3005–3010.

100. Niggli V, and Carafoli E: Interaction of the purified $Ca^{2+} + Mg^{2+}$ ATPase from human erythrocytes with phospholipids and calmodulin. *Acta Biol Med Germ* 40 (1981): 437–442.

101. Niggli V, Adunyah ES, Penniston JR, et al.: Purified $Ca^{2+} + Mg^{2+}$ ATPase of the erythrocyte membrane. Reconstitution and effect of calmodulin and phospho-lipids. *J Biol Chem* 256 (1981): 395–401.

102. Niday E, Wang CS, and Alaupovic P: Studies on the characterization of human erythrocyte acetylcholinesterase and its interaction with antibodies. *Biochim Biophys Acta* 469 (1977):180–193.

103. Ott P, and Brodbeck U: Amphiphile dependency of the monomeric and dimeric forms of acetylcholinesterase from human erythrocyte membrane. *Biochim Biophys Acta* 775 (1984): 71–76.

104. Rosenberry TL, Roberts WL, and Haas R: Glylcolipid membrane-binding domain of human erythrocyte acetylcholinesterase. *Fed Proc* 45 (1986): 2970–2975.

105. Rosenberry TL, and Scoggin DM: Structure of human erythrocyte acetylcholinesterase. Characterization of intersubunit disulfide bonding and detergent interaction. *J Biol Chem* 259 (1984): 5643–5652.
106. Sihotang K: Acetylcholinesterase and its association with lipid. *Eur J Biochem* 63 (1976): 519–524.
107. Moore RB, Manery JF, and Still J: The inhibitory effects of polyoxyethylene detergents on human erythrocyte acetylcholinesterase and Ca^{2+} + Mg^{2+} -ATPase. *Biochem and Cell Biol* 67 (1989): 137–146.
108. Hall ER, and Brodbeck U: Human erythrocyte membrane acetylcholinesterase. Incorporation into the lipid bilayer structure of liposomes. *Eur J Biochem* 89 (1978): 159–167.
109. Ott P, Ariano BH, Binggeli Y, et al.: A monomeric form of human erythrocyte membrane acetylcholinesterase. *Biochim Biophys Acta* 729 (1983): 193–199.
110. Weitz M, Bjerrum OJ, and Brodbeck U: Characterization of an active hydrophilic erythrocyte membrane acetylcholinesterase obtained by limited proteolysis of the purified enzyme. *Biochim Biophys Acta* 776 (1984): 65–74.
111. Cassel D, and Pfeuffer T: Mechanism of cholera toxin action: Covalent modification of the guanyl nucleotide binding protein of the adenylate cyclase system. *Proc Natl Acad Sci USA* 75 (1978): 2669–2673.
112. Nielsen TB, Lad PM, Preston MS, et al.: Characteristics of the quanine nucleotide regulatory component of adenylate cyclase in human erythrocyte membranes. *Biochim Biophys Acta* 629 (1980): 143–155.
113. Cerione RA, Gierschik P, Staniszewski C, et al.: Functional differences in the beta gamma complexes of transducin and the inhibitory quanine nucleotide regulatory protein. *Biochemistry* 26 (1987): 1485–1491.
114. Rasmussen H, Lake W, Gasic G, et al.: Vasoactive hormones and the human erythrocyte. *Prog Clin Biol Res* 1 (1975): 467–490.
115. Brezinski ME, Lefer DJ, Bowker B, et al.: Thromboxane induced red blood cell lysis. *Prostaglandins* 33 (1987): 75–84.
116. Dutta-Roy AK, and Sinha AK: Binding of prostaglandin E1 to human erythrocyte membrane. *Biochim Biophys Acta* 812 (1985): 671–678.
117. Willems C, Stel HV, Van-Aken WG, et al.: Binding and inactivation of prostacyclin (PGI_2) by human erythrocytes. *Br J Haematol* 54 (1983): 43–52.
118. Ghiglieri-Bertez C, Cristol JP, and Bonne C: High affinity binding site for leukotriene C_4 in human erythrocytes. *Biochim Biophys Acta* 879 (1986): 97–102.
119. Michell RH: Inositol phospholipids and cell surface receptor function. *Biochim Biophys Acta* 415 (1975): 81–147.
120. MJ Berridge and RH Michell, eds.: Inositol lipids and transmembrane signalling. *Philosophical transactions of the Royal Society of London*, Ser. B, 320 (1988): 235–436.
121. Berridge MJ: Inositol trisphosphate and diacylglycerol: Two interacting second messengers. *Ann Rev Biochem* 56 (1987): 159–193.
122. Michell RH, King CE, Piper CJ, et al.: Inositol lipids and phosphates in erythrocytes and HL60 cells. In RB Gunn and JC Parker, eds.: *Cell physiology of blood*, pp. 345–355. New York: Rockefeller University Press, 1988.
123. Anderson RA: Regulation of protein 4.1-membrane associations by a phosphoinositide. In P Agre and JC Parker, eds.: *Red blood cell membranes: Structure—Function—Clinical application*, pp. 187–236. New York: Marcel Dekker, 1989.

124. Choquette D, Hakim G, Filoteo AG, et al.: Regulation of plasma membrane Ca^{2+}-ATPases by lipids of the phosphatidylinositol cycle. *Biochem Biophys Res Commun* 125 (1984): 908–915.
125. Nishizuka Y: Studies and perspectives on protein kinase C. *Science* 233 (1986): 305–313.
126. Palfrey HC, and Waseem A: Protein kinase C in the human erythrocyte. *J Biol Chem* 260 (1985): 16021–16029.
127. Cohen CM, and Foley S: Phorbol ester and Ca^{2+}-dependent phosphorylation of human red cell membrane skeletal proteins. *J Biol Chem* 261 (1986): 7701–7709.
128. Faquin WC, Chahwala SB, Cantley C, et al.: Protein kinase C of erythrocytes phosphorylates bands 4.1 and 4.9. *Biochim Biophys Acta* 887 (1986): 142–149.
129. Horne WC, Leto TL, and Marchesi V: Differential phosphorylation of multiple sites in protein 4.1 and protein 4.9 by phorbol ester–activated and cyclic AMP–dependent protein kinases. *J Biol Chem* 260 (1985): 9073–9076.
130. Palfrey HC, and Waseem A: Protein kinase C and its associated substrates in the human erythrocyte: In RB Gunn and JC Parker, eds.: *Cell physiology of blood*, pp. 357–369. New York: Rockefeller University Press, 1988.
131. Witters LA, Vater CA, and Leinhard GE: Phosphorylation of the glucose transporter *in vitro* and *in vivo* by protein kinase C. *Nature* 315 (1985): 777–778.
132. Bennet V, Davis J, Gardner K, et al.: The spectrin-based membrane skeleton: Extensions of the current paradigm. In RB Gunn and JC Parker, eds.: *Cell physiology of blood*, pp. 101–109. New York: Rockefeller University Press, 1988.
133. Eder PS, Soong CJ, and Tao M: Phosphorylation reduces the affinity of protein 4.1 for spectrin. *Biochemistry* 25 (1986): 1764–1770.
134. Axelrod J, and Cohn CK: Methyltransferase enzymes in red blood cells. *J Pharmacol Exper Therap* 176 (1971): 650–654.
135. Hirata F; and Axelrod J: Enzymatic synthesis and rapid translocation of phosphatidylcholine by two methyltransferases in erythrocyte membranes. *Proc Natl Acad Sci USA* 75 (1978): 2348–2352.
136. Moore RB, and Appel SH: Methylation of erythrocyte membrane phospholipids in patients with myotonic and Duchenne muscular dystrophy. *Expter Neurol* 70 (1980): 380–391.
137. Schultz E, Nissinen E, and Kaakkola S: Determination of catechol-o-methyltransferase activity in erythrocytes by high performance liquid chromatography with electrochemical detection. *Biomed Chromatogr* 3 (1989): 64–67.
138. Van Loon JA, Pazmino PA, and Weinshilboum RM: Human erythrocyte histamine-N-methyltransferase: Radiochemical microassay and biochemical properties. *Clin Chim Acta* 149 (1985): 237–251.
139. Keith RA, Otterness DM, Kerremans AL, et al.: S-Methylation of D- and L-penicillamine by human erythrocyte membrane methyltransferase. *Drug Metab Dispos* 13 (1985): 669–676.
140. Keith RA, Abraham RT, Pazmino P, et al.: Correlation of low and high affinity thiolmethyltransferase and phenol methyltransferase activities in human erythrocyte membranes. *Clin Chim Acta* 131 (1983): 257–272.
141. Kim S, Choi J, and Jun GT: Purification of protein methylase II from human erythrocytes. *J Biochem Biophys Methods* 8 (1983): 9–14.
142. Gilbert JM, Fowler A, Bleibaum J, et al.: Purification of homologous protein

carboxylmethyltransferase isozymes from human and bovine erythrocytes. *Biochemistry* 2 (1988): 5227–5233.

143. Barber JR, and Clarke S: Inhibition of protein carboxyl methylation by S-adenosyl-L-homocysteine in intact erythrocytes. *J Biol Chem* 259 (1984): 7115–7122.

144. Hirata F, and Axelrod J: Enzymatic methylation of phosphatidylethanolamine increases erythrocyte membrane fluidity. *Nature* 275 (1978): 219–220.

145. Brunbauer LS, and Clarke S: Methylation of calmodulin at carboxylic acid residues in erythrocytes. A non-regulatory covalent modification? *Biochem J* 236 (1986): 811–820.

146. O'Connor CM, and Clarke S: Carboxyl methylation of cytosolic proteins in intact human erythrocytes. Identification of numerous methyl accepting proteins, including hemoglobin and carbonic anhydrase. *J Biol Chem* 259 (1984): 2570–2578.

147. Galletti P, Paik WK, and Kim S: Selective methyl esterification of erythrocyte membrane proteins by protein methylase II. *Biochemistry* 17 (1978): 4272–4276.

148. Ro JY, DiMaria P, and Kim S: Differential membrane protein carboxyl-methylation of intact human erythrocytes by exogenous methyl donors. *Biochem J* 219 (1984): 743–749.

149. Lou LL, and Clark S: Carboxyl methylation of human erythrocyte band 3 in intact cells. Relation to anion transport activity. *Biochem J* 235 (1986): 183–187.

150. Lou LL, and Clark S: Enzymatic methylation of band 3 anion transporter in intact human erythrocytes. *Biochemistry* 26 (1987): 52–59.

151. Galletti P, Ingrosso D, Nappi A, et al.: Increased methyl esterification of membrane proteins in aged red blood cells. Preferential esterification of ankyrin and band 4.1 cytoskeletal proteins. *Eur J Biochem* 135 (1983): 25–31.

152. O'Connor CM, and Yutzey KE: Enhanced carboxylmethylation of membrane-associated hemoglobin in human erythrocytes. *J Biol Chem* 263 (1988): 1386–1390.

153. Galletti P, Ingrosso D, Iardino P, et al.: Enzymatic basis for calcium-induced decrease of membrane protein methyl esterification in intact erythrocytes. Evidence for an impairment of S-adenosylmethionione systhesis. *Eur J Biochem* 154 (1986): 489–493.

154. Lorand L, Weissmann LB, Epel DL, et al.: Role of the intrinsic transglutaminase in the Ca^{2+}-mediated crosslinking of erythrocyte proteins. *Proc Natl Acad Sci USA* 73 (1976): 4479–4481.

155. Anderson DR, Davis JL, and Carraway KL: Calcium-promoted changes of the human erythrocyte membrane. Involvement of spectrin, transglutaminase, and a membrane-bound protease. *J Biol Chem* 252 (1977): 6617–6623.

156. Lorand L, Siefring GE Jr., and Lowe-Krentz L: Formation of gamma-glutamyl-epsilon-lysine bridges between membrane proteins by a Ca^{2+}-regulated enzyme in intact erythrocytes. *J Supramol Struc* 9 (1978): 427–440.

157. Siefring GE Jr., Apostol AB, Velasco PT, et al.: Enzymatic basis for the Ca^{2+}-induced cross-linking of membrane proteins in intact human erythrocytes. *Biochemistry* 17 (1978): 2598–2604.

158. Palek J, Liu SC, and Liu PA: Crosslinking of the nearest membrane protein neighbors in ATP-depleted, calcium-enriched and irreversibly sickled red cells. *Prog Clin Biol Res* 20 (1977): 75–88.

159. Murayama M: Sickle cell hemoglobin: Molecular basis of sickling phenomenon theory and therapy. *CRC Crit Rev Biochem* 1 (1973): 461–499.

160. White JG: Ultrastructural features of erythrocyte and hemoglobin sickling. *Arch Intern Med* 133 (1974): 545–562.

161. Finch JT, Perutz MF, Bertles JF, et al.: Structure of sickled erythrocytes and of sickle-cell hemoglobin fibers. *Proc Natl Acad Sci USA* 70 (1973): 718–722.

162. Fischer S, Nagel RL, Bookchin RM, et al.: The binding of hemoglobin to membranes of normal and sickle erythrocytes. *Biochim Biophys Acta* 375 (1975): 422–433.

163. Shaklai N, Ranney HM, and Sharma V: Interactions of hemoglobin S with the red cell membrane. *Prog Clin Biol Res* 51 (1981): 1–16.

164. Lessin LS, Kirantsin-Mills J, Wallas C, et al.: Membrane alterations in irreversibly sickled cells: Hemoglobin–membrane interaction. *J Supramol Struct* 9 (1978): 537–554.

165. Eisinger J, Flores J, and Bookchin RM: The cytosol-membrane interface of normal and sickle erythrocytes. Effect of hemoglobin deoxygenation and sickling. *J Biol Chem* 259 (1984): 7169–7177.

166. Bookchin RM, and Lew VL: Red cell membrane abnormalities in sickle cell anemia. In EB Brown, ed.: *Progress in Hematology*, Vol. 8, pp. 1–18. New York: Grune and Stratton, 1983.

167. Goldberg MA, Lalos AT, Himmelstein B, et al.: Effects of red cell membrane on the polymerization of sickle hemoglobin. *Blood Cells* 8 (1982): 237–243.

168. Nash GB, Johnson CS, and Meiselman HJ: Mechanical properties of oxygenated red blood cells in sickle cell (Hb SS) disease. *Blood* 63 (1984): 73–82.

169. Nash GB, Johnson CS, and Meiselman HJ: Influence of oxygen tension on the viscoelastic behavior of red blood cells in sickle cell disease. *Blood* 67 (1986): 110–118.

170. Evans EA, and Mohandas N: Membrane-associated sickle hemoglobin: A major determinant of sickle erythrocyte rigidity. *Blood* 70 (1987): 1443–1449.

171. Mohandas N, Rossi ME, and Clark MR: Association between morphologic distortion of sickle cells and deoxygenation-induced cation permeability increase. *Blood* 68 (1986): 450–454.

172. Horiuchi K, Ballas SK, and Asakura T: The effect of deoxygenation rate on the formation of irreversibly sickled cells. *Blood* 71 (1988): 46–51.

173. Fortier N, Snyder LM, Garver F, et al.: The relationship between *in vivo* generated hemoglobin skeletal protein complex and increased red cell membrane rigidity. *Blood* 71 (1988): 1427–1431.

174. Asakura T, Ohnishi T, Friedman S, et al.: Abnormal precipitation of oxyhemoglobin S by mechanical shaking. *Proc Natl Acad Sci USA* 71 (1974): 1594–1598.

175. Kim HC, Friedman S, Asakura, et al.: Inclusions in red blood cells containing Hb S or Hb C. *Br J Haematol* 44 (1980): 547–554.

176. Asakura T, Minakata K, Adachi K, et al.: Denatured hemoglobin in sickle erythrocytes. *J Clin Invest* 59 (1977): 633–640.

177. Campwala HQ, and Desforges JF: Membrane-bound hemichrome in density-separated cohorts of normal (AA) and sickled (SS) cells. *J Lab Clin Med* 99 (1982): 25–28.

178. Shaklai N, Shviro Y, Rabizadeh E, et al.: Accumulation and drainage of hemin in the red cell membrane. *Biochim Biophys Acta* 821 (1985): 355–366.

179. Kuross SA, Rank BH, and Hebbel RP: Excess heme in sickle erythrocyte inside-out membranes: Possible role in thiol oxidation. *Blood* 71 (1988): 876–882.

180. Liu SC, Zhai S, and Palek J: Detection of hemin release during hemoglobin S denaturation. *Blood* 71 (1988): 1755–1758.

181. Kuross SA, and Hebbel RP: Nonheme iron in sickle erythrocyte membranes: association with phospholipids and potential role in lipid peroxidation. *Blood* 72 (1988): 1278–1285.

182. Heywood JD, and Finch CA: Erythrocyte free globin levels in some anemic states. *Proc Soc Exper Biol Med* 134 (1970): 131–137.

183. Sears DA, and Lewis PC: Measurements of hemoglobin chains bound to the erythrocyte membrane. *J Lab Clin Med* 96 (1980): 318–327.

184. Sears DA, and Luthra MG: Membrane-bound hemoglobin in the erythrocytes of sickle cell anemia. *J Lab Clin Med* 102 (1983): 694–698.

185. Schwarz HP, Kahlke MB, and Dreisbach L: Phospholipid composition of blood plasma, erythrocytes, and "ghosts" in sickle cell disease. *Clin Chem* 23 (1977): 1548–1550.

186. Sasaki J, Waterman MR, Buchanan GR, et al.: Plasma and erythrocyte lipids in sickle cell anaemia. *Clin Lab Haematol* 5 (1983): 35–44.

187. Muskiet FD, and Muskiet FA: Lipids, fatty acids and trace elements in plasma and erythrocytes of pediatric patients with homozygous sickle cell disease. *Clin Chim Acta* 142 (1984): 1–10.

188. Jain SK, and Shohet SB: Red blood cell [14C] cholesterol exchange and plasma cholesterol esterifying activity of normal and sickle cell blood. *Biochim Biophys Acta* 688 (1982): 11–15.

189. Raval PJ, and Allan D: Changes in membrane polypeptides, polyphosphoinositides and phosphatidate in dense fractions of sickle cells. *Biochim Biophys Acta* 856 (1986): 595–601.

190. Rhoda MD, Sulpice JC, Gascard P, et al.: Endogenous calcium in sickle cells does not activate polyphosphoinositide phospholipase C. *Biochem J* 254 (1988): 161–169.

191. Chiu D, Lubin B, and Shohet SB: Erythrocyte membrane lipid reorganization during the sickling process. *Br J Haematol* 41 (1979): 223–234.

192. Lubin B, Chiu D, Bastacky J, et al.: Abnormalities in membrane phospholipid organization in sickled erythrocytes. *J Clin Invest* 67 (1981): 1643–1649.

193. Lubin B, Chiu D, Roelofsen B, et al.: Abnormal membrane phospholipid asymmetry in sickle erythrocytes and its pathophysiologic significance. *Prog Clin Biol Res* 56 (1981): 171–193.

194. Zachowski A, Craescu CT, Galacteros F, et al.: Abnormality of phospholipid transverse diffusion in sickle erythrocytes. *J Clin Invest* 75 (1985): 1713–1717.

195. Franck PF, Chiu DT, Op den Kamp JA, et al.: Accelerated transbilayer movement of phosphatidylcholine in sickled erythrocytes. A reversible process. *J Biol Chem* 258 (1983): 8436–8442.

196. Franck PF, Bevers EM, Lubin BH, et al.: Uncoupling of the membrane skeleton from the lipid bilayer. The cause of accelerated phospholipid flip-flop leading to an enhanced procoagulant activity of sickled cells. *J Clin Invest* 75 (1985): 183–190.

197. Mohandas N, Rossi M, Bernstein S, et al.: The structural organization of skeletal proteins influences lipid translocation across erythrocyte membrane. *J Biol Chem* 260 (1985): 14264–14268.

198. Chiu D, Lubin B, Roelofsen B, et al.: Sickled erythrocytes accelerate clotting *in*

vitro: An effect of abnormal membrane lipid asymmetry. *Blood* 58 (1981): 398–401.

199. Schroitt AJ, Tanaka V, Madsen J, et al.: The recognition of red blood cells by macrophages: Role of phosphatidylserine and possible implications of membrane phospholipid asymmetry. *Biol Cell,* 51 (1984): 227–238.

200. Jain SK, and Shohet SB: A novel phospholipid in irreversibly sickled cells: Evidence for *in vivo* peroxidative membrane damage in sickle cell disease. *Blood* 63 (1984): 362–367.

201. Chiu D, Vichinsky K, Yee M, et al.: Peroxidation, vitamin E and sickle cell anemia. *Ann NY Acad Sci* 393 (1982): 323–335.

202. Jain SK: Evidence for membrane lipid peroxidation during the *in vivo* aging of human erythrocytes. *Biochim Biophys Acta* 937 (1988): 205–210.

203. Jain SK: The accumulation of malonyldialdehyde, a product of fatty acid peroxidation, can disturb aminophospholipid organization in the membrane bilayer of human erythrocytes. *J Biol Chem* 259 (1984): 3391–3394.

204. Herrick JB: Peculiar elongated and sickle-shaped red blood corpuscles in a case of severe anemia. *Arch Intern Med* 6 (1910): 517–521.

205. Bessis M, and Delpech G: Sickle cell shape and structure: Images and concepts (1840–1980). *Blood Cells* 8 (1982): 359–435.

206. Serjeant G, Serjeant B, and Milner P: The irreversibly sickled cell: A determinant of haemolysis in sickle cell anemia. *Br J Haematol* 17 (1969): 527–533.

207. Bertles JF, and Dobler J: Reversible and irreversible sickling: A distinction by electron microscopy. *Blood* 33 (1969): 884–898.

208. Jensen WN, and Lessin LS: Membrane alterations associated with hemoglobino-pathies. *Semin Hematol* 7 (1970): 409–426.

209. Schaeffer K, Brinkley BR, Young JE, et al.: The occurrence of lysosome-like structures in sickling erythrocytes. *Lab Invest* 23 (1970): 297–301.

210. Lux SE, and John KM: Evidence that spectrin is a determinant of shape and deformability in the human erythrocyte. *Prog Clin Biol Res* 17 (1977): 481–491.

211. Rice-Evans C, and Chapman D: Biochemical approach. Red blood cell biomembranes structure and deformability. *Scand J Clin Lab Invest* 156 (1981): 99–110.

212. Durocher JR, and Conrad ME: Erythrocyte membrane proteins in sickle cell anemia. *Proc Soc Exp Biol Med* 146 (1974): 373–375.

213. Ballas SK, and Burka ER: Failure to demonstrate red cell membrane protein abnormalities in sickle cell anemia. *Br J Haematol* 46 (1980): 627–629.

214. Riggs MG, and Ingram VM: Differences in erythrocyte membrane proteins and glycoproteins in sickle cell disease. *Biochem Biophys Res Commun* 74 (1977): 191–198.

215. Rubin RW, Milikowski C, and Wise GE: Organization differences in the membrane proteins of normal and irreversibly sickled erythrocytes. *Biochim Biophys Acta* 595 (1980): 595:1–8.

216. Chun PW, Rennert O, Saffern E, et al.: Polyamines in sickling red blood cells. *Biophys Chem* 6 (1977): 326.

217. Natta CL, and Kremzner LT: Polyamines and membrane proteins in sickle cell disease. *Blood Cells* 8 (1982): 273–280.

218. Ballas SK, Mohandas N, Marton L, et al.: Stabilization of erythrocyte membranes by polyamines. *Proc Natl Acad Sci USA* 80 (1983): 1942–1946.

219. Ballas SK, Mohandas N, Clark MR, et al.: Reduced transglutaminase-catalyzed

cross-linking of exogenous amines to membrane proteins in sickle erythrocytes. *Biochim Biophys Acta* 812 (1985): 234–242.

220. Palek J: Red cell membrane injury in sickle cell anaemia. *Br J Haematol* 35 (1977): 1–9.

221. Palek J, Liu SC, and Liu PA: Crosslinking of the nearest membrane protein neighbors in ATP depleted, calcium enriched and irreversibly sickled red cells. *Prog Clin Biol Res* 20 (1978): 75–91.

222. Liu SC, Fairbanks G, and Palek J: Spontaneous, reversible protein crosslinking in the human erythrocyte membrane. Temperature and pH dependence. *Biochemistry* 16 (1977): 4066–4074.

223. Palek J: Membrane protein and organization in normal and hemoglobinopathic red cells. *Tex Rep Biol Med* 40 (1980–81): 397–416.

224. Palek J, and Liu SC: Alterations of spectrin assembly in the red cell membrane: Functional consequences. *Scand J Clin Lab Invest* 156 (1981): 131–138.

225. Hoover R, Rubin R, Wise G, et al.: Adhesion of normal and sickle erythrocytes to endothelial monolayer cultures. *Blood* 54 (1979): 872–876.

226. Hebbel RP, Moldow CF, and Steinberg MH: Modulation of erythrocyte-endothelial interactions and the vasoocclusive severity of sickling disorders. *Blood* 58 (1981): 947–952.

227. Mohandas N, Evans E, and Kukan B: Adherence of sickle erythrocytes to vascular endothelial cells: Requirement of both cell membrane changes and plasma factors. *Blood* 64 (1984): 282–287.

228. Hebbel RP, Yamada O, Moldow CF, et al.: Abnormal adherence of sickle erythrocytes to cultured vascular endothelium. Possible mechanism for microvascular occlusion in sickle cell disease. *J Clin Invest* 65 (1980): 154–160.

229. Clark LJ, Chan S, Powars DR, et al.: Negative charge distribution and density on the surface of oxygenated normal and sickle red cells. *Blood* 57 (1981): 675–678.

230. Nicolson G, and Painter RG: Anionic sites of human erythrocyte membranes. II: Antispectrin induced transmembrane aggregation of the binding sites for positively charged colloidal particles. *J Cell Biol* 59 (1973): 395–406.

231. Lux SE, John KM, and Karnovsky MJ: Irreversible deformation of the spectrin-actin lattice in irreversibly sickled cells. *J Clin Invest* 58 (1976): 955–963.

232. Lux S: Spectrin-actin membrane skeleton of normal and abnormal red blood cells. *Semin Hematol* 16 (1979): 21–51.

233. Platt OS, Falcone JF, and Lux SE: Molecular defect in the sickle erythrocyte skeleton. Abnormal spectrin binding to sickle inside-out vesicles. *J Clin Invest* 75 (1985): 266–271.

234. Allan D, Limbrick AR, Thomas P, et al.: Release of spectrin-free spicules on reoxygenation of sickled erythrocytes. *Nature* 295 (1982): 612–613.

235. Bookchin RM, Ortiz OE, and Lew VL: Activation of calcium-dependent potassium channels in deoxygenated sickle red cells. *Prog Clin Biol Res* 240 (1987): 193–200.

236. Glader BE, and Nathan DG: Cation permeability alterations during sickling: Relationship to cation composition and cellular hydration of irreversibly sickled cells. *Blood* 51 (1978): 983–989.

237. Glader BE, Lux SE, Mueller-Soyano A, et al.: Energy reserve and cation composition of irreversibly sickled cells *in vivo*. *Br J Haematol* 40 (1978): 527–532.

238. Clark MR, Unger RC, and Shohet SB: Monovalent cation composition and ATP and lipid content of irreversibly sickled cells. *Blood* 51 (1978): 1169–1178.

239. Eaton JW, Skelton TD, Swofford HS, et al.: Elevated erythrocyte calcium in sickle cell disease. *Nature* 246 (1973): 105–106.

240. Eaton JW, Berger E, White JG, et al.: Calcium-induced damage of haemoglobin SS and normal erythrocytes. *Br J Haematol* 38 (1978): 57–62.

241. Steinberg MH, Eaton JW, Berger E, et al.: Erythrocyte calcium abnormalities and the clinical severity of sickling disorders. *Br J Haematol* 40 (1978): 533–539.

242. Palek J: Calcium accumulation during sickling of hemoglobin S (HbSS) red cells. *Blood* 42 (1973): 988.

243. Palek J, Thomae D, and Ozog D: Red cell calcium and transmembrane calcium movements in sickle cell anemia. *J Lab Clin Med* 89 (1977): 1365–1374. ˙

244. Cameron BF, and Smariga P: Calcium exchange and calcium related effects in normal and sickle cell anemia erythrocytes. *Prog Clin Biol Res* 20 (1977): 105–118.

245. Bookchin RM, and Lew VL: Progressive inhibition of the calcium pump and Ca:Ca exchange in sickle red cells. *Nature* 284 (1980): 561–563.

246. Gopinath RH, and Vincenzi FF: (Ca^{2+} + Mg^{2+})-ATPase activity of sickle cell membranes: Decreased activation by red blood cell cytoplasmic activator. *Am J Hematol* 7 (1979): 303–312.

247. Litosch I, and Lee KS: Sickle red cell calcium metabolism: Studies on Ca^{2+} + Mg^{2+}-ATPase and Ca-binding properties of sickle red cell membranes. *Am J Hematol* 8 (1980): 377–387.

248. Dixon E, and Winslow RM: The interaction between (Ca^{2+} + Mg^{2+})-ATPase and the soluble activator (calmodulin) in erythrocytes containing haemoglobin S. *Br J Haematol* 47 (1981): 391–397.

249. Niggli V, Adunyah ES, Cameron BF, et al.: The Ca^{2+}-pump of sickle cell plasma membranes. Purification and reconstitution of the ATPase enzyme. *Cell Calcium* 3 (1982): 131–151.

250. Leclerc L, Girard F, Galacteros F, et al.: The calmodulin-stimulated (Ca^{2+} + Mg^{2+})-ATPase in hemoglobin S erythrocyte membranes: Effects of sickling and oxidative agents. *Biochim Biophys Acta* 897 (1987): 33–40.

251. Shalev O, Lavi V, Hebbel RP, et al.: Erythrocyte (Ca^{2+} + Mg^{2+})-ATPase activity: Increased sensitivity to oxidative stress in glucose-6-phosphate dehydrogenase deficiency. *Am J Hematol* 19 (1985): 131–136.

252. Hebbel RP, Shalev O, Foker W, et al.: Inhibition of erythrocyte Ca^{2+}-ATPase by activated oxygen through thiol- and lipid-dependent mechanisms. *Biochim Biophys Acta* 19 (1985): 131–136.

253. Moore RB, Brummitt ML, and Mankad VN: Hydroperoxides selectively inhibit human erythrocyte membrane enzymes. *Arch Biochem Biophys* 273 (1989): 527–534.

254. Gardös G: The function of calcium in the potassium permeability of human erythrocytes. *Biochim Biophys Acta* 30 (1958): 653–654.

255. Lew VL, Hockaday A, Sepulveda MI, et al.: Compartmentalization of sickle cell calcium in endocytic inside-out vesicles. *Nature* 315 (1985): 586–589.

256. Rhoda MD, Giraud F, Craescu CT, et al.: Compartmentalization of Ca^{2+} in sickle cells. *Cell Calcium* 6 (1985): 397–411.

257. Murphy E, Berkowitz LR, Orringer E, et al.: Cytosolic free calcium levels in sickle red blood cells. *Blood* 69 (1987): 1469–1474.

258. Tosteson DC: The effects of sickling on ion transport. II. The effect of sickling on sodium and cesium transport. *J Gen Physiol* 39 (1955): 55–67.

259. Tosteson DC, Carlson E, and Dunham ET: The effects of sickling on ion transport. *J Gen Physiol* 39 (1955): 31–53.

260. Clark MR, Guatelli JC, White AT, et al.: Study on the dehydrating effect of the red cell Na$^+$/K$^+$ pump in nystatin-treated cells with varying Na$^+$ and water contents. *Biochim Biophys Acta* 646 (1981): 422–432.

261. Joiner CH, Platt OS, and Lux SE: Cation depletion by the sodium pump in red cells with pathologic cation leaks. Sickle cells and xerocytes. *J Clin Invest* 78 (1986): 1487–1496.

262. Ohnishi ST, Horiuchi KY, and Horiuchi K: The mechanism of *in vitro* formation of irreversibly sickle cells and modes of action of its inhibitors. *Biochim Biophys Acta* 886 (1986): 119–129.

263. Brugnara C, Kopin A, Bunn HF, et al.: Regulation of cation content and cell volume in hemoglobin erythrocytes from patients with homozygous hemoglobin C disease. *J Clin Invest* 75 (1985): 1608–1617.

264. Canessa M, Fabry ME, Spalvins A, et al.: Activation of a K:Cl cotransporter by cell swelling in HbAA and HbSS red cells. *Prog Clin Biol Res* 240 (1987): 201–215.

265. Canessa M, Fabry ME, and Nagel RL: Deoxygenation inhibits the volume-stimulated, Cl(−)-dependent K$^+$ efflux in SS and young AA cells: A cytosolic Mg^{2+} modulation. *Blood* 70 (1987): 1861–1866.

266. Canessa M, Fabry ME, Blumenfeld N, et al.: Volume-stimulated, Cl(−)-dependent K$^+$ efflux is highly expressed in young human red cells containing normal hemoglobin or HbS. *J Memb Biol* 97 (1987): 97–105.

267. Nagel RL, Fabry ME, Kaul DK, et al.: Known and potential sources for epistatic effects in sickle cell anemia. *Ann NY Acad Sci* 565 (1989): 228–238.

268. Canessa M, Spalvins A, and Nagel RL: Volume-dependent and NEM-stimulated K$^+$ Cl$^-$ transport is elevated in oxygenated SS, SC and CC human red cells. *FEBS Lett* 200 (1986): 197–202.

269. Tsung K and Palek J: Red cell membrane protein phosphorylation in hemolytic anemias and muscular dystrophies. *Muscle and Nerve* 3 (1980): 55–69.

270. Fairbanks G, Liu A, Dino JE, et al.: Endogenous spectrin kinase activity in sickle cell anemia. *Blood* 52 (1978): 96.

271. Beutler E, Guinte E, and Johnson C: Human red cell protein kinase in normal subjects and patients with hereditary spherocytosis, sickle cell disease and autoimmune hemolytic anemia. *Blood* 48 (1976): 887–898.

272. Hosey MM, and Tao M: Altered erythrocyte membrane phosphorylation in sickle cell disease. *Nature* 263 (1976): 424–425.

273. Hosey MM, Plut DA, and Tao M: Inhibition of protein phosphorylation and induction of protein cross-linking in erythrocyte membranes by diamide. *Biochim Biophys Acta* 506 (1978): 211–220.

274. Dzandu JK, and Johnson RM: Membrane protein phosphorylation in intact normal and sickle cell erythrocytes. *J Biol Chem* 255 (1980): 6382–6386.

275. Delaunay J, Galand C, and Boivin P: Erythrocyte membrane phosphorylation in sickle cell disease. *Nouv Rev Fr Hematol* 24 (1982): 227–230.

276. Fairbanks G, Palek J, Dino JE, et al.: Protein kinases and membrane protein phosphorylation in normal and abnormal human erythrocytes: Variation related to mean cell age. *Blood* 61 (1983): 850–857.

277. Johnson RM, Dzandu JK, and Warth JA: The phosphoproteins of the sickle erythrocyte membrane. *Arch Biochem Biophys* 244 (1986): 202–210.

278. Johnson RM, and Dzandu JK: Calcium and ionophore A23187 induce the sickle cell membrane phosphorylation pattern in normal erythrocytes. *Biochim Biophys Acta* 692 (1982): 218–222.

279. Ramachandran M, Nair CN, and Abraham EC: Increased membrane-associated phorbol-12,13 dibutyrate (PDBu) receptor function in sickle red cells. *Biochem Biophys Res Commun* 147 (1987): 56–64.

280. Ponnappa BC, Greenquist AC, and Shohet SB: Calcium-induced changes in polyphosphoinositides and phosphatidate in normal erythrocytes, sickle cells and hereditary pyropoikilocytosis. *Biochim Biophys Acta* 598 (1980): 494–501.

281. Rhoda MD, Sulpice JC, Gascard P, et al.: Endogenous calcium in sickle cell does not activate polyphosphoinositide phospholipase C. *Biochem J* 254 (1988): 161–169.

282. Ro JY, Neilan B, Magee PN, et al.: Reduced erythrocyte membrane protein methylation in sickle cell anemia. *J Biol Chem* 256 (1981): 10572–10576.

283. Green GA, Sikka SC, and Kalra VK: Differential turnover of methyl groups on methyl-accepting membrane proteins of irreversibly sickled erythrocytes. *J Biol Chem* 258 (1983): 12958–12966.

284. Ro JY, Neilan B, and Kim S: Further investigation of methylation on sickle erythrocyte membranes. *Biochem Med* 30 (1983): 342–348.

285. Manna C, Hermanowicz N, Ro JY, et al.: Abnormal membrane protein methylation and merocyanine 540 fluorescence in sickle erythrocyte membranes. *Biochem Med* 31 (1984): 362–370.

286. Piau JP, Delaunay J, Fischer S, et al.: Human red cell membrane adenylate cyclase in normal subjects and patients with hereditary spherocytosis, sickle cell disease and unidentified hemolytic anemias. *Blood* 56 (1980): 963–968.

287. Raval PJ, and Allan D: Sickling of sickle erythrocytes does not alter phospholipid asymmetry. *Biochem J* 203 (1984): 555–557.

4

Interactions of Blood Cells and Vascular Endothelium in Sickle Cell Disease: Eicosanoids as Signals and Modulators

Gesina L. Longenecker

The basis and pathophysiology of sickle cell disease (SCD), as well as its consequences and management, have been covered in many excellent reviews (1–7). The basics of SCD are described very briefly here: Additional information may be obtained from the Reference List.

The primary defect in sickle cell disease (SCD) is known to be a simple amino acid substitution in the β-chain of hemoglobin. This modification results in behavioral changes in the hemoglobin itself (e.g., polymerization under conditions of low oxygen) as well as the red blood cells (RBC) in which the altered hemoglobin is contained (abnormal shape and deformability). It is increasingly recognized that other cell types may also be involved in the overall pathophysiology of SCD. It is also increasingly recognized that these other cell types and their products may significantly influence RBC behavior. The purpose of this chapter is to review changes in SCD in two cell types of the vascular system, namely platelets and vascular endothelium, and some of their intercellular signals, especially those derived from lipids (e.g., eicosanoids, or products of arachidonic acid metabolism, and parallel products). Additional purposes are to show how these types of interactions may extend to RBC, with significant consequences, and to create a working model for interactions among platelets, RBC, and endothelium, in general, and in SCD in particular.

PLATELETS: FUNCTION, REGULATION AND MONITORING

Several excellent, recent articles and monographs have reviewed aspects of the physiology, biochemistry, pharmacology, and pathophysiology of platelet function (8–14). These should be consulted for details of aspects covered in the

brief overview of platelet function that follows below. The overview is presented
as an introduction to changes in platelets that have been reported for SCD.

Function

Platelets are numerous, circulating, excitable fragments of megakaryocyte
cytoplasm. The release of platelets by megakaryocytes is under hormonal control
via the kidney-produced, circulating hormone thrombopoietin (15). Circulating
numbers of platelets are also influenced by splenic function (decreased function
results in increased numbers) (16). The excitable responses that platelets undergo
fall into two general categories, namely, adhesive responses (*aggregation,* or
sticking of platelets to one another, and *adhesion,* or sticking of platelets to
nonplatelet surfaces) and release responses (of both stored and de novo synthesized materials). Both types of responses may be elicited simultaneously in
metabolically intact, drug-free platelets by a variety of stimuli, including thrombin, collagen, ADP, epinephrine, vasopressin (17), arachidonic acid, and platelet
activating factor (PAF) (see reference 18). For many stimuli, the responses are
initiated by the interaction of the stimulus with a specific class of platelet receptor,
for example, epinephrine with α_2-adrenoceptors (19). The signal is then transmitted via a coupled G (N) protein and transduced by increases in intraplatelet
calcium (Ca^{++}; phospholipase C-phosphoinositol mediated and/or via receptor-
operated channels [20–22]). The response may then be amplified by the release
of platelet stimulatory mediators by the platelets. The latter may include ADP
from dense granules (exocytosis) and additional products such as *de novo* synthesized thromboxane A_2 (TxA) (see reference 23 and Figure 4.1). Surface
glycoprotein adhesive receptors involved in aggregation are also exposed in
response to stimulation. For example, glycoprotein IIb/IIIa complex is exposed
after ADP or thrombin stimulation, allowing fibrinogen, in plasma or released
from platelet α granules, to attach to the platelets (24). Recently, the exposure
of fibrinogen binding sites has been shown to involve the cleavage of a surface
protein, aggregin, secondary to increases in intraplatelet calcium and the activation of proteases (calpains) (25). Thrombin-stimulated platelets expose and
release a lectin that may be a cleavage product of fibrinogen (26, 27): This lectin
agglutinates RBC and may also be involved in platelet adhesive responses.

From the list of stimuli and adhesive-type responses characteristic of platelets
it can be seen that they are uniquely suited to their documented role in hemostasis.
The latter role is also influenced by the presence on platelet surfaces of adsorbed
coagulation factors that can be activated early in the sequence of platelet stimulation (28), by the release of phospholipid (PF3), and possibly by additional
procoagulant effects resulting from plasma lipid oxidation (29). The presence
of additional platelet surface adhesive receptors (e.g., glycoproteins Ia, Ib, IIb,
IIIa, and IIIb [IV] [11]) allows the adhesion of platelets not only to each other
(through fibrinogen, as mentioned above) but also to surfaces on which macromolecules such as collagen (subendothelium) and von Willebrand factor (fac-

tor VIII:vWF; endothelial cells) occur (11, 30, 31). Indeed, a lack of these receptors is associated with major defects in platelet adhesive responses, such as Bernard-Soulier disorder (lack of subendothelial adhesion; GPIb deficiency) and Glanzmann's thrombosthenia (lack of aggregation, multiple stimuli; GPIIb/ IIIa deficiency).

Regulation

Platelet responsiveness is regulated *in vivo* both by levels or availability of stimuli (see previous section above) and by the presence and levels of inhibitory hormones or drugs, as well as by plasma proteins (32). For stimuli, addition or synergy is possible, even with compounds that are inactive alone (33–35). Desensitization also occurs and can lead to platelet refractoriness on subsequent stimulus exposure. Epinephrine, in amounts insufficient to cause observable aggregation responses, can reverse the refractoriness/inhibition caused by other agents as well as facilitate responses to other agents in general (19). Angiotensin II can also facilitate responses to other agents (36–38).

Prostacyclin (PGI) is one of the best known and most potent hormone inhibitors of platelet function (23, 39). It is an end-product of arachidonic acid metabolism in endothelial (and some other) cells (see Figure 4.1) and is potently inhibitory to platelet aggregation: Platelet adhesion is also inhibited by PGI. Control of platelet reactivity by the balance between PGI and TxA has been suggested (23, 40). PGI acts on specific receptors coupled to adenylyl cyclase, most likely through a G protein(s) (41), and thus increases intraplatelet levels of cyclic adenosine monophosphate (cAMP): cAMP basically antagonizes the effects of intraplatelet Ca^{++} (20). PGI has been proposed as a local regulator only of platelet responsiveness because of its low concentrations and short half-life in blood (42–44). PGI's duration of action is considerably longer than its half-life, however, suggesting that cumulative effects can occur and persist and that PGI effects are probably more than just local. A decreased endothelium production of PGI has been associated with several pathologic states in which platelet dysfunction also occurs. Other endothelial factors in addition to PGI may also be involved in platelet regulation.

Another endothelial product in the platelet regulatory hormone category is endothelium-derived relaxant factor (EDRF), which currently is identified as nitric oxide (45). EDRF, like PGI, is a potent and short-lived inhibitor of platelet responses (46); it may even be more effective than PGI in limiting platelet adhesion. A synergy between PGI and EDRF has been suggested (47), and, although co-release has been observed (47), it is apparently possible to release (or inhibit release of) each somewhat selectively (48): The evaluation of co-release and independent release may be complicated by an ability of PGI to release EDRF (49).

Adenosine, which is present in blood in variable amounts (≤ 0.3 μM), determined in part by its formation from substrates at RBC and endothelial surfaces

(50), also inhibits platelets via action on specific receptors (P_1) coupled to adenylyl cyclase (51–55), and is transported by them (52, 56, 57). Thus, adenosine is another possible hormonal factor involved in platelet regulation.

Drug inhibition of platelet function can be accomplished by several mechanisms. The most straightforward is the specific antagonism of stimulatory receptors, for example, thrombin receptors by hirudin (58) or epinephrine/α_2 adrenoceptors (19) by phentolamine (nonspecific α blockade) or yohimbine (α_2-selective blockade). Other approaches include the simulation of natural inhibitors. For example, PGI is mimicked by its stable analogue, iloprost, which also increases platelet cAMP. Elevation of cAMP by inhibition of its breakdown by an inhibitor (I) of one or more cyclic nucleotide phosphodiesterases (PDE) is also an effective way of reducing platelet responsiveness. Indeed, cyclase stimulation together with phosphodiesterase inhibition can be an especially effective antiplatelet strategy (59, 60): Dipyridamole, as a function of concentration, may achieve both by blocking adenosine uptake (prolonging its action) (56, 57) and acting as a phosphodiesterase inhibitor (PDEI) (56, 61). Dipyridamole may also increase PGI release (62–65).

Interference with the de novo synthesis of TxA is also an effective platelet inhibitory strategy. This can be accomplished with nonsteroidal antiinflammatory drugs (NSAID; e.g., aspirin, indomethacin), which inhibit the initial oxygenation (by cyclooxygenase) of arachidonic acid liberated from phospholipids in response to stimulation, or with thromboxane synthase inhibitors (TxSI; e.g., dazoxiben) (see reference 23 and Figure 4.1). TxSI actually act indirectly and are only effective *in vivo*. This is due to the release (leak) of the TxA precursor (PGH_2) from platelets: The leaked precursor is then available for conversion to inhibitory PGI by endothelium. In humans, conversion to PGD_2, another platelet-inhibitory compound, by serum albumin also occurs (66). Involvement of platelet-inhibitory PG in the effects of TxSI is supported by synergy between TxSI and PDEI (67). *In vitro*, PGH_2 persists and acts on TxA receptors, resulting in platelet activation, and no inhibition by TxSI can be detected. Thus, while the NSAID inhibit synthesis of *all* intermediates and end products of the cyclooxygenase pathway, even endothelial PGI (an exception may be ibuprofen [68]), the TxSI act only on Tx-synthesizing systems and inhibit *only* TxA synthesis.

Polymers can also influence platelet function. Heparin, for example, activates platelets (enhancing TxA [69, 70] and/or antagonizing PGI [71]). Dextran may directly inhibit platelets or produce a refractory state (72–74). Other expanders (Fluosol/Pluronic F68) result in inhibition (75, 76), possibly by surface effects or by inhibiting phospholipase A_2 (77).

Monitoring

Platelet responsiveness can be assessed *in vivo* or *in vitro*. Some general descriptions have been provided in a brief review (78). *In vivo* assessment usually involves indirect observations such as changes in platelet number (manual or

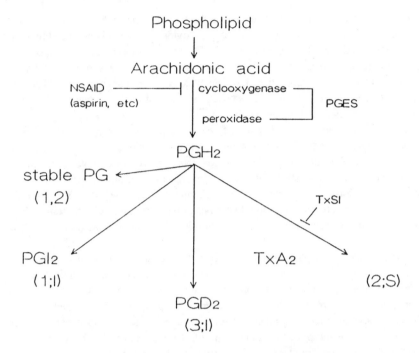

Figure 4.1. Schematic representation of the liberation (by phospholipase[s]) and conversion of arachidonic acid to its various end products via the cyclooxygenase-initiated pathway: 1 = conversion occuring mainly in vascular endothelium; 2 = conversion occuring mainly in platelets; 3 = conversion occurring via serum albumin; I = inhibitor of platelet responses; S = stimulator; PG = prostaglandin(s); Tx = thromboxane; PGES = prostaglandin endoperoxide synthase (combined activity of cyclooxygenase and peroxidase). The points of inhibition of two classes of drugs, NSAID (nonsteroidal antiinflammatory drugs) and TxSI (thromboxane synthase inhibitors) are shown. *In vivo*, the use of TxSI may result in the diversion of PGH$_2$ to PGI$_2$ and PGD$_2$. Not shown is the potential parallel formation of PAF (platelet activating factor) from lysophospholipid, from which arachidonic acid is liberated.

electronic counting; blood or platelet-rich plasma); occurrence or presence of microaggregates (79), platelet products in plasma—for example, TxA metabolites (TxB, 11-dehydro-TxB) (80)—or α granule products—for example, β-thromboglobulin (BTG) (81) and platelet factor 4 (PF4) (81, 82). Survival or production times for platelets can be estimated by monitoring platelet radioactivity subsequent to the injection of radiolabelled platelets (83) or by determining the recovery time for cyclooxygenase product formation from aspirin inhibition (84).

In vitro assessment can be done purely for the use of platelets as an assay system (e.g., quantitation of PGI, direct testing of drug effects; [78, 85, 86]) or to assess the consequences of *in vivo* exposures (e.g., disease, drugs, or experimental manipulations [87]). One caveat for the latter is that the loss of some *in vivo* exposure effects can occur if an influencing agent(s) is labile, provided the agent is produced by non-blood cells, and the effects are reversible: PGI, for example, is labile and produced by endothelium, *and* its effects reverse over times as short as 30–60 minutes, which is about the usual preparation time for platelets to be used in aggregometry. Thus, to include consideration of labile agents present *in vivo* but not being generated *in vitro* may require special handling protocols.

The most commonly used *in vitro* test system for platelet responsiveness is nephelometric aggregometry, although potentiometric (whole blood) aggregometry is also used (34, 88). Platelets (suspended in autologous, or even heterologous, plasma or buffer) are warmed and stirred and responses are observed and recorded over time after the addition of stimulus/test agents. Complete dose-response data can be obtained for several stimuli using small volumes of blood or platelets. The standardization of *in vitro* aggregometry protocols is absolutely essential to the accrual of valid data.

Biochemical responses of platelets can be monitored in parallel with aggregometry responses (in the same samples, and occasionally at the same time), or independently of aggregation. Specialized aggregometers (Lumi-aggregometers) use infrared, rather than visible, light for nephelometric measurements and are also equipped to detect light emission due to platelet release of ATP (luciferase assay; components are added to platelet suspension prior to stimulation) (89). Similar approaches have been taken for Ca^{++}, using the simultaneous monitoring of calcium-sensitive dye fluorescence. A more usual procedure is to stimulate the platelet sample, allow the response to occur for some period of time, and then stop any further response, including the biochemical one of interest, by adding a specific inhibitor. This approach has been used for TxA (68), BTG (90), PF4, and even serotonin (5-hydroxytryptamine or 5HT) if platelets are preloaded with radiolabelled 5HT.

The platelet content (rather than the releasable quantity) of preformed materials (such as ADP and 5HT [91]) can also be measured directly. Compounds for which uptake occurs can be studied for change in the kinetics of uptake (see, e.g., reference 92).

Most of the monitoring methods described above have been used to assess platelet function in SCD. These data are reviewed in the following section.

PLATELET FUNCTION IN SCD

Platelet Numbers, Survival Time, and Circulating Microaggregates

Circulating numbers of platelets in steady state SCD are somewhat elevated compared with control populations (see references 93 and 94 and also Figure 4.2). Platelet survival time in SCD may be shortened (83) although production time has been cited as normal (95). These data are especially interesting in view of the observations that (1) healthy Africans may have somewhat lower platelet

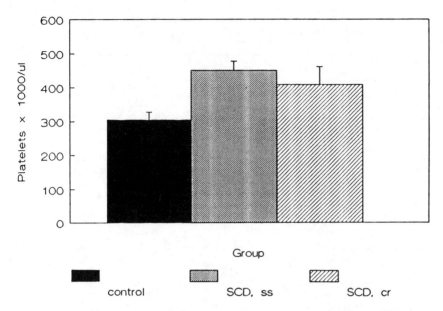

Figure 4.2.   Platelet numbers in controls, sickle cell disease steady state (SCD, ss),
and (in the same patient population) sickle cell disease crisis (SCD, cr;
24–36 hours after initial hospital admission for pain). SCD platelet
numbers are elevated with respect to control and decrease some during
crisis.

counts (96) than in other groups and (2) other conditions that decrease the survival
times of platelets in general do so more significantly in blacks (97). The relatively
increased platelet numbers in steady state SCD may result from release of thrombopoietin secondary to anemia or renal ischemia. Thrombopoietin levels may
also be directly increased in response to increased platelet consumption and
shorter life span. Another possibility is decreased splenic function, since this is
common in SCD (98): Splenectomy has been reported to result in (temporary)
thrombocytosis (94, 99, 100). Interestingly, secondary thrombocytosis, as might
occur in SCD, is usually *not* associated with decreased platelet function (101),
in contrast to primary thrombocytosis (myeloproliferative disorders).

Platelet numbers may decrease in crisis (93, 102; see also Figure 4.2), although
this is not universally reported. Thrombocytopenia, when noted, does not *usually*
occur to a dangerous level. In crisis, platelet survival time is significantly shortened (103). A period of relative thrombocytosis may follow the crisis, with a
peak at about 2 weeks (93, 104). An increase in the number of circulating platelet
microaggregates has been reported during crises (105), suggesting increased
platelet stimulation at these times. Ongoing stimulation may also occur, as
increased microaggregates have also been reported in steady state (106, 107):

Gesina L. Longenecker

Table 4.1
Platelet α Granule Protein Levels in Sickle Cell Disease

	β-TG,ng/ml		
Controls	Steady State	Crisis	Reference
36 ± 1.6*	50 ± 3.6	55 ± 5.9	(109)
29 ± 6	55 ± 9	276 ± 154	(108)
38**	83**	-	(106)
29 ± 19	70 ± 30	-	(106)
69.9± 10.7	83.4± 5.6	110.1± 13***	(110)
	PF₄,ng/ml		
6 ± 0.8	10 ± 1.2	9.3 ± 2.3	(109)
13**	34**	-	(106)

Notes:
  β-TG = Beta-Thromboglobulin.
  PF₄ = Platelet Factor 4.
  * Average ± SEM.
  **Data shown are medians; average ± SEM not available.
  ***Twenty-four hours afer crisis initiation; $p<0.05$ compared with either controls or steady
    state.

However, the increase in steady state may also be another consequence of decreased splenic function (107).

Biochemical Indices

Biochemical indices of platelet stimulation in SCD present a mixed picture. BTG, for example, is consistently elevated in both steady state *and* crisis (83, 106, 108, 109), but in most studies there is no statistically significant difference between steady state and crisis. Our data support these observations, but additionally show a significance of differences (see Table 4.1 and reference 110). It has also been reported that releasable BTG, namely, the amount released by specifically stimulated platelets in a controlled exposure, is unchanged (106). Levels of another platelet α granule substituent, PF4, which is considered by some scientists to be a more reliable and specific marker of platelet release (especially if done in parallel with BTG measurements; [82]), have also been reported to be elevated in steady state (83, 106, 108, 109) and crisis, with the latter again not differing from the elevated steady state levels (109). In one report, BTG but not PF4 was elevated. This, together with a positive correlation between platelet number and BTG/PF4 levels and no change in dense granule contents (see below and reference 109), was suggested to indicate artefactual platelet stimulation. Our data also show a significant correlation between platelet number and BTG, but only for steady state SCD and not for controls or crisis

Table 4.2
Thromboxane Levels in Sickle Cell Disease

Basal Controls	Steady State	Crisis	Reference
≈90	≈175	≈89	(113)
60[**]	81[**]		(106)
44.6 ± 5.4	30.2 ± 3.1	31.2 ± 4.8	(110)
Maximal (serum)			
259 ± 145	326 ± 165	-	(106)
110.1± 5.4	67.8 ± 3.5[***]	62.5 ± 8.2	(110)
Per Platelet			
0.21 ± 0.004	0.09 ± 0.2[***]	0.07 ± 0.02[**]	(110)
	0.10 ± 0.03	0.09 ± 0.02[***]	

*Values estimated by author from graphical data.
**Data shown are medians; average ± SEM not availble.
***p<0.05 compared with controls.
+ Value twenty-four hours after crisis intitiation.
+ + Seventy-two hours and seven days after crisis event, respectively.

SCD (110). Such a pattern is equally consistent with ongoing stimulation in steady state and crisis SCD. In crises, a broader range of values due to platelet exhaustion and replacement can be anticipated.

Platelet dense granule contents of ATP and ADP appear unchanged in SCD (109). Dense granule 5HT content has been reported to be unaltered in both steady state and crisis (109). Releasable 5HT (i.e., the amount released per platelet by specifically stimulated platelets in a controlled setting) has likewise been reported to be no different from control values (106). However, in situations with increased platelet turnover, as reported for SCD, a greater number of platelets are young and large (94, 111); since large platelets have a significantly higher 5HT content (111), it is possible that determinations on "average" (unfractionated) populations may include extremes that do not provide an accurate picture. Thus, in SCD there could be a large population of older and smaller (or previously stimulated) platelets, with respectively lower granule contents, balanced by a large population of young, larger platelets with higher granule contents. This is a possibility that should be carefully examined, especially since *many* other properties of platelets, including reactivity, are also influenced by size, age, and prior agonist exposure (112, 113).

Levels and release of de novo synthesized TxA (TxB) have been reported to be unchanged (106), higher (114), or decreased in both steady state and crisis (115, 110). In the first and last cases, platelet number was taken into account; in other words, the amount per platelet, in addition to total amount, was examined. Available data is summarized in Table 4.2.

Adhesive Responses

Adhesive reactions of platelets have been examined in SCD, with mixed outcome. Decreased *in vitro* aggregation responses are frequently reported for several initiators in steady state—ADP (higher concentrations only) (105, 106, 116, 117), epinephrine (105, 116), collagen (116), and ristocetin (116)—and in crisis—ADP (117, 118). However, responses in the near normal range have also been reported (95), as have increased responses, at least with respect to ADP threshold (106, 107). For the latter, decreased splenic function may be involved, as similar changes were noted for platelets from splenectomized patients (99, 107). Platelet adhesion responses in SCD have been less often examined, with no change or a decrease reported for crisis state (see references 118 and 119, respectively).

Changes in Factors Influencing Platelets

RBC

A number of factors with potential influence on platelet function are altered in SCD in general and may change further in crisis. For example, RBC undergoing sickling or hemolysis under mechanical stress may release ADP (52, 120) and other contents (e.g., 2,3-DPG; 2,3-diphosphoglycerate). The former is a direct stimulant of platelets and, in sufficient amounts, may lead to irreversible platelet aggregation; in sub-maximal amounts, however—even those that induce only minimal aggregation and essentially no release—ADP may lead to desensitization (refractoriness) of platelets: ADP-scavenging systems can reverse this desensitization (121). The latter may prove important to test on SCD platelets demonstrating reduced aggregation responses. 2,3-DPG has been reported to enhance platelet aggregation responses, and to enhance or inhibit TxA synthesis and release, under some conditions (122).

The deformability of S-RBC is decreased. "Stiff" S-RBC may thus mechanically initiate platelet aggregation in SCD as reported for the "stiff" RBC of diabetes (123). RBC-induced platelet aggregation, while mechanically initiated, may involve platelet amplification by the release of ADP, PAF, and TxA (123). RBC, in general, may be involved in platelet stimulation in the circulation (120). There is a direct correlation between the degree of platelet adhesion and the number of RBC. Under some flow conditions, platelet adhesion increases up to fivefold as the hematocrit increases from 10 to 40 and then plateaus (124); the altered flow shows monotonic adhesion (and thrombus formation) as the hematocrit increases from 10 to 70. The mechanisms of these relationships are unknown but their occurrence could have import for SCD patients.

In addition to the stimuli already mentioned, platelets respond to immunoglobulins (125) and complement activation (C3a in particular) (126). Although not documented to have any role for RBC-platelet interactions in SCD, it is worthwhile to note that S-RBC, in contrast to C-RBC, can surface-bind significant amounts of IgG, and that surface binding increases with deoxygenation and sickling (127) as well as with increased RBC age (128).

RBC in SCD may generate significant quantities of superoxide anion (SO; O_2) or other active oxygen species (AOS) (129–131). There are reports of oxygen species altering platelet function, including aggregation (132–135): Platelet aggregation is usually enhanced if exposure to submaximal aggregating agent occurs first, followed by AOS (H_2O_2, SO), but inhibited if the order of exposure is reversed. Whether SO/AOS influence platelets in SCD to any significant degree is unknown but clearly possible.

In summary, then, it is possible, but undocumented, that the combined rigidity (mechanical), surface phenomena (IgG), and leak of platelet-active biochemical agents (ADP, 2,3-DPG, SO/AOS) associated with S-RBC render them highly interactive with platelets.

Coagulation Factors

SCD crises may be precipitated or exacerbated by ongoing coagulation (93; for review, see 136). Fibrinogen levels may be normal (93, 116, 136) or elevated in SCD in steady state and decrease during crisis (93; also see Figure 4.3), possibly in proportion to thrombin generation and activity (137). (In our studies, increased fibrinogen occurred or recurred late in crises; see Figure 4.3). Thrombin generation could thus lead to platelet stimulation in parallel with fibrinogen consumption. *Direct* enhancing effects of increased fibrinogen on platelet function are not likely, although indirect effects are possible. Elevated fibrinogen (and fibrin) levels may lead to elevated split (degradation) products, which can influence platelet function (usually inhibiting it, perhaps by preventing platelet-fibrinogen binding by competition; [138]). It should be noted that fibrinolysis may be decreased in SCD (136).

Other pro-coagulant (pro-thrombotic) changes in SCD may contribute to platelet stimulation. For example, Factor X/Xa has been suggested both to enhance platelet function (32) and to depress thromboxane synthesis (139). Also, S-RBC membranes may undergo lipid remodeling, which promotes coagulation (140), as a result of sickling.

Factor VIII is increased in SCD, including factors VIII antigen (VIII:Ag), procoagulant (VIII:c), and von Willebrand factor (VIII:vWF; vWF; 83, 116, 141). In a study of plasma factors contributing to increased circulating platelet microaggregates, vWF was identified as a major contributor (32). Not only is vWF elevated in SCD, the predominant multimeric forms may be shifted to very large multimers (ULvWF) (141), possibly as a result of ongoing endothelial stimulation. While at first glance this would seem to facilitate platelet agglutination responses (ristocetin aggregation/agglutination), it has been proposed that a high VIII:c, Ag/VIII:vWF ratio may account for the aforementioned defective ristocetin agglutination observed in SCD (116). This is supported by the observation that ristocetin responsiveness of SCD platelets can be restored by

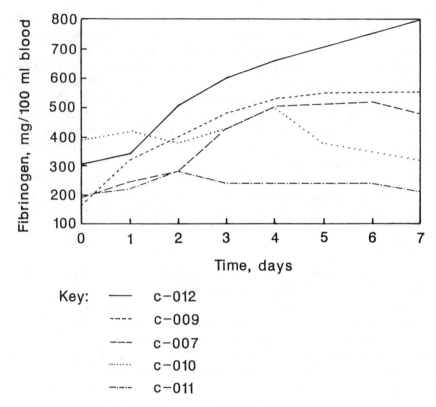

Figure 4.3. Figrinogen levels for five sickle cell patients as a function of time after admission for pain crisis. Increases, sometimes dramatic (O12), were observed as the crisis resolved.

washing and resuspension in control plasma with normal VIII component levels and ratios, or with the use of very high concentrations of ristocetin. It has also been shown that platelets from blacks in general respond less to lower ristocetin concentrations (and more comparably at higher ristocetin) and that plasma from blacks can reduce nonblacks' platelet responses to ristocetin (142). These data are consistent with a competitive circumstance in SCD for various components of factor VIII but indicate that this may also occur to some extent in blacks in general.

Anti-platelet Activity of Drugs Used in SCD

It is not a purpose of this chapter to review drug therapy of SCD (see reviews 5 and 143). However, it is worthwhile to note that quite a few of the drugs that have been found beneficial in either limiting the number of crises or crisis severity, or that have *in vitro* activities strongly suggesting utility, also have antiplatelet effects.

Aspirin, perhaps the classic antiplatelet drug, when used alone and in low doses, did not reduce the frequency of crises (144). However, in other studies, aspirin alone and together with dipyridamole was found to reduce symptoms significantly (50%) and improve blood indicators of crisis as well (93, 145). RA–233, a phosphodiesterase inhibitor of the pyrimido-pyrimidine class (mopidamole, an analogue of dipyridamole) with the ability to inhibit platelets, reportedly increases RBC deformability (146); data from the author's laboratory indicates that dipyridamole also inhibits RBC adhesion to endothelium (see the section on Mechanisms under: Interactions of Platelets and Endothelium with RBC). Piracetam, which reduces both platelet adhesive (147) and release (148) responses, limits RBC adhesion (149, 150) and has antisickling properties (151). Perfluorocarbon compounds have been suggested to be useful in SCD based on their ability to increase RBC deformability and improve rheologic behavior (152): Perfluorocarbons are also antiplatelet (75–77). Cetiedil, a relatively new agent with proposed benefits in SCD (153), including antisickling effects (154) and improved RBC deformability (155), inhibits platelet aggregation and thromboxane formation (156). Ticlopidine, a well-known antiplatelet agent, (157–159), has been used in a very brief (one month) clinical trial in SCD (83), with mixed results. An experimental compound, RMI 11071A, from a series of compounds with antiplatelet activity, has been shown to also have antisickling effects (160).

Recent data suggests that calcium channel blockers (CCB), some of which influence platelets, may be therapeutically useful in SCD, primarily by reducing small vessel tone (161). It has also been shown that CCB reduce stimulated release of vWF from endothelium (162): This could theoretically reduce platelet (and RBC; see below) adhesion as well, indicating another potential area of benefit from CCB in SCD. There are a number of additional examples of SCD drugs that also have antiplatelet effects (e.g., chloroquine [163, 164]; pentoxifylline [165], and oxypentoxifylline [155]): Whether agents with multiple activities, including antiplatelet effects, offer greater clinical utility than those without, remains to be seen.

ENDOTHELIAL FUNCTION IN SCD

The function of the vascular endothelium may be significantly altered in SCD, although data to document this are not abundantly available. The approach taken in this section is to describe known changes in SCD and show that additional changes may be expected based on data for other states.

The endothelium is the source of circulating vWF (166) and thus is the ultimate source of the ULvWF multimers already mentioned, although some amount of the multimers may also be formed *after* endothelial release (167). ULvWF are thought to be important to abnormal adhesion of S-RBC to endothelium (141;

also see below). Moreover, vWF promotes platelet adhesion, and its large multimers may be required for platelet-initiated hemostatic plug formation (168).

Endothelium produces two important fibrinolytic hormones, namely, tissue
plasminogen activator (tPA) and urokinase: The release of each is regulated
(169). It should be noted that platelets contain and release both vWF (ULvWF)
and tPA, which they take up from the plasma: Changes in platelet levels of these
proteins should thus parallel changes in plasma.

Endothelium is the site of thrombomodulin, a receptor for thrombin and protein
C, which facilitates the activation of the latter substance (170). Protein C, which
enhances fibrinolysis and limits the amounts of activated factors V and VIII:c,
is decreased in SCD (171). It should also be noted that the interaction of thrombin
with thrombomodulin limits thrombin stimulation of both platelets and
coagulation.

Endothelium is the source of PGI (and EDRF), a modulator(s) of platelet
function *in vivo;* adequate production of this hormone is held to be requisite for
normal platelet responsiveness. Endothelium also releases, responds to, and
transports adenosine (50, 52, 172), which can also affect platelet reactivity (53).
Endothelium is involved in regulating the responsiveness of the blood vessels.
The net tone of blood vessels is determined by levels of relaxants like PGI,
EDRF, and adenosine, in combination with levels of constrictive factors like
TxA, epinephrine, 5HT, vasopressin, angiotensin II, and so on. Any circumstance that changes the balance in favor of the constrictors could thus increase
vessel tone and potentially lead to a low flow condition, namely ischemia or
crisis.

Ischemia as a Model

Situations that may be analogous to certain aspects of SCD are known to
change PGI release and/or levels. Ischemia and hypoxia induced by the occlusion
of the superior mesenteric artery (SMAO), in addition to producing a profound
and frequently lethal shock state, decreases the release of PGI from subsequently
isolated vascular rings (86). *In vivo,* there is usually a significant acute *increase*
in PGI (stable metabolite) in the circulation in transient ischemic states. The
increase results in part from increased Ca^{++} availability (ATP depletion, Na^+
loading, increased Na^+-Ca^{++} exchange) and thus phospholipase stimulation
(arachidonic acid release and metabolism). Ischemia-induced increases in substances that act on endothelial receptors to increase PGI, for example, bradykinin
(173), may also contribute. Stimulated PGI release is followed by a refractory
("exhausted") state, as described above for the vascular rings taken from ischemia-induced shock animals. Autocatalytic destruction of cyclooxygenase and/
or PGI synthase could contribute to refractoriness (173, 174), although other
desensitization phenomena, including substrate depletion and receptor down-
regulation, may be involved.

In SCD there may be ongoing low-level ischemia coupled with poor oxygen-

Table 4.3
Prostacylin Levels in Sickle Cell Disease

Controls	Steady State	Crisis	Reference
40 ± 14[*]	446 ± 89	-	(183)
21.3 ± 10.3	30.3 ± 9.7	14.3 ± 6.5	(182)
67.0 ± 27.9	11.6 ± 2.3	-	(181)
31.7 ± 5.0	20.4 ± 2.5[***]	12.2 ± 2.0[****]	(110)
1.6 ng/ml[**]	2.4 ng/ml[**]	-	(106)

*Average ± SEM, pg/ml.
**Data shown are medians; average ± SEM not available.
***$p < 0.05$ with respect to controls.
****Twenty-four hours after crisis initiation; $p < 0.05$ with respect to steady state.

carrying capacity, as well as intermittent, acute ischemia and hypoxemia (i.e., crisis). Such conditions would be expected to lead to an ongoing stimulation *and* a relative refractory state, with spikes of additional stimulation followed by greater refractoriness and, possibly, partial recovery. Based on this description, lower than usual PGI, on average, would be anticipated, with acute variations also probable.

SCD

There are data to further support the expectation of decreased PGI in SCD, including decreased levels of plasma PGI releasing factor in SCD (175; see also 176–178). ADP, which may be leaked from RBC (and released from platelets, as discussed previously), can release PGI (but possibly not EDRF) from endothelium (48, 50, 52, 179). Thus, ADP could contribute to ongoing and acute endothelial stimulation as well as to refractoriness. AOS reportedly stimulate PGI release (see the end of the section on vasoconstrictors), thus increased production and release of AOS by S-RBC could contribute to ongoing stimulation and refractoriness also. In addition to the factors already described, some co-agulation factors (such as Xa and Va) may inhibit PGI release (180), in contrast to thrombin, which stimulates it. Curiously, X/Xa likewise depresses thromboxane synthesis (139) but also enhances platelet function, as previously mentioned (32).

Vasodilators

PGI.   The actual data available for PGI in SCD are mixed, with both increases and decreases reported (110, 114, 181–183; see also Table 4.3). In both cases where significantly increased steady state PGI was noted (114, 183), increased levels were also noted during crises. In another report, steady state levels were not significantly different from controls, while in crisis significant decreases were found (182). Our data indicates significant decreases in steady state, with an additional significant decrease early in crisis (110, 115, 181). Whether the disparities in the collective data are a function of different types or intensity of crises, slightly different timing of sampling, degree of prior and/or current vascular damage, or differences in levels of vasostimulators that release PGI from endothelium (including ADP, epinephrine, and even S-RBC adhesion [184]) is unknown at present. Verification of RIA data, which can be problematic (44), by GC-MS-MS (gas chromatography–tandem mass spectroscopy) and highly specific ELISA (enzyme-linked immunosorbent assay) is currently in progress. In addition, mechanisms of altered PGI in SCD are currently under investigation, including comparisons of plasma and RBC binding of PGI. Changes in plasma binding of PGI may be important since albumin binding of PGI stabilizes it (185), and it is known that the degree of binding changes in response to fatty acid levels (via diet and other changes) and disease (186).

EDRF.   The vascular release of EDRF has not been examined in SCD. However, several observations would indicate a significant probability of alteration. Hemoglobin and hemolysate have been suggested to inactivate EDRF (45, 187), so that in *any* state where free hemoglobin is present, a decreased effectiveness of EDRF might be anticipated. EDRF can also be destroyed by AOS (SO; 45, 46) and, as previously noted, S-RBC produce significant quantities of SO (129). Thus, EDRF may be destroyed by both free hemoglobin/hemolysate and intact S-RBC (SO). The action of nitrovasodilators, which act through NO (EDRF) generation, may also be reduced in SCD.

Summary.   Taken in aggregate, endothelial production of important vasodilator and platelet inhibitory compounds is probably decreased in SCD. In addition, other thrombosis or coagulation-preventing functions may be decreased. The consequences may include increased platelet aggregation and adhesion responsiveness as well as increased vascular tone. An additional activity of PGI may also be reduced: Since PGI stimulates fibrinolysis, clot lysis may take place more slowly as a result of reduced PGI (188–190). The latter is consistent with the reduced fibrinolysis previously mentioned for SCD (136; as is reduced protein C [171]). Vascular tone could be affected by other changes also, as described in the next section.

Vasoconstrictors—Platelet Stimulatory Products

Platelets—TxA.   During periods of platelet stimulation and release, vasoactive substances are released, including TxA, an extremely potent vasoconstrictor agent, and 5HT. Monoamines other than 5HT are also stored and released by platelets, including dopamine, norepinephrine, and even epinephrine: The amounts stored and released reflect circulating levels. Release may thus be contributory to local vasoocclusion as well as widespread vascular tone changes.

Epinephrine.   Another interplay may involve epinephrine (norepinephrine), which is a potent, direct stimulator of platelets and which is vasoactive (and cardio-stimulant). Epinephrine (and norepinephrine) levels increase in response to stress (possibly including stress caused by pain) and may modify platelet (191–193) as well as vascular responses, probably by synergistic action with other agents, as previously discussed (19). Norepinephrine, like epinephrine, has an ability to increase platelet reactivity. It also increases platelet numbers (194), although the latter has been proposed as a splenic effect (splenic function is decreased in SCD). The experience of pain itself during crisis could thus be a significant contributor to platelet recruitment and to increased tone in some vascular beds. Both the latter may be somewhat attenuated by the epinephrine-induced release of PGI, presuming the endothelium is capable of release.

Epinephrine, and *many* other vasoactive substances, particularly vasopressin, may also release vWF from endothelium (195), with consequences for RBC (and platelet) adhesion. Epinephrine also may decrease RBC deformability (196).

Curiously, levels and/or changes in levels of catecholamines in SCD, both steady state or crisis, have not been reported. This may be a significant oversight in attempts to explore mechanisms of SCD pathophysiology. Indeed, observation of a panel of platelet and endothelial/vasoactive hormones in SCD as a function of status could prove enlightening and useful.

Other Vasoconstrictors. Hemoglobin (heme, hemin) exposure may have additional endothelial consequences. Hemolysate significantly reduces vascular relaxant responses, or even converts relaxation to contraction, for a number of hormones and drugs, most likely by reducing PGI (EDRF) release (187). In addition, the exposure of endothelial cells in culture to either S-RBC or hemin seems to be harmful, resulting in a significant, albeit reversible, inhibition of growth and division, thymidine uptake, and so on (197): Heme is a component of multiple cellular entities and a known regulator of many cellular processes, including the activity of the P450 monoxygenase system (198). The presence of hemin (labile Fe) in culture media could cause the formation of AOS, which may be one mechanism of action (199). AOS, which are generated biochemically, have been reported to cause similar damage to EC in culture (200). The effects of AOS, in particular H_2O_2, on PGI are variable and may be dose-dependent (low stimulates—high inhibits) (201–205). Endothelium may be exposed to significant quantities of AOS, including SO, from S-RBC (as previously noted), from excess heme/hemoglobin, and even from WBC/PMN. Since these exposures would occur via plasma, it is important to note that plasma has little to no inactivation capacity for SO or other AOS.

Another index of vascular endothelial damage in SCD is an increase in the number of circulating endothelial cells (206). Similar increases are noted in smokers and even in individuals passively exposed to smoke (207).

INTERACTIONS OF PLATELETS AND ENDOTHELIUM WITH RBC

Some interactions among the platelets, endothelium, and RBC have been described in previous sections, for example, the potential for stiff RBC to mechanically and biochemically activate platelets and effects of RBC-released contents on platelets (2, 3-DPG, ADP) and endothelium (ADP, hemoglobin/heme). In the following sections, the effects of platelet and endothelial products on RBC, as well as some effects of the RBC on those products, are described.

Prior to the discovery of the unstable and highly active arachidonic acid products PGI and TxA, attention focused (necessarily) on stable metabolites, for example, prostaglandins (PG) E_2, $F_{2\alpha}$, D_2, and E_1. The latter is not an arachidonic acid product (all of which can easily be identified by the numeric subscript 2), but rather is a product of cyclooxygenase-initiated metabolism of another, much less abundant fatty acid, dihomogammalinolenic acid (C18:3n6) (208). Stable PG are produced by *many* cells, including platelets and endothelium (23). They are significantly bioactive (for reviews see references 209 and 210), causing vasoconstriction (e.g., $F_{2\alpha}$) or relaxation (E_1, PGI), uterine stimulation (E_2, $F_{2\alpha}$), and platelet inhibition (E_1, D_2, PGI) or facilitation ($F_{2\alpha}$) (211).

RBC Deformability

The property of RBC most often examined for effects by PG is deformability: The ability to deform is necessary for RBC passage through capillaries. As noted, S-RBC are less deformable than control RBC, for a number of reasons (15). Deformability has been assessed by two general means, namely, positive or negative pressure-induced filtration through capillary pore membranes (212–220) and degree of entry of RBC membrane into a micropipette under variable negative pressure (221–223).

Increases in RBC deformability (control RBC as well as RBC made less deformable by disease (such as systemic sclerosis or peripheral vascular disease) or by calcium loading have been reported for E_1 (224–227) and PGI (224, 228, 229). Decreases have been reported for E_2 (196, 225, 226, 230–232), A_1 (230), E_1 (230), and even PGI (233), as well as for RBC isolated after *in vivo* aspirin treatment (234). Indeed, sickle crisis precipitation has also been suggested for E_2 (231, 232) and $F_{2\alpha}$ (235). A total lack of effect on deformability has also been reported for both E_1 and E_2 (236).

Ion Balance

The general topic of RBC ion balance has been reviewed recently (237), and also for SCD (238). Briefly, RBC contain four basic transport systems involving Na^+, K^+, Cl^- and Ca^{++}: (1) the Na^+, K^+-transport ATPase, (2) a Cl^--dependent Na^+, K^+-cotransport system, (3) a Ca^{++}-activated K^+ channel and (4) a Cl^--dependent K^+ transport system. In S-RBC, sickling has been associated with RBC dehydration and K^+ loss (paralleled by Na^+ gain), as well as with increased Ca_i^{++} (239, 240): Increased K^+ loss appears to be related to systems (3) and (4) and possibly to (1), but not to (2). Decreased RBC deformability has also been associated with increased Ca^{++} (241).

Electrolyte balance changes in RBC may also be effected by PG, although, again, reports are contradictory. Both increased RBC K^+ loss *and* increased Ca^{++} accumulation have been reported for PGE_2 (242, 243). However, PGE_1, E_2, A_1, A_2, and $F_{2\alpha}$ have also been reported to have *no* effect on RBC electrolyte transport (244). A regulatory interaction may also exist between PGE_1 and Ca^{++}: In the presence of Ca^{++}, PGE_1 can be incorporated into membranes, which then become permeable to divalent, but not monovalent, cations (245). Recently, PGI has been reported to stimulate, and cAMP to inhibit, (bumetanide-sensitive) Na^+,K^+-cotransport (but not ouabain-sensitive Na^+,K^+-ATPase) (246), although this cotransport system does not appear to be involved in S-RBC dehydration (238). However, LTB_4 (leukotriene B_4, a 5-lipoxygenase metabolite of arachidonic acid) increased (ouabain- and bumetanide-resistant) K^+ flux (246), suggesting it could favor S-RBC dehydration and sickling.

Lipids

Other membrane effects have also been reported for PG. For example, PGE_1 increased the "fluidity" of RBC ghost and intact RBC membranes (225, 247). PGE_1 may also effect a separation of sphingomyelin and phosphatidylcholine in situations of cholesterol enrichment (248). This PGE_1–cholesterol effect appears to be associated with *de*creased membrane fluidity. Changes in the occurrence and/or ratios of other phospholipids by PG, especially in SCD, have not been reported. Such changes could be important since the process of sickling apparently changes the composition of the outer RBC membrane to favor exposure of procoagulant phosphatidyl serine (140).

Release

TxA and its stable analogues, carbocyclic TxA and prostaglandin endoperoxide intermediate (U46619), release hemoglobin from RBC in a concentration-dependent manner (249). This appears to be a receptor-mediated event, as TxA-induced hemoglobin release can be prevented with the TxA receptor antagonist BM 13505. Platelet activation resulting in TxA formation and release could thus amplify changes in RBC, with the consequent establishment of a positive feed-back cycle (RBC ADP release by TxA was not examined but is probable in situations in which hemoglobin is released). Platelet activating factor (PAF) is a potent, lipid-derived mediator formed by platelets, endothelium, and, particularly, polymorphonuclear leukocytes, and is also a potent platelet stimulus (18); it has recently been shown to cause RBC release of ATP and ADP (250). Thus, platelet stimuli may elicit a simultaneous RBC response and also contribute to a positive feedback cycle.

Adhesion

Recently, S-RBC were shown to adhere to endothelium to a significant degree (251–259; for review, see 2); control RBC adhere very little and significantly less than S-RBC. One factor involved in promoting S-RBC adhesion is ULvWF (141). Anti-vWF antibody can reduce (while desmopressin, which releases vWF from endothelial cells, can increase) adhesion (260). Antibodies against GPIb or GPIIb/IIIa also inhibit S-RBC adhesion (261). In view of these data, the observation that platelets can promote conversion of low- to mid-range vWF to ULvWF is particularly significant (262).

The adhesion of S-RBC to endothelial cells in culture caused the culture's release of PGI (184), although inhibition of endothelial PGI synthesis (flurbiprofen) had little effect on S-RBC adhesion. These data would seem to indicate that endothelial PGI is not involved in the regulation of S-RBC adhesion. However, we have recently shown that iloprost (Schering), a stable analogue of PGI, can significantly reduce S-RBC adhesion (259) at very low concentrations ($\leq$ 200 nM). Endothelial PGI could have an effect on circulating RBC that is not mimicked by PGI released in response to adhesion (i.e., PGI may act on preadherent but not on postadherent cells). In SCD, where PGI may be continuously low or cycle through very low periods, effects on RBC adhesion would be anticipated to be reduced or absent either all or part of the time. In addition, in SCD *in vivo,* endothelium may or may not be able to respond (fully or in part) to RBC adhesion with PGI release. Regardless of which, if any, of these scenarios apply, it appears that pharmacologic levels of iloprost/PGI can reduce S-RBC adhesion; importantly, these same doses of iloprost could simultaneously reduce platelet responsiveness, as well as (possibly) decrease vascular tone and increase fibrinolysis, all of which could be useful in SCD crisis management and prevention.

Other lipid-derived mediators may also influence RBC adhesion. For example, PAF dose dependently enhances S- (but not C-) RBC adhesion (263), as may leukotriene B_4 (unpublished data).

Other Effects of Prostaglandins

A number of miscellaneous bits of data suggest additional roles of importance for PG in SCD. These include erythropoietic effects (for a review see reference 264) and hemoglobin-oxygen affinity effects (PGE_2 may increase affinity slightly [265]).

Mechanisms

The mechanism(s) by which eicosanoids initiate signaling and transduction in RBC have only been examined briefly. PGE_1 binds to both high- and low-affinity sites on human RBC (266). Curiously, this binding is displaced by cAMP or cold PGE_1 very effectively but less effectively by PGI and ineffectively by other agents (266). Binding is decreased by neuraminidase or trypsin exposure, also supporting receptor involvement. Binding of PGI to RBC has also been observed but was not characterized (184, 267). Our data indicates binding of PGI (PGE_1) to S-RBC, but binding to C-RBC is nearly identical and neither appears saturable (268).

In many systems, including platelets (see initial sections), receptors for inhibitory PG are coupled to cAMP/adenylyl cyclase, while stimulatory eicosanoids receptors are coupled to Ca^{++}. These generalities may also apply to RBC: S-RBC have higher cyclase than control RBC, possibly as a result of the younger average age of S-RBC (269), and may also have altered ion transport/levels, as already mentioned. In control RBC, no increase in cAMP was elicited by β-adrenergic stimulation (isoproterenol) or PGE_2 (270), although NaF does increase cyclase activity (269) in controls, hereditary spherocytosis, and S-RBC. In the latter study, PGE_1 effected a small increase in cAMP in control and spherocytosis RBC, but data was not reported for S-RBC. We have shown an iloprost-induced increase in S-RBC cAMP that is significantly greater than that in C-RBC (268).

Levels of ATP, the substrate for cyclase for cAMP generation, may be involved in regulation of protein behavior in RBC (e.g., phosphorylation status of spectrin). ATP added to either spherocytosis or S-RBC resulted in protein kinase-mediated membrane phosphorylation (271), part of which was moderately increased by cAMP and (a different) part of which was strongly enhanced by EGTA (Ca^{++} removal). Phosphorylation status, particularly of spectrin, has been suggested to be involved in RBC shape control (272). To date, changes in phosphorylation in S-RBC under various manipulations or treatments have not been reported but can be anticipated to vary from control based on data for other disease states. An additional means by which eicosanoids may modulate cAMP/ATP-Ca^{++} in RBC is suggested by data from avian RBC, in which PGA_1 has been found to inhibit cAMP export (273, 274). Whether this type of export occurs in human cells is unknown, but remains an intriguing possibility.

In support of an involvement of cAMP in eicosanoids effects on RBC, some effects of AAM can be mimicked by cAMP. For example, the membrane fluidity changes due to PGE_1 can be duplicated by external RBC treatment with cAMP (and also cGMP) (247). RBC Na^+,K^+-cotransport can be inhibited by treatment with cAMP, and the inhibition can be further increased by addition of IBMX (isobutylmethyl xanthine; PDE inhibitor). Our data indicate that the inhibition of S-RBC adhesion by iloprost can also be mimicked with dibutyryl cAMP (a lipid soluble analogue of cAMP). Furthermore, the effects of sub-maximal iloprost can be enhanced by (submaximal) dipyridamole, an inhibitor of PDE (dipyridamole alone is also inhibitory) (259). These data, when taken in aggregate, indicate an active and potentially important interaction between eicosanoids and cyclic nucleotides in S-RBC. Studies are in progress to fully characterize iloprost (PGI) binding and interactions with adenylyl cyclase in S-RBC. Recently, studies involving another second messenger, namely Ca^{2+}, especially in its relationship to PAF effects on adhesions of S-RBC to endothelium, have been initiated (275).

Effects of RBC on Eicosanoids

RBC may also influence the levels of some AAM. It has been suggested, albeit not universally supported, that PGI that is bound to RBC is more rapidly degraded (267, 276). This contrasts with the binding of PGI to albumin, which "protects" it and significantly increases its half-life (seconds versus minutes for free and bound, respectively [185, 277]): Our data indicates no difference in either binding or half-life of PGI for SCD versus controls (278). Exactly how PGI is inactivated while bound to RBC has not been documented; however, it should be noted that both PG-9-keto reductase and PG-15-dehydrogenase are present in RBC. Other eicosanoids intermediates may also undergo metabolism by exposure to RBC. For example, RBC apparently have LTA_4 hydrolase activity and can thus convert LTA_4, which perhaps is leaked from PMNs, to LTB_4. The latter enhances RBC K^+ flux, as mentioned previously, but is best known for its effects on PMN, which include aggregation, degranulation, and SO and PAF generation. Since most SCD patients have higher than usual WBC (PMN), this activity of RBC could represent yet another positive feedback cycle, directly for RBC and PMN, but potentially also involving platelets via PAF.

SUMMARY

Changes in the function of platelets and endothelium in sickle cell disease clearly occur and probably contribute to the overall symptoms of the disease, especially those of crisis. The initiating factors for platelet function changes are numerous and can be tied to changes in red cells, endothelium, and coagulation. Red cells can chemically (ADP, 2, 3-DPG) and mechanically stimulate platelets: Platelet products, in turn, can influence red cells (e.g., thromboxane releases hemoglobin and platelet activating factor releases ATP/ADP and results in shape change), as well as the vasculature (increases tone) and the coagulation system (procoagulant). Under some conditions (thrombin stimulation), platelets may even expose/release a lectin-like activity. Ongoing and periodic acute stimulation of endothelium (ADP, thrombin, mechanical, vasoactive substances [including platelet thromboxane and serotonin]) may increase the release of factor VIII:vWF (especially large multimers) and thus promote both platelet function and red cell-endothelial cell adhesion; a partially exhausted or refractory state for prostacyclin could also result. Since prostacyclin is antiplatelet, promotes fibrinolysis, and may regulate red cell deformability and adhesion, decreases in its availability may be significant. Hemoglobin release (stimulated or by hemolysis) may also limit the effectiveness of endothelium-derived relaxing factor, another platelet (and vascular) regulatory hormone. Increased vascular tone may also result from decreases in prostacyclin and endothelium-derived relaxing factor (and may be worsened by an increased availability of vasoconstrictors), contributing to vasoocclusion. Attention to identifying the role of the interactions described or suggested herein, and to identifying additional interactions, can lend significantly to the understanding of global pathology in sickle cell disease and, thereby, its rational management.

REFERENCES

1. Whitten CF, and Bertles JF: Sickle cell disease, Ann NY Acad Sci (special issue) (1989).
2. Hebbel RP: Beyond hemoglobin polymerization: The red blood cell membrane and sickle disease pathophysiology. Blood 77 (1991): 214–237.
3. Murphy RC Jr, and Shapiro S: The pathology of sickle cell disease. Ann Intern Med 23 (1945): 376–397.
4. Vichinsky EP, and Lubin BH: Sickle cell anemia and related hemoglobinopathies. Ped Clin N Amer 27 (1980): 429–447.
5. Mathur LR: Sickle cell anemia: New approaches to therapy. Res Resources Rep 7 (1983): 1–4.
6. Overturf G, and Powars D: Infections in sickle cell anemia: Pathogenesis and control. Tex Rep Biol Med 40 (1980): 283–292.
7. Brewer, GJ: Detours on the road to successful treatment of sickle cell anemia. In ED Garber, ed.: Genetic perspectives in biology and medicine, pp. 273–295. Chicago: University of Chicago Press, 1985.
8. MacIntyre E, and Gordon J: Platelets in biology and pathology. Amsterdam: Elsevier, 1987.
9. Gerrard JM: Platelet aggregation: Cellular regulation and physiologic role. Hosp Pract (Off) 23 (1988): 89–108.
10. Longenecker GL: The platelets: Physiology and pharmacology. Orlando, FL: Academic Press, 1985.
11. McGregor JL, and Clemetson KJ: Biochemistry of the platelet membrane. Curr Stud Hematol Blood Transf 55 (1988): 5–31.
12. Remaly AT, Kennedy JM, and Laposata M: Utility of platelet aggregation studies. Am J Hematol 31 (1989): 188–193.
13. Lusher JM, Mammen EF, McCoy LE, et al.: Factor VIII/vWF and platelet formation and function in health and disease: A tribute to Marion Barnhart, Ann. NY Acad Sci 509 (special issue) (1987).
14. Oates JA, Hawiger J, and Ross R: Interaction of platelets with the vessel wall. Bethesda, MD: American Physiological Society, 1985.
15. McGregor JL, and Clemetson KJ: Regulation of megakaryocytopoiesis by thrombopoietin. Ann NY Acad Sci 509 (1987): 1–24.
16. Bessler H, Mandel EM, and Djaldetti M: Role of the spleen and lymphocytes in regulation of the circulating platelet number in mice. J Lab Clin Med 91 (1978): 760–768.
17. Haslam RJ, and Rosson GM: Aggregation of human blood platelets by vasopressin. Am J Physiol 223 (1972): 958–967.
18. Snyder F: Biochemistry of platelet-activating factor: A unique class of biologically active phospholipids (42839). Proc Soc Exper Biol Med 190 (1988): 125–135.

19. Kerry R, and Scrutton MC: Platelet adrenoceptors. In GL Longenecker, ed.: *The platelets: Physiology and pharmacology*, pp. 113–157. Orlando, FL: Academic Press, 1985.

20. Feinstein MB, Zavoico GB, and Halenda SP: Calcium and cyclic AMP: Antagonistic modulators of platelet function. In GL Longenecker, ed.: *The platelets: Physiology and pharmacology*, pp. 237–269. Orlando, FL: Academic Press, 1985.

21. Feinstein MB, and Halenda SP: Arachidonic acid mobilization in platelets: The possible role of protein kinase C and G-proteins. *Experientia* 44 (1988): 101–104.

22. Smith CD, Cox CC, and Snyderman R: Receptor-coupled activation of phosphinositide-specific phospholipase C by an N protein. *Science* 232 (1986): 97–100.

23. Longenecker GL: Platelet arachidonic acid metabolism. In GL Longenecker, ed.: *The platelets: Physiology and pharmacology*, pp. 159–185. Orlando, FL: Academic Press, 1985.

24. Hawiger J, Kloczewiak M, and Timmons S: Platelet-receptor mechanisms for adhesive macromolecules. In JA Oates, J Hawiger, and R Ross, eds.: *Interaction of platelets with the vessel wall*, pp. 1–19. Baltimore, MD: Waverly Press, 1985.

25. Puri RN, Zhou FX, Bradford H, et al.: Thrombin-induced platelet aggregation involves an indirect proteolytic cleavage of aggregin by calpain. *Arch Biochem Biophys* 271 (1989): 346–358.

26. Gartner TK, Williams DC, and Minion FC: Thrombin-induced platelet aggregation is mediated by a platelet plasma membrane-bound lectin. *Science* 200 (1978): 1281–1283.

27. Gartner TK, Phillips DR, and Williams DC: Expression of thrombin-enhanced platelet lectin activity is controlled by secretion. *FEBS Lett* 113 (1980): 196–200.

28. Ehrman M, Toth E, and Frojmovic M: A platelet procoagulant activity associated with platelet shape change. *J Lab Clin Med* 92 (1978): 393–401.

29. Barrowcliffe TW, Edwards SJ, Gray E, et al.: Procoagulant activity of platelet arachidonic acid metabolism. *Br J Pharmacol* 92 (1987): 129–132.

30. Hawiger J: Macromolecules that link platelets following vessel wall injury. *Ann NY Acad Sci* 509 (1987): 131–141.

31. Meyer D, Fressinaud E, Sakariassen KS, et al.: Role of von Willebrand factor in platelet vessel wall interactions. *Ann NY Acad Sci* 509 (1987): 118–130.

32. Neri Serneri GG, Abbate R, Mugnaini C, et al.: Increased platelet aggregation due to a plasma aggregating activity: Identification of responsible factors. *Haemostasis* 9 (1980): 941–956.

33. Kinlough-Rathbone RL, Packham MA, and Mustard JF: Synergism between platelet aggregating agents: The role of the arachidonate pathway. *Thromb Res* 11 (1977): 567–580.

34. Adams GA: Platelet aggregation. In GL Longenecker, ed.: *The platelets: Physiology and pharmacology*, pp. 1–14. Orlando, FL: Academic Press, 1985.

35. Grant JA, and Scrutton MC: Positive interaction between agonists in the aggregation response of human blood platelets: Interaction between ADP, adrenaline and vasopressin. *Br J Haematol* 44 (1980): 109–125.

36. Ding Y-A, MacIntyre DE, Kenyon CJ, et al.: Potentiation of adrenaline-induced platelet aggregation by angiotensin II. *Thromb Haemostas* (Stuttgart) 54 (1985): 717–720.

37. Worowski K, Poplawski A, Prokopowicz J, et al.: The effect of angiotensin II on the clotting and fibrinolytic system in dogs. *Coagulation* 2 (1969): 237–239.

38. Poplawski A: The effect of angiotensin II on the platelet aggregation induced by adenosine diphosphate, epinephrine and thrombin. *Experientia* 26 (1970): 86.

39. Moncada S: Prostacyclin—Discovery and biological importance. In GL Longenecker and SW Schaffer, eds.: *Prostaglandins: Research and clinical update*, pp. 1–39. Minneapolis: Alpha Editions, 1985.

40. Bunting S, Moncada S, and Vane JR: The prostacyclin–thromboxane A_2 balance: Pathophysiological and therapeutic implications. *Br Med Bull* 39 (1983): 271–276.

41. Freissmuth M, Casey PJ, and Gilman AG: G proteins control diverse pathways of transmembrane signaling. *FASEB J* 3 (1989): 2125–2131.

42. FitzGerald GA, Brash AR, Falardeau P, et al.: Estimated rate of prostacyclin secretion into the circulation of normal man. *J Clin Invest* 68 (1981): 1272–1276.

43. Steer ML, MacIntyre DE, Levine L, et al.: Is prostacyclin a physiologically important circulating anti-platelet agent? *Nature* 283 (1980): 194–195.

44. Longenecker, GL: Correspondence problems in prostacyclin levels by different methods. In GL Longenecker, and S Schaffer, eds.: *Prostaglandins: Research and clinical update*, pp. 341–347. Minneapolis, MN: Alpha Editions, 1985.

45. Ignarro LJ: Biological actions and properties of endothelium-derived nitric oxide formed and released from artery and vein. *Circ Res* 65 (1989): 1–21.

46. Radomski MW, Palmer RMJ, and Moncada S: Comparative pharmacology of endothelium-derived relaxing factor, nitric oxide and prostacyclin in platelets. *Br J Pharmacol* 92 (1987): 181–187.

47. D'Orleans-Juste P, de Nucci G, and Vane JR: Kinins act on B1 or B2 receptors to release conjointly endothelium-derived relaxing factor and prostacyclin from bovine aortic endothelial cells. *Br J Pharmacol* 96 (1989): 920–926.

48. Boulanger C, Hendrickson H, Lorenz RR, et al.: Release of different relaxing factors by cultured porcine endothelial cells. *Circ Res* 64 (1989): 1070–1078.

49. Shimokawa H, Flavahan N, Lorenz RR, et al.: Prostacyclin releases endothelium-derived relaxing factor and potentiates its action in coronary arteries of the pig. *J Vasc Med Biol* 1 (1989): 115.

50. Gordon JL: Extracellular ATP: Effects, sources and fate. *Biochem J* 233 (1986): 309–319.

51. Reimers, H-J: Adenine nucleotides in blood platelets. In GL Longenecker, ed.: *The platelets: Physiology and pharmacology*, pp. 85–112. Orlando, Academic Press, 1985.

52. Luthje J: Origin, metabolism and function of extracellular adenine nucleotides in the blood. *Klin Wochenschr* 67 (1989): 317–327.

53. Mills DCB, and Smith JB: The influence on platelet aggregation of drugs that affect the accumulation of adenosine-3',5'-monophosphate in platelets. *Biochem J* 121 (1971): 185–196.

54. Agarwal KC, and Parks RE Jr: 5'-methylthioadenosine and 2',5'-dideoxyadenosine blockade of the inhibitory effects of adenosine on ADP-induced platelet aggregation by different mechanisms. *Biochem Pharmacol* 29 (1980): 2529–2532.

55. Jakobs KH, Saur W, and Johnson RA: Regulation of platelet adenylate cyclase by adenosine. *Biochim Biophys Acta* 583 (1979): 409–421.

56. Summers A, Subbarao K, Rucinski B, et al.: The effect of dipyridamole on adenosine uptake by platelets ex vivo. *Thromb Res* 11 (1977): 611–618.

57. Lips JPM, Sixma JJ, and Trieschnigg AC: Inhibition of uptake of adenosine into human blood platelets. *Biochem Pharmacol* 29 (1980): 43–50.

58. Tam SW, Fenton JW II, and Detwiler RC: Dissociation of thrombin from platelets by hirudin. *J Biol Chem* 254 (1979): 8723–8725.

59. Smith JB: Effects of thromboxane synthase inhibitors on platelet function: Enhancement by inhibition of phosphodiesterase. *Thromb Res* 28 (1982): 471–485.

60. Bult H, Fret HRL, Jordaens FH, et al.: Dipyridamole potentiates the anti-aggregating and vasodilator activity of nitric oxide. *Eur J Pharmacol* 199 (1991): 1–8.

61. Vigdahl RL, Mongin J, and Marquis NR: Platelet aggregation IV: Platelet phosphodiesterase and its inhibition by vasodilators. *Biochem Biophys Res Commun* 42 (1971): 1088–1094.

62. Jackson CA, Greaves M, and Preston FE: A study of the stimulation of human venous prostacyclin synthesis by dipyridamole. *Thromb Res* 27 (1982): 563–573.

63. Boeynaems JM, Van Coevorden A, and Demolle D: Dipyridamole and vascular prostacyclin production. *Biochem Pharmacol* 35 (1986): 2897–2902.

64. Neri Serneri GG, Masotti G, Abbate R, et al.: Enhanced prostacyclin production and decreased thromboxane formation by dipyridamole. *Int Congr Ser, Excerpta Med* 491 (1979): 489–494.

65. Blass K-E, Block H-U, Forster W, et al.: Dipyridamole: A potent stimulator of prostacyclin (PGI_2) biosynthesis. *Br J Pharmacol* 68 (1980): 71–73.

66. Watanabe T, Narumiya S, Shimizu T, et al.: Characterization of the biosynthetic pathway of prostaglandin D_2 in human platelet rich plasma. *J Biol Chem* 257 (1982): 14847–14853.

67. Smith JB: Effect of thromboxane synthetase inhibitors on platelet function: Enhancement by inhibition of phosphodiesterase. *Thromb Res* 28 (1982): 477–485.

68. Longenecker GL, Swift IA, Bowen RJ, et al.: Kinetics of ibuprofen effect on platelet and endothelial prostanoid production. *Clin Pharm Ther* 37 (1985): 343–350.

69. MacIntyre DE, Handin RI, Rosenberg R, et al.: Heparin opposes prostanoid and non-prostanoid platelet inhibitors by direct enhancement of aggregation. *Thromb Res* 22 (1981): 167–175.

70. Cofrancesco E, Colombi M, Fowst C, et al.: Heparin-induced platelet aggregation and its inhibition by antagonists of the thromboxane pathway. *Thromb Res* 42 (1986): 867–868.

71. Eldor A, and Weksler BB: Heparin and dextran sulfate antagonize PGI_2 inhibition of platelet aggregation. *Thromb Res* 16 (1979): 617–628.

72. Bygdeman S, and Johnsen O: Effect of dextrans on platelet function. *Acta Med Scand* 525-suppl. (1971): 249–252.

73. Tiffany M, and Penner J: Heparin and other sulfated polyanions: Their interaction with the blood platelet. *Ann NY Acad Sci* 370 (1981): 662–667.

74. Longenecker GL, Horton TJ, Kase C, et al.: Dextran 40 (D40) and platelet function. *Trans SE Pharm Soc* 5 (1984): 17.

75. Colman RW, Chang LK, Mukherji B, et al.: Effects of a perfluoro erythrocyte substitute on platelets in vitro and in vivo. *J Lab Clin Med* 95 (1980): 553–562.

76. Benner K, Gaehtgens P, and Frede K: Aggregation of human red blood cells (RBC) and platelets and its reversal by a surface-active substance (Pluronic F68). *Bibl Anat* 12 (1973): 208–215.

77. Shakir KM, and Williams TJ: Inhibition of phospholipase A_2 activity by Fluosol, an artificial blood substitute. *Prostaglandins* 23 (1982): 919–927.

78. Rosenberg JC, and Sell TL: In vitro evaluation of inhibitors of platelet release and aggregation. *Arch Surg* 110 (1975): 981–983.

79. Wu KK, and Hoak JC: Spontaneous platelet aggregation in arterial insufficiency: Mechanisms and implications. *Thromb Haemostas* (Stuttgart) 35 (1976): 702–711.

80. Granstrom E, Westlund P, and Kumlin M. Measurement of platelet eicosanoid compounds. In GL Longenecker, ed.: *The platelets: Physiology and pharmacology*, pp. 441–461. Orlando, FL: Academic Press, 1985.

81. Zahavi J, and Kakkar VV: Beta-thromboglobulin—A specific marker of in vivo platelet release reaction. *Thromb Haemostasis* (Stuttgart) 43 (1980): 23–29.

82. Niewiarowski S, and Holt JC: Platelet alpha-granule proteins: Biochemical and pathological aspects. In GL Longenecker, ed.: *The platelets: Physiology and pharmacology*, pp. 49–83. Orlando, FL: Academic Press, 1985.

83. Semple MJ, Al-Hasani SF, Kioy P, et al.: A double-blind trial of ticlopidine in sickle cell disease. *Thromb Haemostas* (Stuttgart) 51 (1984): 303–306.

84. Hamberg M, Svensson J, and Blomback M: A method for measurement of platelet regeneration in man. *Prostaglandins Med* 1 (1978): 455–460.

85. Longenecker, GL: Bioassay of prostacyclin by platelet aggregometry. In GL Longenecker, and S Schaffer, eds.: *Prostaglandins: Research and clinical update*, pp. 333–339. Minneapolis, MN: Alpha Editions, 1985.

86. Longenecker GL, Bowen RJ, Eddy LJ, et al.: Aortic prostacyclin release is lowered by superior mesenteric artery occlusion (SMAO) shock in pigs. *Circ Shock* 9 (1981): 393–401.

87. Longenecker GL, and Glenn TM: Alterations in pig platelets after a shock-inducing procedure. *Circ Shock* 7 (1980): 309–315.

88. Glazier J: Measurement of platelet aggregation in whole blood. *Am Clin Prod Rev* 6 (1987): 26–30.

89. Feinman RD, Detwiler TC, and Ingerman-Wojenski C: The lumi-aggregometer as a research and clinical tool. In GL Longenecker, ed.: *The platelets: Physiology and pharmacology*, pp. 429–440. Orlando, FL: Academic Press, 1985.

90. Longenecker GL, Bowen RJ, Swift IA, et al.: Increased beta-thromboglobulin in the serum of smokers occurs because of increased platelet counts. *Res Comm Sub Abuse* 5 (1984): 147–152.

91. Rao GHR, and White JG: An improved method for measuring endogenous serotonin in platelets. *Thromb Res* 51 (1988): 225–227.

92. Oei HH, Hughes WE, Schaffer SW, et al.: Platelet serotonin uptake during myocardial ischemia. *Am Heart J* 106 (1983): 1077–1081.

93. Alkjaersig N, Fletcher A, Joist H, et al.: Hemostatic alterations accompanying sickle cell pain crises. *J Lab Clin Med* 88 (1976): 440–449.

94. Freedman ML, and Karpatkin S: Short communication: Elevated platelet count and megathrombocyte number in sickle cell anemia. *Blood* 46 (1975): 579–582.

95. Buchanan GR, and Holtkamp CA: Platelet aggregation, malondialdehyde generation and production time in children with sickle cell anaemia. *Thromb Haemostas* (Stuttgart) 46 (1981): 690–693.

96. Bain BJ, and Seed M: Platelet count and platelet size in healthy Africans and West Indians. *Clin Lab Haematol* 8 (1986): 43–48.

97. Thomas LC, Giles TD, Stuckey WJ, et al.: Racial differences in platelet survival time in patients with symptomatic coronary atherosclerosis. *Arteriosclerosis* 3 (1983): 138–140.

98. Pearson HA: The kidney, hepatobiliary system, and spleen in sickle cell anemia. *Ann NY Acad Sci* 565 (1989): 120–125.

99. Nagasue N, Inokuchi K, Kobayashi M, et al.: Platelet aggregability after splenectomy in patients with normosplenism and hypersplenism. *Am J Surg* 136 (1978): 260–264.

100. Schwartz AD: The splenic platelet reservoir in sickle cell anemia. *Blood* 40 (1972): 678–683.

101. Ginsburg AD: Platelet function in patients with high platelet counts. *Ann Intern Med* 82 (1975): 506–511.

102. Allen U, MacKinnon H, Zipursky A, et al.: Severe thrombocytopenia in sickle cell crisis. *Ped Hematol Oncol* 5 (1988): 137–141.

103. Haut MJ, Cowan DH, and Harris JW: Platelet function and survival in sickle cell disease. *J Lab Clin Med* 82 (1973): 44–53.

104. Van der Sar A: The sudden rise in platelets and reticulocytes in sickle cell crises. *Trop Geogr Med* 22 (1970): 30–40.

105. Mehta P, and Mehta J: Abnormalities of platelet aggregation in sickle cell disease. *J Ped* 96 (1980): 209–213.

106. Westwick J, Watson-Williams EJ, Krishnamurthi S, et al.: Platelet activation during steady state sickle cell disease. *J Med* 14 (1983): 17–36.

107. Kenny MW, George AJ, and Stuart J: Platelet hyperactivity in sickle-cell disease: A consequence of hyposplenism. *J Clin Pathol* 33 (1980): 622–625.

108. Mehta P: Significance of plasma B-thromboglobulin values in patients with sickle cell disease. *J Ped* 97 (1980): 941–944.

109. Buchanan GR, and Holtkamp CA: Evidence against enhanced platelet activity in sickle cell anaemia. *Br J Haematol* 54 (1983): 595–603.

110. Longenecker GL, Beyers BJ, and Mankad VN: Platelet regulatory prostanoids and platelet release products in sickle cell disease. *Am J Hematol* 40 (1992): 12–19.

111. Thompson CB, Eaton KA, Princiotta SM, et al.: Size dependent platelet subpopulations: Relationship of platelet volume to ultrastructure, enzymatic activity, and function. *Br J Haematol* 50 (1982): 509–519.

112. Jakubowski JA, Thompson CB, Vaillancourt R, et al.: Arachidonic acid metabolism by platelets of different size. *Br J Haematol* 53 (1983): 503–511.

113. Martin JF, Trowbridge EA, Salmon G, et al.: The biological significance of platelet volume: Its relationship to bleeding time, platelet thromboxane B_2 production and megakaryocyte nuclear DNA production. *Thromb Res* 32 (1983): 443–460.

114. Buchanan GR, and Holtkamp CA: Plasma levels of platelet and vascular prostaglandin derivatives in children with sickle cell anaemia. *Thromb Haemostasis* (Stuttgart) 54 (1985): 394–396.

115. Mankad VN, Williams JP, Harpen M, et al.: Magnetic resonance imaging, percentage of dense cells and serum prostanoids as tools for objective assessment of pain crises: A preliminary report. In R Nagel, ed.: *Pathophysiological aspects of sickle cell vaso-occlusion*, pp. 337–359. New York: Alan R. Liss, 1987.

116. Sarji KE, Eurenius K, Fullwood CO, et al.: Abnormalities of platelet aggregation in sickle cell anemia: Presence of a plasma factor inhibiting aggregation by ristocetin. *Thromb Res* 14 (1979): 283–297.

117. Gruppo RA, Glueck HI, Granger SM, et al.: Platelet function in sickle cell anemia. *Thromb Res* 10 (1977): 325–335.

118. Stuart MJ, Stockman JA, and Oski FA: Abnormalities of platelet aggregation in the vaso-occlusive crisis of sickle-cell anemia. *J Ped* 85 (1974): 629–632.

119. Gupta VL, Dube GK, Chaubey BS, et al.: Platelet function, fibrinogen and misfi—

An immunohaematological study in sickle cell crisis. *J Assoc Phys India* 29 (1981): 183–187.

120. Born GVR: Fluid mechanical and biochemical interactions in hemostasis. *Br Med Bull* 33 (1977): 193–197.

121. Rozenberg MC, and Holmsen H: Adenine nucleotide metabolism of blood platelets IV: Platelet aggregation response to exogenous ATP and ADP. *Biochim Biophys Acta* 157 (1968): 280.

122. Iatridis PG, Hadd H, Kotrotsou M, et al.: The combined effects of 2,3-DPG and sodium arachidonate on platelet aggregation and on TxA2 formation. *Thromb Res* 42 (1986): 177–185.

123. Juhan-Vague I, Chignard M, Poisson C, et al.: Possible participation of adenosine 5'-diphosphate, arachidonic acid and PAF-acether in the platelet pro-aggregating effect of uncontrolled insulin-dependent diabetic erythrocytes in vitro. *Thromb Res* 38 (1985): 83–89.

124. Turitto VT, and Weiss HJ: Red blood cells: Their dual role in thrombus formation. *Science* 207 (1980): 541–543.

125. Becker EL, and Henson PM: In vitro studies of immunological-induced secretion of mediators from cells and related phenomena. *Adv Immunol* 17 (1973): 93.

126. Becker S, Meuer S, Hadding U, et al.: Platelet activation: A new biological activity of guinea pig C3a anaphylatoxin. *Scand J Immunol* 7 (1978): 173–180.

127. Green GA, and Kalra VK: Sickling-induced binding of immunoglobulin to sickle erythrocytes. *Blood* 71 (1988): 636–639.

128. Mohandas N, and Groner W: Cell membrane and volume changes during red cell development and aging. *Ann NY Acad Sci* 554 (1989): 217–224.

129. Chiu D, and Lubin B: Oxidative hemoglobin denaturation and RBC destruction: The effect of heme on red cell membranes. *Semin Hematol* 26 (1989): 128–135.

130. Hebbel RP, Eaton JW, Balasingam M, et al.: Spontaneous oxygen radical generation by sickle erythrocytes. *J Clin Invest* 70 (1982): 1253–1259.

131. Hebbel RP: Auto-oxidation and a membrane-associated "Fenton Reagent": A possible explanation for development of membrane lesions in sickle erythrocytes. *Clin Haematol* 14 (1985): 129–140.

132. Iatridis SG, Iatridis PG, Kyrkou KA, et al.: Platelet aggregation following exposure of phospholipase-treated platelet rich plasma to hydrogen peroxide. *Thromb Res* 15 (1979): 733–741.

133. Handin RI, Karabin R, and Boxer GJ: Enhancement of platelet function by superoxide anion. *J Clin Invest* 59 (1977): 959–965.

134. Canoso RT, Rodvien R, Scoon KL, et al.: Hydrogen peroxide and platelet function. *Blood* 43 (1974): 645–656.

135. Holmsen H, and Robkin L: Hydrogen peroxide lowers ATP levels in platelets without altering adenylate energy charge and platelet function. *J Biol Chem* 252 (1977): 1752–1757.

136. Rickles FR, and O'Leary DS: Role of coagulation system in pathophysiology of sickle cell disease. *Arch Intern Med* 133 (1974): 635–641.

137. Leichtman DA, and Brewer GJ: Elevated plasma levels of fibrinopeptide A during sickle cell anemia pain crisis—Evidence for intravascular coagulation. *Am J Hematol* 5 (1978): 183–190.

138. Hantgan RR: Fibrin protofibril and fibrinogen binding to ADP-stimulated platelets: Evidence for a common mechanism. *Biochim Biophys Acta* 968 (1988): 24–35.

139. Sinha AK, Rao AK, Willis J, et al.: Inhibition of thromboxane A_2 synthesis in human platelets by coagulation factor Xa. *Proc Natl Acad Sci USA* 80 (1983): 6086–6090.

140. Chiu D, Lubin B, Roelofsen B, et al.: Sickled erythrocytes accelerate clotting in vitro: An effect of abnormal membrane lipid asymmetry. *Blood* 58 (1981): 398–401.

141. Wick TM, Moake JL, Udden MM, et al.: Unusually large von Willebrand factor multimers increase adhesion of sickle erythrocytes to human endothelial cells under controlled flow. *J Clin Invest* 80 (1987): 905–910.

142. Buchanan GR, Holtkamp CA, and Levy EN: Racial differences in ristocetin-induced platelet aggregation. *Br J Haematol* 49 (1981): 455–464.

143. Luskey KL, Schechter AN, and Hercules JI: New approaches to the therapy of sickle cell disease. *Tex Rep Biol Med* 40 (1980): 305–312.

144. Greenberg J, Ohene-Frempong K, Halus J, et al.: Trial of low doses of aspirin as prophylaxis in sickle cell disease. *Ped Pharmacol Ther* 102 (1983): 781–784.

145. Chaplin H Jr, Alkjaersig N, Fletcher AP, et al.: Aspirin-dipyridamole prophylaxis of sickle cell disease pain crises. *Thromb Haemostas* (Stuttgart) 43 (1980): 218–227.

146. Ambrus JL, Bannerman RM, Sills RH, et al.: Studies on the vasoocclusive crisis of sickle cell disease III. In vitro and in vivo effect of the pyrimido-pyrimidine derivative, RA-233: Studies on its mechanism of action. *J Med* 18 (1987): 165–198.

147. Bick RL: In-vivo platelet inhibition by piracetam. *Lancet* 2, no. 8145 (1979): 752.

148. Henry RL, Nalbandian RM, Herman GE, et al.: Release of PF4 and BTG from platelets and inhibition by piracetam. *Blood* 52-suppl. (1978): 163.

149. Nalbandian RM, Henry RL, Burek CL, et al.: Diminished adherence of sickle erythrocytes to cultured vascular endothelium by piracetam. *Am J Hematol* 15 (1983): 147–151.

150. Nalbandian RM, Henry RL, Fleischman JA, et al.: Erythrocyte-endothelial cell adherence in sickle cell disease, diabetes mellitus, and falciparum malaria: Adverse effects reversed with piracetam. *Med Hypotheses* 8 (1982): 155–162.

151. Asakura T, Ohnishi ST, Adachi K, et al.: Effect of piracetam on sickle erythrocytes and sickle hemoglobin. *Biochim Biophys Acta* 668 (1980): 397–405.

152. Reindorf CA, Kurantsin-Mills J, Allotey JB, et al.: Perfluorocarbon compounds: Effects on the rheological properties of sickle erythrocytes in vitro. *Am J Hematol* 19 (1985): 229–236.

153. Benjamin LJ, Kokkini G, and Peterson CM: Cetiedil: Its potential usefulness in sickle cell disease. *Blood* 55 (1980): 265–270.

154. Asakura T, Ohnishi ST, Adachi K, et al.: Effect of cetiedil on erythrocyte sickling: New type of antisickling agents that may affect erythrocyte membranes. *Proc Natl Acad Sci USA* 77 (1980): 2955–2959.

155. Stuart J, Stone PCW, Bilto YY, et al.: Oxpentifylline and cetiedil citrate improve deformability of dehydrated sickle cells. *J Clin Pathol* 40 (1987): 1182–1186.

156. Yamaguchi A, Asakura T, Tanoue K, et al.: Effect of cetiedil on platelet aggregation and thromboxane synthesis. *Thromb Res* 37 (1985): 391–400.

157. O'Brien JR: *Ticlopidine: A promise for the prevention and treatment of thrombosis and its complications.* Basel: Karger, 1983.

158. Panak E, Maffrand JP, Picard-Fraire C, et al.: Ticlopidine: A promise for the

prevention and treatment of thrombosis and its complications. *Haemostasis* 13-suppl. 1 (1983): 1–54.

159. Akashi A, Hashizume T, Tanaka M, et al.: Pharmacological studies on ticlopidine, a new platelet aggregation inhibitor, part II: General pharmacological properties. *Arzneim-Forsch/Drug Res* 30 (1980): 415–419.

160. Mackenzie RD, Gleason EM, Schatzman GL, et al.: In vitro inhibition of the rate of erythrocyte sickling by RMI11071A and its possible mechanism (40652). *Proc Soc Exper Biol Med* 162 (1979): 224–226.

161. Rodgers GP, Roy MS, Noguchi CT, et al.: Is there a role for selective vasodilation in the management of sickle cell disease? *Blood* 71 (1988): 597–602.

162. Musumeci V, Cardillo C, Baroni S, et al.: Effects of calcium channel blockers on the endothelial release of von Willebrand factor after exercise in healthy subjects. *J Lab Clin Med* 113 (1989): 525–531.

163. Massabi M: Maternal chloroquine prophylaxis and sickle cell anemia. *Lancet* no. 1 (1983): 1046.

164. Nurse GT: Maternal chloroquine prophylaxis and sickle-cell anemia. *Lancet* no. 1 (1983): 1271.

165. Manrique R: Sickle cell anemia. Pathophysiological role of increased intracorpuscular calcium and changes during treatment with pentoxifylline. *La Ricerca Clin Lab* 17 (1987): 355–362.

166. Kawai Y, and Montgomery RR: Endothelial cell processing of von Willebrand proteins. *Ann NY Acad Sci* 509 (1987): 60–70.

167. Tsai HM, Nagel RL, Hatcher VB, et al.: Multimeric composition of endothelial cell-derived von Willebrand factor. *Blood* 73 (1989): 2074–2076.

168. Brinkhous KM: Development and present status of concentrate therapy for hemophilia and von Willebrand's disease. *Wien Klin Wochenschr* 94 (1982): 509–514.

169. Levin EG, and Loskutoff DJ: Regulation of plasminogen activator production by cultured endothelial cells. *Ann NY Acad Sci* 40 (1982): 184–194.

170. Comp PC: Clinical implications of the protein C/protein S system. *Ann NY Acad Sci* 509 (1987): 149–155.

171. Terkonda R, Ebbinghaus S, Willoughby TL, et al.: Protein C levels in sickle cell diseases. *Ann NY Acad Sci* 565 (1989): 430–431.

172. Kroll K, Kelm MK, Burrig KF, et al.: Transendothelial transport and metabolism of adenosine and inosine in the intact rat aorta. *Circ Res* 64 (1989): 1147–1157.

173. Stalcup SA, Davidson D, and Melins RB: Endothelial cell functions in the hemodynamic responses to stress. *Ann NY Acad Sci* 401 (1982): 117–131.

174. Marnett LJ, Dix TA, Siedlik PH, et al.: Hydroperoxide metabolism and oxidant generation in platelets. In GL Longenecker, ed.: *The platelets: Physiology and pharmacology*, pp. 187–200. Orlando, FL: Academic Press, 1985.

175. Stuart MJ, and Sills RH: Deficiency of plasma prostacyclin or PGI_2 regenerating ability in sickle cell anaemia. *Br J Haematol* 48 (1981): 545–550.

176. Deckmyn H, Zoja C, Arnout J, et al.: Partial isolation and function of the prostacyclin regulating plasma factor. *Clin Sci* 69 (1985): 383–393.

177. Vergara-Dauden M, Balconi G, Breviario F, et al.: Further studies on the mechanism of action of human plasma in stimulating prostacyclin production by rat smooth muscle cells. *Thromb Haemostasis* 53 (1985): 372–376.

178. Snopko R, Guffy T, Rafelson ME, et al.: Serum stimulation of prostacyclin synthesis

in aortically, venously and microvascularly derived endothelial cells. *Clin Physiol Biochem* 5 (1987): 70–76.

179. Needham L, Cusack NJ, Pearson JD, et al.: Characteristics of the P2 purinoceptor that mediates prostacyclin production by pig aortic endothelial cells. *Eur J Pharmacol* 134 (1987): 199–209.

180. Sinha AK, Dutta-Roy AK, Chiu HC, et al.: Coagulant factor Xa inhibits prostacyclin formation in human endothelial cells. *Arteriosclerosis* (1985): 244–249.

181. Longenecker GL, and Mankad V: Decreased prostacyclin levels in sickle cell disease. *Pediatrics* 71 (1983): 860–861.

182. Koren-Kurlat A, and Halevi R: Decreased prostacyclin levels in sickle cell disease. *Ped Hematol Oncol* 6 (1989): 67–69.

183. Mehta P, and Albiol L: Prostacyclin and platelet aggregation in sickle cell disease. *Pediatrics* 70 (1982): 354–356.

184. Wautier J-L, Pintigny D, Maclouf J, et al.: Release of prostacyclin after erythrocyte adhesion to cultured vascular endothelium. *J Lab Clin Med* 107 (1986): 210–215.

185. Purdon AD, and Rao AK: Interaction of albumin, arachidonic acid and prostanoids in platelets. *Prostaglandins Leukotrienes Essen Fatty Acids* 1989; 35:213–218.

186. Lucas FV, Skrinska VA, Chisolm GM, et al.: Stability of prostacyclin in human and rabbit whole blood and plasma. *Thromb Res* 43 (1986): 379–387.

187. Toda N: Hemolysate inhibits cerebral artery relaxation. *J Cereb Blood Flow Metab* 8 (1988): 46–53.

188. Crutchley DJ, Conanan LB, and Maynard JR: Stimulation of fibrinolytic activity in human skin fibroblasts by prostaglandins E_1, E_2 and I_2. *J Pharm Exp Ther* 222 (1982): 544–549.

189. Holloway DS, Zuckerman L, Vagher JP, et al.: The effects of prostacyclin on the coagulation of whole blood. *Thromb Haemostas* (Stuttgart) 50 (1983): 671–675.

190. Szczeklik A, Kopec M, Sladek K, et al.: Prostacyclin and the fibrinolytic system in ischemic vascular disease. *Thromb Res* 29 (1983): 655–660.

191. Gordon JL, Bowyer DE, Evans DW, et al.: Human platelet reactivity during stressful diagnostic procedures. *J Clin Pathol* 26 (1973): 958–962.

192. Haft JI, and Fani K: Stress and the induction of intravascular platelet aggregation in the heart. *Circulation* 48 (1973): 164–169.

193. Sorkin RP, Tokarsky JM, Huber-Smith MJ, et al.: In vivo platelet aggregation and plasma catechoamines in acute myocardial infarction. *Am Heart J* 104 (1982): 1255–1261.

194. Sloand JA, Hooper M, and Izzo JL Jr: Effects of circulating norepinephrine on platelet, leukocyte and red blood cell counts by alpha$_1$-adrenergic stimulation. *Am J Cardiol* 63 (1989): 1140–1142.

195. Kraus KH, Turrentine MA, and Johnson GS: Multimeric analysis of von Willebrand factor before and after desmopressin acetate (DDAVP) administration intravenously and subcutaneously in male beagle dogs. *Am J Vet Res* 48 (1987): 1376–1379.

196. Allen JE, and Rasmussen H: Human red blood cells: Prostaglandin E_2, epinephrine, and isoproterenol alter deformability. *Science* 174 (1971): 512–514.

197. Weinstein R, Wenc K, and Zhou M: *Endothelial cell alteration by sickle erythrocytes and hemin.* Paper presented at the 14th annual Sickle Cell Centers' Conference, 1989: abstract 83.

198. Dwarki VJ, Francis VNK, Bhat GJ, et al.: Regulation of cytochrome P-450 messenger RNA and apoprotein levels by heme. *J Biol Chem* 262 (1987): 16958–16962.

199. Gutteridge, JMC: Lipid peroxidation: Some problems and concepts. In B Halliwell, ed.: *Oxygen radicals and tissue injury*, pp. 9–19. Bethesda, MD: Upjohn/FASEB, 1988.

200. Ody C, and Junod AF: Effect of variable glutathione peroxidase activity on H_2O_2-related cytotoxicity in cultured aortic endothelial cells (42150). *Proc Soc Exp Biol Med* 180 (1985): 103–111.

201. Panganamala RV, Karpen CW, and Merola AJ: Peroxide mediated effects of homocysteine on arterial prostacyclin synthesis. *Prostaglandins, Leukotrienes Med* 22 (1986): 349–356.

202. Jackson RM, Chandler DB, and Fulmer JD: Production of arachidonic acid metabolites by endothelial cells in hyperoxia. *J Appl Physiol* 61 (1986): 584–591.

203. Yamaja Setty BN, Jurek E, Ganley C, et al.: Effects of hydrogen peroxide on vascular arachidonic acid metabolism. *Prostaglandins, Leukotrienes Med* 14 (1984): 205–213.

204. Harlan JM, and Callahan KS: Role of hydrogen peroxide in the neutrophil-mediated release of prostacyclin from cultured endothelial cells. *J Clin Invest* 74 (1984): 442–448.

205. Rampart M, Jose PJ, and Williams TJ: Leukocytes activated by C5a des Arg promote endothelial prostacyclin (PGI_2) production via release of oxygen species in vitro. *Agents Actions* 16 (1985): 21–22.

206. Sowemimo-Coker SO, Meiselman HJ, and Francis RB Jr: Increased circulating endothelial cells in sickle cell crisis. *Am J. Hematol* 31 (1989): 263–265.

207. Davis JW, Shelton L, Watanabe IS, et al.: Passive smoking affects endothelium and platelets. *Arch Intern Med* 149 (1989): 386–389.

208. Longenecker, GL: Dietary manipulation of eicosanoid production and platelet reactivity. In GL Longenecker and S Schaffer, eds.: *Prostaglandins: Research and clinical update*, pp. 239–274. Minneapolis, MN: Alpha Editions, 1985.

209. Moskowitz MA, and Coughlin SR: Basic properties of the prostaglandins. *Stroke* 12 (1981): 696–701.

210. Ogburn PL Jr, and Brenner WE: *The physiologic actions and effects of prostaglandins*, pp. 1–41 Kalamazoo, MI: Upjohn, 1981.

211. Longenecker GL: Effects of prostaglandin $F_{2\alpha}$ on submaximal ADP-induced aggregation of canine platelets. *Thromb Res* 18 (1980): 369–374.

212. Hanss M: Erythrocyte filterability measurement by the initial flow rate method. *Biorheology* 20 (1983): 199–211.

213. Jones JG, Holland BM, Humphrys J, et al.: The flow of blood cell suspensions through 3 μm and 5 μm Nuclepore membranes: A comparison of kinetic analysis with scanning electron microscopic examinations. *Br J Haematol* 59 (1985): 541–546.

214. Reid HL, Barnes AJ, Lock PJ, et al.: A simple method for measuring erythrocyte deformability. *J Clin Pathol* 29 (1976): 855–858.

215. Reinhart WH, Usami S, Schmalzer EA, et al.: Evaluation of red blood cell filterability test: Influences of pore size, hematocrit level, and flow rate. *J Lab Clin Med* 104 (1984): 501–516.

216. Teitel P: Basic principles of the "filterability test" (FT) and analysis of erythrocyte flow behavior. *Blood Cells* 3 (1977): 55–70.

217. Evans E, and Fung Y-C: Improved measurements of the erythrocyte geometry. *Microvasc Res* 4 (1972): 335–347.

218. Leblond P, and Coulombe L: The measurement of erythrocyte deformability using micropore membranes. *J Lab Clin Med* 94 (1979): 133–143.

219. Cokelet GR: Dynamics of erythrocyte motion in filtration tests and in vivo flow. *Scand J Clin Lab Invest* 41, suppl. 156 (1981): 77–82.

220. Acquaye C, Walker EC, and Schechter AN: The development of a filtration system for evaluating flow characteristics of erythrocytes. *Microvasc Res* 33 (1987): 1–14.

221. Hochmuth RM: Solid and liquid behavior of red cell membrane. *Ann Rev Biophys Bioeng* 11 (1982): 43–55.

222. Meiselman HJ, Evans EA, and Hochmuth RM: Membrane mechanical properties of ATP-depleted human erythrocytes. *Blood* 52 (1978): 499–504.

223. Evans EA, and La Celle PL: Intrinsic material properties of the erythrocyte membrane indicated by mechanical analysis of deformation. *Blood* 45 (1975): 29–43.

224. Dowd PM, Kovacs IB, Bland CJH, et al.: Effect of prostaglandins I_2 and E_1 on red cell deformability in patients with Raynaud's phenomenon and systemic sclerosis. *Br Med J* 283 (1981): 350.

225. Kury PG, Ramwell PW, and McConnell HM: The effect of prostaglandins E_1 and E_2 on the human erythrocyte as monitored by spin labels. *Biochem Biophys Res Commun* 56 (1974): 478–483.

226. Allen JE, and Valeri CR: Prostaglandins in hematology. *Arch Intern Med* 133 (1974): 86–96.

227. Clifford PC, Martin MFR, Sheddon EJ, et al.: Treatment of vasospastic disease with prostaglandin E_1. *Br Med J* 281 (1980): 1031–1034.

228. Kovacs IB, and O'Grady J: Prostacyclin increases filterability of normal and rigidified human red blood cells in vitro. *Agents Actions* 14 (1984): 306–310.

229. Galanti G, Paoli G, Albanese B, et al.: Effetto della prostaciclina sulla deformabilita. *La Ricerca Clin Lab* 13-suppl. (1983): 445–450.

230. Johnston CC, Dowers SL, and Urbanski RJ: Examination of the filterability of oxygenated erythrocytes (containing normal, trait or sickle cell disease type hemoglobins) in the presence of L-epinephrine, D,L-isoproterenol or prostaglandins (PG) A_1, A_2, E_1, E_2, $F_{1\alpha}$, or $F_{2\alpha}$. *Prostaglandins* 13 (1977): 281–309.

231. Johnson M, Rabinowitz I, Willis AL, et al.: Detection of prostaglandin induction of erythrocyte sickling. *Clin Chem* 19 (1973): 23–26.

232. Shine I, and Lal S: Prostaglandin E_2 and sickling. *N Engl J Med* 289 (1973): 1040.

233. Belch JJF, Lowe GDO, Drummond MM, et al.: Prostacyclin reduces red cell deformability. *Thromb Haemostasis* (Stuttgart) 45 (1981): 189.

234. Kovacs IB, and O'Grady J: Impaired red blood cell deformability after oral administration of aspirin in man. *Biomed Biochim Acta* 43 (1984): S395–S398.

235. Willis AL, Johnson M, Rabinowitz I, et al.: Prostaglandin $F_{2\alpha}$ may induce sickle-cell crisis. *N Engl J Med* 286 (1972): 783.

236. Jay AWL, Rowlands S, and Skibo L: Red blood cell deformability and the prostaglandins. *Prostaglandins* 3 (1973): 871–877.

237. Diez, J., Braquet, P., Nazaret, C., et al.: The effect of cyclic nucleotides and eicosanoids on $Na+$ and $K+$ transport systems in human red cells and mouse macrophages. In P Greengard, et al., eds.: *Advances in cyclic nucleotide and protein phosphorylation research,* Vol. 17, pp. 621–630. New York: Raven Press, 1984.

238. Brugnara C, Bunn HF, and Tosteson DC: Ion content and transport and the regulation of volume in sickle cells. *Ann NY Acad Sci* 565 (1989): 96–103.

239. Palek J: Red cell membrane injury in sickle cell anaemia. *Br J Haematol* 35 (1977): 1–9.

240. Rubin E, Schlegel RA, and Williamson P: Endocytosis in sickle erythrocytes: A mechanism for elevated intracellular Ca^{2+} levels. *J Cell Physiol* 126 (1986): 53–59.

241. Dreher KL, Eaton JW, Breslawec KP, et al.: Calcium-induced erythrocyte rigidity. *Am J Pathol* 101 (1980): 543–556.

242. Gruber CA, and Gilbertson TJ: The effect of prostaglandin E_2-induced echinocytic transformation on the potassium loss, viscosity and osmotic fragility of normal and sickle cell erythrocytes. *Prostaglandins* 15 (1978): 429–436.

243. Rabinowitz IN, Wolf PL, Berman S, et al.: Prostaglandin E_2 effects on cation flux in sickle erythrocyte ghosts. *Prostaglandins* 9 (1975): 545–555.

244. Dunn MJ, and Howe D: Prostaglandins lack a direct inhibitory action on electrolyte and water transport in the kidney and the erythrocyte. *Prostaglandins* 13 (1977): 417–429.

245. Bergel'son LD, Bezuglov VV, Manevich EM, et al.: Interaction of prostaglandins with phospholipid vesicles, serum lipoproteins and erythrocytes. *Biomed Biochim Acta* 43 (1984): 121–124.

246. Garay R, Nazaret C, Diez J, et al.: The effect of cyclic nucleotides and icosanoids on Na+ and K+ transport in human red cells. *Biomed Biochim Acta* 42 (1983): S53–S57.

247. Kury PG, and McConnell HM: Regulation of membrane flexibility in human erythrocytes. *Biochemistry* 14 (1975): 2798–2803.

248. Manevich EM, Lakin KM, Archakov AI, et al.: Influence of cholesterol and prostaglandin E_1 on the molecular organization of phospholipids in the erythrocyte membrane. A fluorescent polarization study with lipid-specific probes. *Biochim Biophys Acta* 815 (1985): 455–460.

249. Brezinski ME, Lefer DJ, Bowker B, et al.: Thromboxane-induced red blood cell lysis. *Prostaglandins* 33 (1987): 75–84.

250. Joseph R, Welch KMA, D'Andrea G, et al.: Platelet-activating factor and red blood cells. *Thromb Res* 53 (1989): 629–633.

251. Hoover R, Rubin R, Wise G, et al.: Adhesion of normal and sickle erythrocytes to endothelial monolayer cultures. *Blood* 54 (1979): 872–876.

252. Hebbel RP, Yamada O, Moldow CF, et al.: Abnormal adherence of sickle erythrocytes to cultured vascular endothelium. *J Clin Invest* 65 (1980): 154–160.

253. Hebbel RP, Boogaerts MAB, Koresawa H, et al.: Erythrocyte adherence to endothelium as a determinant of vasoocclusive severity in sickle cell disease. *Trans Assoc Amer Phys* 93 (1980): 94–99.

254. Hebbel RP, Boogaerts MAB, Eaton JW, et al.: Erythrocyte adherence to endothelium in sickle-cell anemia. *N Engl J Med* 302 (1980): 992–995.

255. Hebbel RP, Eaton JW, Steinberg MH, and White JG: Erythrocyte/endothelial interactions and the vasoocclusive severity of sickle cell disease. *Prog Clin Biol Res* 55 (1981): 145–157.

256. Mohandas N, and Evans E: Adherence of sickle erythrocytes to vascular endothelial cells: Requirement for both cell membrane changes and plasma factors. *Blood* 64 (1984): 282–287.

257. Smith BD, and La Celle PL: Erythrocyte-endothelial cell adherence in sickle cell disorders. *Blood* 68 (1986): 1050–1054.

258. Hebbel RP, Schwartz RS, and Mohandas N: The adhesive sickle erythrocyte: Cause and consequence of abnormal interactions with endothelium, monocytes/macrophages and model membranes. *Clin Haematol* 14 (1985): 141–161.

259. Longenecker GL, Beyers BJ, and McMullan E: Red cell–endothelial cell adhesion: role and modulation in sickle cell disease. In G Rubanyi, and P Vanhoutte, eds.: *Endothelium-Derived Relaxing Factors,* pp. 281–290. Basel: Karger, 1990.

260. Kaul D, Sussman II, Tsai HM, et al.: *Anti–von Willebrand factor antibodies inhibit and desmopressin enhances adhesion of SS cells to the endothelium in flow conditions.* Paper presented at the 14th annual Sickle Cell Centers' Conference, 1989: #38.

261. McIntire LV, Wick TM, Moake JL, et al.: Role of ULVWF in sickle/endothelial cell adhesion under venous flow conditions. Paper presented at the 14th Annual Sickle Cell Centers' Conference, 1989: abstract #94.

262. Ferri A, Guerra S, Gemmati D, et al.: Evidence for a factor promoting the conversion of vWF from low and intermediate to high molecular mass polymers in the platelet membrane. *FEBS Lett* 249 (1989): 363–366.

263. Longenecker GL, and Beyers BJ: Platelet-activating factor (PAF) increases sickle red cell–endothelium adhesion. *The Pharmacologist* 32 (1990): 170.

264. Fisher JW, and Hagiwara M: Effects of prostaglandins on erythropoiesis. *Blood Cells* 10 (1984): 241–260.

265. Rabinowitz I, Wolf PL, Shikuma N, et al.: Prostaglandin E_2 effects on oxygen affinity by sickle erythrocytes. *Prostaglandins* 7 (1974): 309–317.

266. Dutta-Roy AK, and Sinha AK: Binding of prostaglandin E_1 to human erythrocyte membrane. *Biochim Biophys Acta* 812 (1985): 671–678.

267. Willems C, Stel HV, Van Aken WG, et al.: Binding and inactivation of prostacyclin (PGI_2) by human erythrocytes. *Br J Haematol* 54 (1983): 43–52.

268. Longenecker L, and Longenecker GL: Iloprost binding to human red blood cell ghosts. *Blood* 74-suppl. 1 (1989): 300a.

269. Piau JP, Delaunay J, Fischer S, et al.: Human red cell membrane adenylate cyclase in normal subjects and patients with hereditary spherocytosis, sickle cell disease and unidentified hemolytic anemias. *Blood* 56 (1980): 963–968.

270. Rasmussen H, Lake W, and Allen JE: The effect of catecholamines and prostaglandins upon human and rat erythrocytes. *Biochim Biophys Acta* 411 (1975): 63–73.

271. Beutler E, Guinto E, and Johnson C: Human red cell protein kinase in normal subjects and patients with hereditary spherocytosis, sickle cell disease, and autoimmune hemolytic anemia. *Blood Cells* 3 (1977): 135–152.

272. Shohet SB, and Greenquist AC: Possible roles for membrane protein phosphorylation in the control of erythrocyte shape. *Blood Cells* 3 (1977): 115–133.

273. Kyle V, and Hazleman B: Prostaglandin E_1 and peripheral vascular disease. *Lancet* no. 1 (1983): 282.

274. Heasley LE, Azari J, and Brunton LL: A glutathione adduct of prostaglandin A_1 acts intracellularly to elevate cyclic AMP by inhibiting its extrusion. *J Cyclic Nucleotide Prot Phosphoryl Res* 10 (1985): 3–8.

275. Longenecker GL, and Beyers BJ: Calcium channel blockers (CCB) modify sickle red blood cell (S-RBC) adhesion to endothelium. *J Clin Pharmacol* 31 (1991): 852.

276. Ward RHT, Fairweather DVI, and Modell B: Inactivation of prostacyclin (PGI_2) by erythrocytes. *Br J Haematol* 54 (1983): 658–660.

277. Pifer DD, Cagen LM, and Chesney CM: Stability of prostaglandin I_2 in human blood. *Prostaglandins* 21 (1981): 165–175.
278. Longenecker LL, McNeil A, and Longenecker, GL: Plasma protein binding and biologic half life of prostacyclin sickle cell disease. *Thromb Res* 64 (1991): 751–756.

5

Anatomical Lesions in Sickle Cell Hemoglobinopathies

Lemuel W. Diggs

The morphological characteristics of the lesions that occur in individuals with the various types of sickle cell diseases and conditions vary depending on the age of the patient and the age of the lesions. Since the number of autopsies that have been performed and studied by this author and reported and illustrated in the literature are limited for each age group, the incidence of specific pathological abnormalities will be stated in general rather than in statistical terms. The atrophic, vascular occlusive and fibrotic lesions that occur in all types of sickle cell disease are similar in many respects. Sickle cell anemia will be used as a prototype. Unless otherwise stated, the anatomical aberrations are those that have been observed in patients with homozygous sickle cell anemia (Hb SS). The peculiarities of tissue changes that occur in patients with heterozygous S-hemoglobinopathies will be presented separately. General references include monographs and selected medical publications (1–10). From these a more complete bibliography can be obtained.

PATHOPHYSIOLOGY

When erythrocytes that contain molecules of sickle cell hemoglobin are exposed to hypoxic environments, the hemoglobin molecules are converted to linear polymers which combine to form parallel bundles that distort the elastic membranes of the red cells, producing elongated and multipointed cells (Chapter 2). Recently formed sickle cells rapidly revert to discoid cells when reoxygenated. Red cells that have been sickled for long periods become irreversibly sickled (Chapter 3). These cells are elongated, narrow and double-pointed, and, as a rule, curved (Figure 5.1).

Sickled erythrocytes of all types are less elastic (less deformable, less pliable,

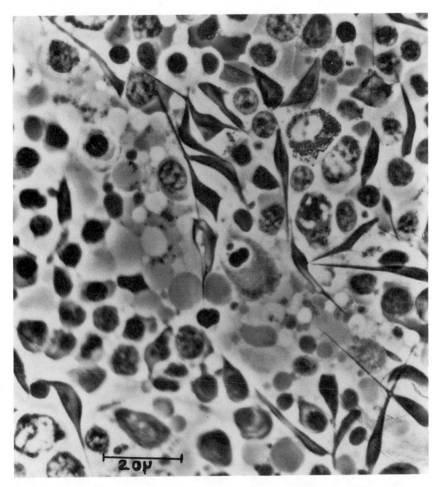

Figure 5.1. Sickled cells in moist, unstained preparation of air-exposed bone marrow aspirate

and more rigid) than are nonsickled cells. Red cells that are sickled enter capillaries with difficulty at the bifurcation points. Sickled cells that do gain entry may be entrapped and hemolyzed or else move slowly and in single file. Plasma often separates individual cells. Due to hypoxic injury to the endothelial cells, plasma escapes into the tissue spaces. The perivascular edema compresses the capillaries and is an additional factor in impeding the flow of blood. Retardation or stoppage of blood flow in a given network of capillaries is followed by distension of pre-capillary arterioles which become engorged by "log-jams" of sickled erythrocytes. Blood that cannot get into small capillaries is forced under arterial pressure into larger arterial capillaries in marginal areas in order to detour around the infarcts. The arteriovenous shunts and the post-capillary venules adjacent to necrotic areas are filled by entangled mats of sickled cells. Injury to blood cells as well as parenchymal cells within infarcted areas causes the release of the clot-activating tissue thromboplastin and is followed by intravascular coagulation. The clots that form in the blood that no longer flows extend in a retrograde manner to the nearest patent arteriole or artery and in a forward manner into arteriovenous shunts, venules, and veins.

The membranes of red cells are altered as they sickle and unsickle in the circulating blood. Sickled cells are readily phagocytosed. As the result of increased erythrocyte destruction, hemolysis, and phagocytosis there is jaundice of the hemolytic type which is characterized by a yellowish discoloration of the conjunctiva, hyperbilirubinemia, and an increase in urobilinogen in the feces and urine.

Hemosiderin, which is derived from the pigmented heme portion of hemoglobin molecules, is demonstrable in the form of brown granules in the Kupffer cells of the liver and in other phagocytic cells. Hemosiderin also is demonstrable in large quantities in the hepatic cord cells and juxta-glomerular epithelial cells of kidney tubules and in small quantities in the glomerular tissues and the urinary sediment. When stained by the prussian blue method, the hemosiderin particles are dark blue.

The survival time of erythrocytes in sickle cell disease is decreased. An imbalance between the rate of blood destruction and the formation and delivery of red cells from the bone marrow into the blood stream results in chronic anemia, in response to which there occurs marrow hyperplasia. The proliferation of hemopoietic cells includes leukocytes and megakaryocytes as well as erythrocytic cells.

The hyperplasia of the marrow in occasional patients may be manifested by nodular masses of extra-medullary hematopoiesis, which most frequently are located near the spine in the thoracic or lumbar region (11, 12).

THE BODY AS A WHOLE

The abnormality that is consistently demonstrable by light microscopy in sections of tissues fixed in formalin or gluteraldehyde solutions is the presence of erythrocytes that are narrow and long with tapering round or pointed ends. In addition, there are red cells with multiple points and fin-like marginal protrusions (Figure 5.2). Erythrocytes in thin sections of fixed tissues examined by electron microscopy are identified by the presence of linear Hb S polymers in their cytoplasm as well as by their characteristic shapes (Figure 5.3).

Due to chronic anemia and the unremitting impairment in the flow of blood in terminal vascular channels, there are progressive atrophic changes. All organs are involved. The withering or wasting away process is similar to that which takes place in normal individuals as they age. In patients with sickle cell diseases the atrophy occurs at a faster rate than normal. In addition to generalized atrophy,

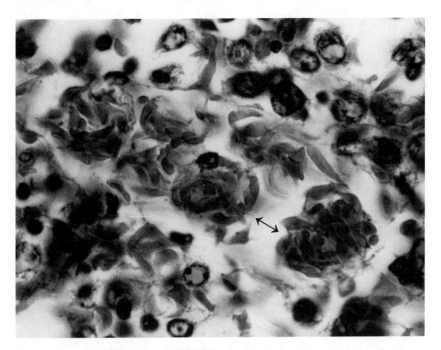

Figure 5.2.   Maternal blood (Hb AS) in a formalin-fixed placenta. Aggregates of
sickled red cells (double-pointed arrow).

there are also focal areas of infarction and the replacement of parenchymal cells
by fibrous tissue.

Ischemic infarcts are most likely to develop in stationary organs that have
numerous oxygen-demanding cells, such as the bone marrow, brain, and kidney.
Focal areas of necrosis seldom develop in the heart and skeletal striated muscles
or in gastrointestinal organs in spite of their high oxygen uptake because these
organs have numerous vascular channels that are freely communicating and
because contraction and relaxation have a milking action that favors the rapid
ingress of oxygenated arterial blood, a rapid egress of deoxygenated blood, and
the clearance of metabolic waste products. Splenic infarcts are due to the entrapment of sickled erythrocytes in the reticular spaces of red pulp areas. Vascular
occlusive lesions that occur in the lungs are due to emboli in the pulmonary
arterial system.

The parts of organs, with the exception of the lungs, that are most likely to
develop focal areas of ischemia and necrosis are the capillary areas, where the
circulation is terminal and hypoxemia maximal. The anatomical sites where
occlusion of small and terminal blood vessels by sickled erythrocytes is most
likely to occur are:

Tubular bones of the hands and feet in young children
Capital epiphysis of the femur, humerous and fibula

Cerebral cortex
Periphery of the retina
Red pulp of the spleen
Renal cortex
Renal papilla
Tip of the papillary heart muscle
Skin of the lower leg

Ischemic infarcts may occur in lymph nodes, ovaries, testes, and endocrine organs but infarcts in these organs are infrequent, in spite of the latter's high cellularity, because they are small and have numerous anastomatic vascular channels. Vascular occlusive lesions are least likely to occur in fatty and fibrous tissues because fat cells and fibrocytes require minimal amounts of oxygen to meet their metabolic needs. Ischemic and necrotic lesions are infrequent in the walls of blood vessels, the gall bladder, and the urinary bladder, or in heart valves, articular ligaments, tendons, and calcific bones because these tissues have low oxygen requirements. Peripheral nerves and synovial membranes have

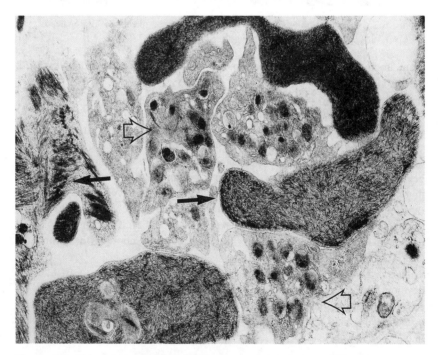

Figure 5.3.   Electronic microscopic view of a section of a glomerulus. Sickled erythrocytes (arrows), showing hemoglobin S polymer.

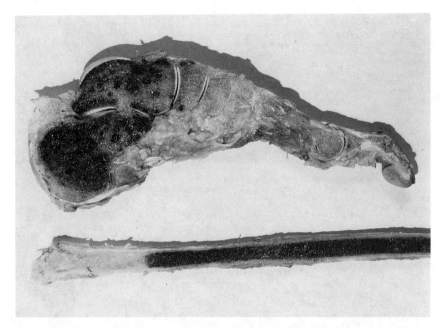

Figure 5.4. Section of a foot and a fibula, showing cellular marrow in cuboidal bones and in shaft of fibula, fibrosis of upper end of fibula.

relatively few parenchymal cells and numerous blood vessels which are freely communicating. In those organs, focal ischemia and necrosis seldom occur.

It is not possible for infarcts to develop in avascular cartilaginous areas, intervertebral discs, corneae, teeth, or nails. Anatomical abnormalities that are demonstrable in these structures are due to vascular occlusive lesions in closely adjacent tissues.

BONES AND JOINTS

During the first few years of life the bone marrow is hematopoietic in all bones of normal individuals as well as those with all types of S-hemoglobinopathies. The red and cellular marrow of all individuals gradually and progressively recedes from the cold and tubular bones of the hands and feet, but in patients with sickle cell diseases, the marrow continues to be hyperplastic during the preschool years.

The red and cellular marrow of normal individuals also gradually recedes from the tubular and cuboidal bones of the wrists, hands, ankles, and feet and from the shafts of the long bones of the arms and legs. This is in contrast to patients with sickle cell anemia in which the marrow spaces retain blood cell progenitors and relatively little fat (Figure 5.4).

The marrow in the warm and cancellous bones of the axial skeleton (head and trunk) throughout life is red and the intertrabecular spaces are filled mainly with

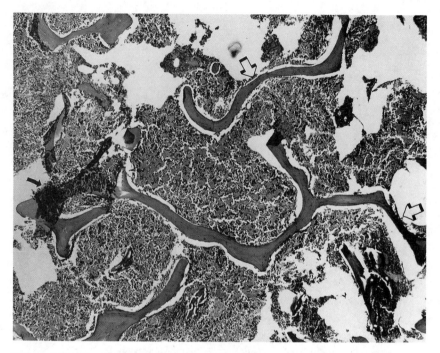

Figure 5.5.   Vertebral body, showing cellular marrow, stasis of blood in sinusoids. Trabeculae (open arrows) are atrophic.

hemopoietic cells (Figure 5.5). Marrow hyperplasia in infants with Hb SS is associated with a slight widening of the medullary spaces and a thinning of trabeculae and cortices. There is a significant increase in the width of the skull and maxillary bones in a few patients (see the sections on the skull and the facial bones). The oxygen requirement of cellular marrow is high and the flow of blood in wide sinusoids and tissue spaces is slow. The stage, therefore, is set for the sickling of erythrocytes, hemostasis, necrosis, and the development of painful and febrile vascular occlusive bone crises. When small focal marrow infarcts heal, the necrotic tissue is usually replaced by an ingrowth of new blood cells.

Small necrotic areas in marrow spaces may be surrounded by shells of calcific fibrous tissue. Sections of these geode-like lesions are revealed as nonpigmented narrow rims around amorphous material. Radiologists designate these opaque rings as ''doughnut'' lesions.

Much of our knowledge of anatomical lesions in the bones and joints as well as in other organs has been obtained not by gross and microscopic examinations but by imaging procedures. For information and additional references related to technical devices, the excellent and scholarly monographs by Reynolds (2), Bohrer (13), and the articles by various authors in *Seminars in Roentgenology, Sickle Cell Anemia,* edited by Felson and Wiot (76), are recommended.

Bones of the Hands and Feet

The tubular bones of the hands and feet of young children contain a predominance of oxygen-demanding blood cells and only a few fat cells. The presence of fetal hemoglobin (Hb F) in high concentrations and relatively low concentrations of Hb S in erythrocytes at the time of birth and the first few months afterwards aids in preventing the formation of sickled cells. After the first four months and during the next four to six years, sickling of erythrocytes in the bones that are most distant from the lungs and least well oxygenated may be of a degree sufficient to cause ischemia and marrow necrosis. Hypoxemia is favored by vasoconstriction due to chilling and the shunting of arterial blood into veins, thus depriving the tubular bones of adequate oxygen.

An infarct in a given tubular bone usually involves the entire shaft. Following the death of marrow tissue and cortical bone there is periosteal separation (Figure 5.6) and soft tissue swelling. Multiple bones may be affected simultaneously, and recurrent episodes during the preschool years are common. Infarcts usually heal without deformity, but in occasional patients there may be thickening and shortening of one or more of the tubular bones.

Necrotizing lesions involving the hands and feet due to the sickling of erythrocytes do not occur in older children, adolescents, or adults because the bone marrow spaces are filled with fat and connective tissue cells which can survive in relatively anoxic environments.

Long Bones

The shafts, as well as the ends, of the long bones of the arms and legs contain bone marrow that is red and hypercellular, and infarcts may occur in any and in all areas. Ischemic necrosis is usually limited to medullary spaces, without the death of cortical bone. When the cortex as well as the medulla are deprived of an adequate supply of oxygenated blood, there is death of osteocytes in cortical canals. Osteonecrosis is followed by soft tissue swelling (edema) and periosteal separation.

Following the separation of the periosteum from a given cortical shell, new bone is formed by periosteal osteoblasts, thus causing the cortex to be thickened. The degree of thickening in different areas is highly variable. Fibrous tissue and/ or cellular marrow may form between the layers of new periosteal bone and the old cortex. Noncalcified structures appear in longitudinal sections of long bones as dark and narrow fissures of varying lengths and in radiographs as radiolucent lines between two opaque linear and marginal structures (''tram-lines'').

The cellular marrow in the diaphyses of long bones of the extremities is supplied with blood by nutrient arteries as well as by capillaries that enter the intertrabecular spaces through the periosteum. In between these two afferent arterial systems, hypoxemia, sickling of erythrocytes, hemostasis, fibrosis, and the replacement of marrow cells by endosteal new bone are maximal. As a result,

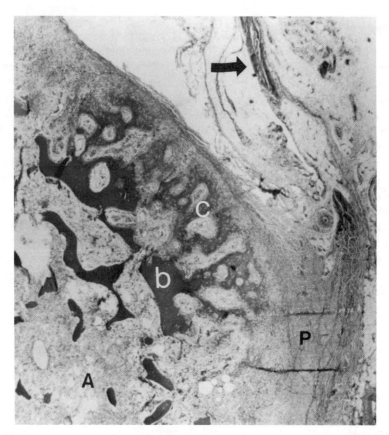

Figure 5.6.   Midshaft of proximal phalanx of an infant. Marrow necrosis (A); partial
necrosis of cortical bone (B); dead cortical bone (C); periosteum (P);
periosteal separation (arrow).

Courtesy Dr. A. G. Weinberg.

"bones within bones" may develop in the marrow spaces at the arterial junction
sites. The cylinders of new bone are inside of and parallel to the cortex. On
cross-section, these cylindrical, boney structures appear as ill-formed light gray
rings. In longitudinal sections the cylinders are revealed as pale gray and narrow
linear structures of varying lengths (Figure 5.7). In X-ray plates the new calcific
bone areas appear as opaque lines parallel to and inside the cortex.

Extremely large infarcts in the marrow spaces of long bones remain as avascular, amorphous, and necrotic areas that have a yellow-gray color and a soft,
gelatinous consistency. The lower ends of femurs and upper ends of tibias, which
are supplied with blood by the metaphyseal and epiphyseal, as well as by the
diaphyseal, arteries, tend to be widened, producing the so-called "Erlenmeyer

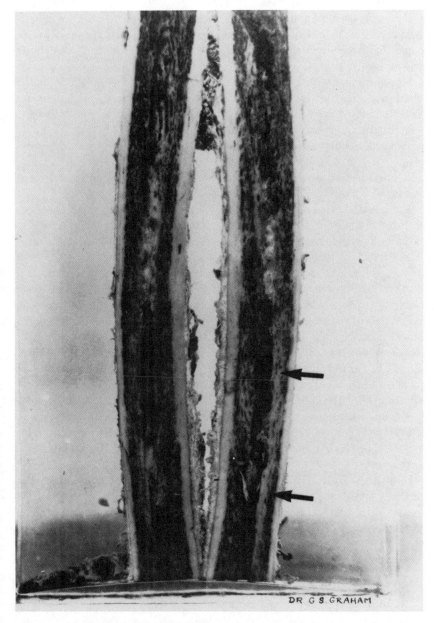

Figure 5.7. Longitudinal section of femur, showing cellular marrow, bone-within-bone formation (arrows).

Source: G. S. Graham, A case of sickle cell anemia with necropsy, *Arch Intern Med* 34 (1924), p. 785, Fig. 3. Copyright 1924, American Medical Association. Used by permission.

flask'' abnormality. As patients age, the blood supply to the capital epiphysis of the femur becomes progressively less adequate. Chronic circulatory impairment results in death of bone adjacent to the synovial cartilage (Figure 5.8). As a rule, the ischemic infarcts are focal, but in some cases the entire epiphysis may be involved.

Movement and weight bearing are followed by the disruption and fragmentation of cartilage. The joint fluid contains cellular debris. Older lesions are characterized by injury to the acetabulum, and in some cases there is ankylosis. Associated with degenerative and destructive lesions in the hip joint are proliferative peri-articular arthritic lesions. There is roentgenologic evidence that degenerative changes in the head of the femur begin during childhood. Early lesions, as a rule, are not associated with pain or disability, while older and more destructive lesions may result in severe disability.

The capital epiphysis of the humerus of older patients is subject to vascular occlusive changes similar to those that occur in the head of the femur. The degree of disability related to the shoulder and knee are less marked than in the hip.

Infarcts of the long bones adjacent to the synovial cartilage of the knee and elbow cause pain in these joint areas. The onset is usually sudden, and the pain is exaggerated by movement. The joint areas are characterized by soft tissue swelling, redness, warmth, pressure tenderness and exaggeration of pain on movement. In some cases there is a significant increase in synovial fluid and a widening of the joint spaces. Fluids aspirated from the knees and elbows of patients with sickle cell anthropathies are aseptic. These fluids usually have a yellowish color and are slightly cloudy. The viscosity is normal, and the leukocyte count is variable. As a rule, there is a moderate leukocytosis with a predominance of neutrophils. The concentration of sugar is normal, and crystals are not demonstrable. Biopsies of synovial membranes taken at the time of knee or joint effusions reveal an engorgement of the numerous blood vessels by sickled erythrocytes. There is no evidence of ischemic necrosis or cellular inflammatory reaction (14).

Disabilities due to Hb S arthropathies involving the knee and elbow areas generally disappear spontaneously within a few days or several weeks after the onset of pain, but there is considerable variation in the clinical course depending on the degree of degenerative changes and superimposed conditions.

Vertebrae

The medullary spaces of spinal bones, like all other cancellous and warm bones of the head and trunk, are filled with marrow that is red and cellular. The cortical shells are thin, and the trabeculae are narrow and widely spaced. As the result of weight bearing, the osteoporotic vertebral bodies are flattened (15).

In the central portions of the vertebral bodies where the circulation is terminal and hypoxemia and hemostasis due to sickled erythrocytes are maximal, the growth of bones is less than in the lateral areas, where the blood flow is more

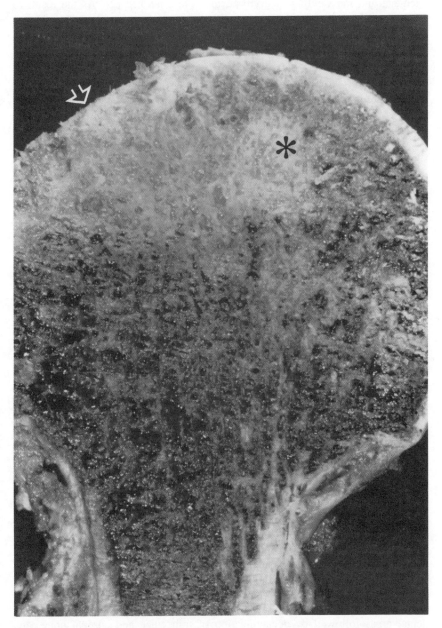

Figure 5.8. Avasulcar necrosis of the head of a femur, showing replacement of cellular marrow by fibrous tissue (asterisk), focal loss of articular cartilage (open arrow).

adequate and the sickling of erythrocytes is less marked (2). As the result of faulty central growth, the vertebral bodies are depressed by vertebral discs (Figure 5.9). These central depressions often are irregularly shaped cones with flattened (truncated) tops. When viewed in sections or in X-ray plates, some of the indentations have trapezoid rather than crescentric shapes. Consequently, the terms "fish vertebrae" or "fish mouth vertebrae" are inappropriate.

Focal areas of necrosis in the vertebral bodies can cause severe and disabling back pain. Infarcts are most likely to occur in the lumbar vertebrae. In rare instances, there is a collapse of a vertebral body. When the infarcts heal, there is replacement of hemopoietic marrow by fibrous tissue (Figure 5.10).

Skull

The bone marrow of the skull is hyperplastic, and roentgenographic examination reveals varying degrees of granularity and osteoporosis. In approximately 5 percent of patients there is a significant increase in the width of diploe, a thinning of the outer cortex, and striking "hair-on-end" or "porcupine quill" trabecular striations (Figure 5.11). The skull thickening involves mainly the frontal and parietal bones. Diploic widening and abnormal trabecular patterns that occur in infancy persist throughout life (16).

The skull abnormalities are not specific for sickle cell diseases. Similar lesions also occur in patients with thalassemia major, hereditary spherocytosis, and severe iron deficiency. As patients age, the marrow of the skull becomes progressively more sclerotic. Residual islands of cellular marrow surrounded by calcific bone are revealed on roentgenological examination as round focal areas of lucency which simulate the osteolytic lesions that occur in patients with multiple myeloma and metastatic malignancy.

Facial Bones

Due to marrow hyperplasia there is, in a few patients, a significant increase in the size of maxillary bones and overriding of the upper jaw. This type of gnathopathy may result in protrusion of the incisor teeth beyond the closed lips (7). Hyperplasia of the marrow in mandibular bones is revealed in roentgenographs by increased translucency and a lacy trabecular pattern. The trabeculae between the teeth have a horizontal or step-ladder pattern. Mandibular infarcts in the region of the mental foramen may cause periosteal edema and pressure on the nerve at this site. Sensory nerve stimulation is clinically manifested by a burning sensation and numbness of the lower lip (17). Aseptic necrosis in dental areas followed by decalcification of trabeculae and cortical bone, and associated with pain, fever, and lower jaw swelling, may be mistaken for osteomyelitis and the needless removal of healthy teeth. Infarcts that occur in the bone of the forehead and upper face are manifested by soft tissue swelling. The periosteal edema may be sufficient to cause the closure of the eye. As a rule,

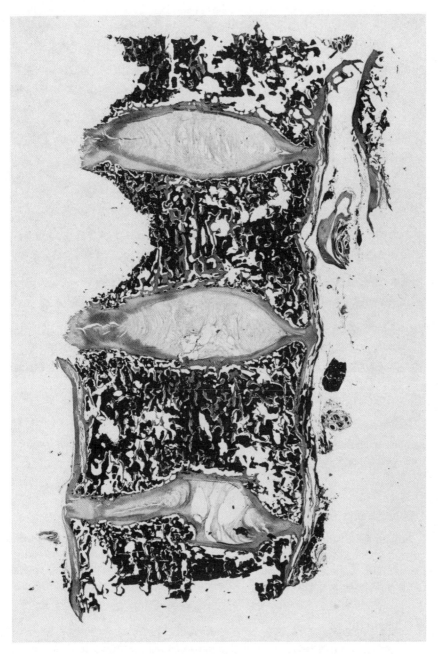

Figure 5.9. Section of bodies of lumbar vertebrae, with central depressions by cartilaginous disc.

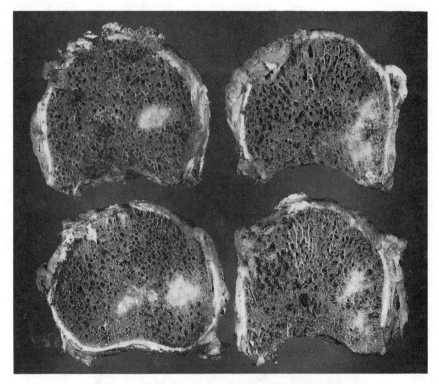

Figure 5.10.   Sections of vertebral bodies, showing focal areas of fibrosis following infarcts.

pain associated with infarcts of the upper face is minimal, and the facial swelling usually disappears in a few days without deformity.

Other Bones

In addition to the bones described above, focal infarcts may develop in the cuboidal bones of the wrists and ankles, the ribs, and the pelvic bones, and in the sternum, scapula, and patella. The tarsal bone that is most frequently involved is the heel bone (calcaneous).

Osteomyelitis

Osteomyelitis is a frequent complication in patients with sickle cell disease. Bone infections may be caused by various types of organisms but are usually due to Salmonella and other enteric bacteria which are thought to gain entrance into the bloodstream from the intestines and to lodge in areas of bone marrow ischemia and necrosis.

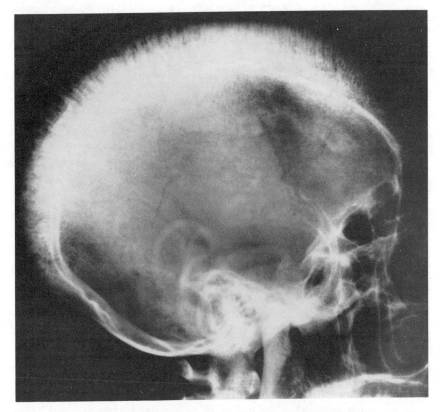

Figure 5.11. X-ray of skull, showing diploic thickening and hair-on-end
trabeculations.

Gout

Due to the increased destruction of red cells there is an increase in serum
urate in many patients with Hb S diseases. There is, in association with the
progressive reduction in nephron units, a decreased secretion of urates. Older
patients develop manifestations of gout more frequently than do non-Hb S individuals of comparable ages. The pain, redness, warmth, swelling, and extreme
tenderness due to superimposed gout are likely to involve multiple joint areas
simultaneously, and especially the joints of the hands and feet. Synovial fluids
may reveal urate crystals in phagocytic cells.

SPLEEN

The spleens of infants during the later months of the first year of life are
enlarged due to the engorgement of red pulp areas by sickled erythrocytes. The

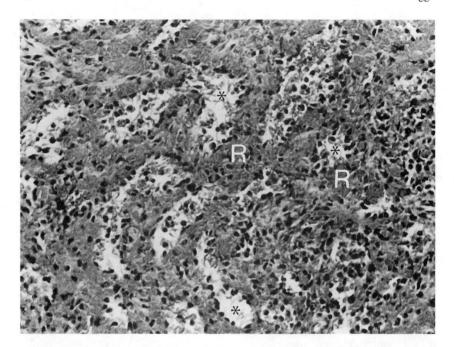

Figure 5.12. Splenic arterio-venous shunts (astericks). Red pulp areas are engorged
by sickled erythrocytes (R).

enlargement continues during the early childhood years. The size of the spleen
is slightly and temporarily increased at the time of painful and febrile crises.
With advancing years the spleen undergoes progressive fibrosis and atrophy.

Enlarged spleens are firm and rubbery. The surface is smooth and the color
is a dark purplish red. Microscopic examination reveals an engorgement of the
reticular spaces of red pulp areas. The stasis of blood is maximal within and at
the margins of the lymph nodules where the blood in terminal arterioles under
arterial pressure meets with resistance due to the blockade of the splenic cords
by sickled erythrocytes. The arterioles in the white pulp areas are distended, and
the trabeculae and splenic corpuscles are widely spaced.

In most congested spleens the venules are compressed and invisible, but in
some microscopic fields there are endothelial-lined spaces that are empty or
contain only a few sickled erythrocytes. These thin-walled and dilated blood
vessels, from which the red cells have escaped, are arterio-venous shunts (Figure
5.12). The bypassing of red pulp areas by means of direct vascular connections
between the arterioles of the lymph nodules and the splenic veins is confirmed
by the failure of injected radioactive material to be visualized. Another evidence
of the *functional asplenia* of enlarged spleens is the presence of nuclear fragments
(Howell-Jolly bodies) in erythrocytes (18). A normally functioning spleen removes nuclear remnants from red cells as they pass through narrow reticular
spaces and fenestrations in the walls of splenic venules.

When children less than five years of age are exposed to etiological factors that favor the systemic sickling of erythrocytes, there is a rapid increase in the size of the spleen due to the entrapment of sickled cells in red pulp areas. The elasticity of trabeculae and the capsule of early spleens make marked expansion possible. The pooling of erythrocytes is not limited to the spleen but also occurs in the sinusoids of the liver and bone marrow. The sequestration of red cells in these organs causes a precipitous decrease in erythrocyte values (sequestration crisis), hypovolemia, and circulatory failure (19). In response to the decrease in the oxygen-carrying capacity of the blood, there is a regenerative marrow response characterized by an increase in reticulocytes and nucleated red cells in the peripheral blood. The sequestration syndrome is life-threatening, and death may occur within a few hours after the onset of clinical manifestations.

At the time of autopsy, the dark color of a congested spleen is in sharp contrast to the extreme pallor of the stomach and intestines. The spleen resembles "a bag of blood." Patients with severe sequestration syndromes, in effect, bleed to death into the spleen and other organs. Sequestration splenic crises do not occur in older patients because their spleens are atrophic, fibrotic, and inelastic.

During the early stages of splenic fibrosis, the spleens are firm and the color, slate blue. The surface is wrinkled and there are depressed areas at the sites of healed infarcts that are near the capsule. When fibrotic spleens are sectioned, the knife meets with resistance and the cut sections are dry.

The organization of hemorrhages in the tissue spaces of white pulp areas (Malpighian bodies, lymph follicles) results in the formation of siderofibrotic nodules (Gamma-Gandy bodies; see Figure 5.13). These structures are grossly visible in cut sections as brown, pin-head sized areas which resemble "granules of rust" or "flecks of tobacco."

Microscopic examinations of well-developed and classical sidero-fibrotic nodules in the spleen at the sites of lymphoid nodules reveal colorful conglomerates of structures with highly variable characteristics (20, 21). These include fibrocytes, macrophages which contain phagocytosed brown hemosiderin particles, multinucleated giant cells, and green and yellow crystals of varying sizes and shapes. Some of the crystals have bamboo-like configurations. Other crystals are encased in ill-formed shells of iron and calcium that appear, in tissue sections, as black rings. Reticular fibers in the walls of arteries and in the trabeculae are encrusted by iron and calcium and, when stained by hematoxylin and eosin, appear as narrow, elongated, black lines. In some connective tissue areas the fibers are segmented and branching and superficially resemble fungi.

Sidero-fibrotic nodules are not demonstrable in children with sickle cell diseases during the first few years of life, but in older children and in adults these nodules, combined with the presence of sickled erythrocytes, are the hallmark of sickle cell diseases. The presence of sidero-fibrotic nodules in adults excludes the sickle cell trait. During the early stages of the organization of hemorrhages in the white pulp areas, the sidero-fibrotic structures are most marked in subcapsular areas where the circulation is terminal. These nodules are least likely

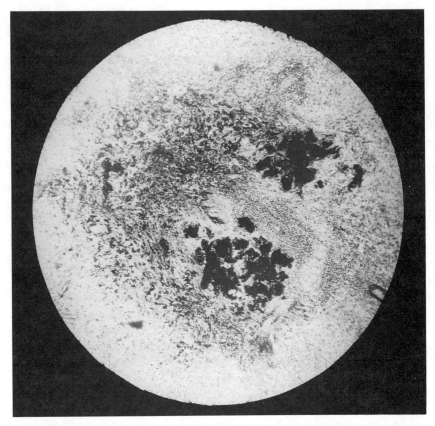

Figure 5.13.   Splenic sidero-fibrotic nodule prepared using Prussian blue iron stain.

to occur in the hilar regions where the blood vessels enter and the circulation is maximal (Figure 5.14).

During the late intermediate stages of atrophy, the weight of the spleen is in the 10–25 gram range. The general shape of the spleen is maintained. The color of small spleens is dull gray. There may be small, residual, spherical areas of red pulp. Well-defined sidero-fibrotic nodules are no longer demonstrable but heme pigments, iron, and calcium encrustations of connective tissue fibers are in a scrambled array (Figure 5.15). The sub-intimal and medial layers of the arteries may contain aggregates of calcium and iron (Monckeberg arteriosclerosis).

At the end stage, the spleen is reduced to a nubbin or mummy of its former self. All that is left is a small mass of fibrous tissue that contains no minimal depositions of mineral salts and/or pigments. The progressive and relentless change from kilograms to milligrams in the final stage may result in the complete disappearance of the spleen as a gross or microscopically identifiable organ.

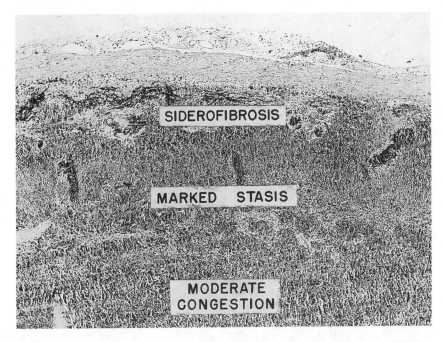

Figure 5.14. Section of an enlarged spleen of a patient with Hb SC disease. Sidero-fibrotic changes are most marked in sub-capsular area.

LIVER

The livers of children, adolescents, and young adults are enlarged and firm. The surfaces, as a rule, are smooth and glistening, and the color is various shades of reddish-brown. Surfaces of cut sections usually reveal normal and homogeneous structural patterns (22).

Microscopic examination of stained sections of blocks of liver that were fixed in formalin or gluteraldehyde solutions consistently reveal sickled erythrocytes that fill the hepatic sinusoids (Figure 5.16). The endothelial cells that line the sinusoids (Kupffer cells) in some cases are prominent and may contain phagocytosed sickled red cells. These phagocytic cells also contain amorphous debris and granules of hemosiderin. Hemosiderin is demonstrable in the liver cord cells.

The hepatic cells of patients who die as the result of diseases that are not associated with the manifestations of liver involvement disclose varied atrophic and degenerative changes. Descriptions include indistinct nuclear and cytoplasmic margins, vacuoles, abnormal granules, and alterations in mitochondria and in endoplasmic reticulum. Abnormal dense bodies are demonstrable in thin sections examined by electron microscopy. In some cases there is evidence of thickening and irregularities in connective tissues (23).

Many patients with sickle cell anemia (estimated at approximately 10% of

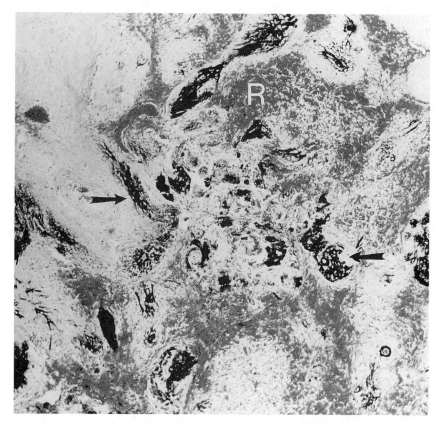

Figure 5.15. Intermediate stage of splenic sidero-fibrosis, showing residual red pulp
(R), calcium- and iron-encrusted reticular fibers (arrows).

those who seek ambulatory medical care) have, in addition to jaundice of the
hemolytic type, a mild degree of obstructive jaundice. The symptoms are vague
and include general malaise, loss of appetite, and indigestion. The edge of the
liver is usually palpable and there is right-upper-quadrant tenderness. The serum
bilirubin is increased in the 10 to 30 mg/100 ml range. Bile as well as an increase
in urobilirubin are demonstrable in the urine. The episodes of obstructive jaundice
of a mild type are usually self-limiting, and there is no information concerning
anatomical abnormalities at the time of transient episodes of mild jaundice. On
the basis of combined symptoms, signs, and laboratory tests it is evident that
there are minor degenerative hepatic lesions and cholestasis (intrahepatic obstructive jaundice).

Occasionally there are patients who die following an acute illness characterized
by deep jaundice with total serum bilirubin values greater than 30 mg per 100
ml and, in rare instances, greater than 80 mg. The symptoms and signs are
similar to those associated with viral hepatitis. One major difference is that there

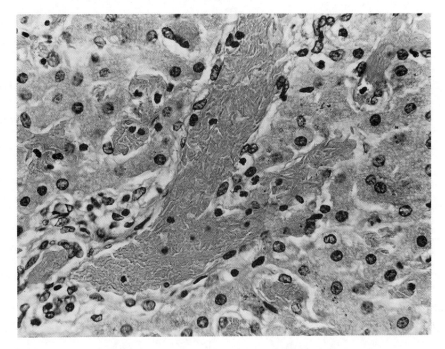

Figure 5.16.   Engorgement of hepatic sinusoids by sickled erythrocytes.

is a neutrophilic leukocytosis in patients with severe sickle cell hepatic crises, whereas in viral hepatitis there is leukopenia with a relative and, in some cases, absolute increase in lymphocytes and plasmocytes. At the time of autopsy there are focal and confluent areas of necrosis (Figure 5.17) which involve all parts of the liver. There is stasis of bile in canaliculi, and lymphocytic infiltration is minimal.

The degree of hepatic fibrosis that is demonstrable at the time of autopsy is highly variable. It is not possible, on the basis of the limited information that is now available, to state for each age group the percentage of livers that reveal nodular cirrhotic changes or to differentiate between fibrosis due to sickled cells and post-necrotic sclerotic and nodular changes due to viral infections, chemical toxicities, cardiac dysfunction, alcoholism, and other etiologic agents.

THE GALLBLADDER, THE BILE DUCTS, AND GALLSTONES

Due to the increased destruction of erythrocytes, there is an increase in plasma bilirubin and hemoglobin excretion of heme pigments by the liver. Bile that contains increased concentrations of pigments is dark, thick, and granular (inspissated) (24). Aggregates of precipitated bile pigments intermingled with other

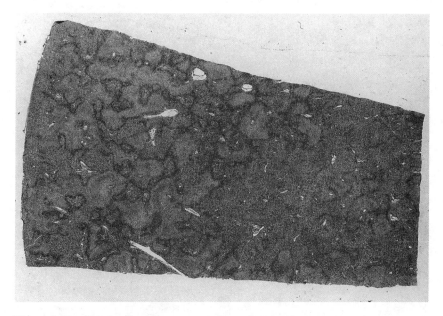

Figure 5.17. Focal and confluent areas of hepatic necrosis.

bile constituents favor the formation of multiple stones in the gall bladder (Figure 5.18).

The gallstones are usually small, soft, and spherical, but they may be faceted. The color of most stones is greenish-black. As a rule, they are calcified and are demonstrable when X-ray plates of the abdomen are examined. The incidence of cholelithiasis in children varies from 10 to 20 percent. With advancing years, the percent of patients with gallstones progressively increases. The incidence in patients 30 years of age or older has been estimated by various investigators to be in the 50 to 70 percent range.

The walls of the gallbladder, as a rule, do not reveal significant anatomical abnormalities. Pericholecystic adhesions, which are indicative of a chronic inflammatory reaction, are usually present in association with gallstones.

LUNGS

Infants and young children have an increased susceptibility to bacterial and viral infectious agents. Sepsis, including bacterial pneumonia, is the most frequent cause of death in children less than 5 years of age, although this is changing rapidly due to preventive measures. Adults with sickle cell disease of all types are subject to the embolic occlusions of pulmonary arteries (25).

There are three types of embolic masses. The most frequently occuring emboli

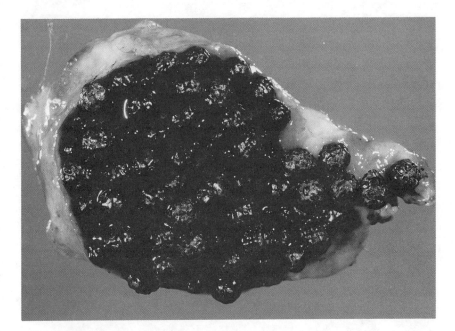

Figure 5.18.   Multiple pigmented gall stones.

are preformed in systemic venules and veins adjacent to infarcts. These emboli consist mainly of entangled mats of sickled erythrocytes mixed in a homogeneous manner with leukocytes, thrombocytes, and a few fibrin strands. Portions of these aggregates, after dislodgement, are transported like tumble weeds to the right heart chambers and from there to the pulmonary arteries. It is to be recalled that the pulmonary arteries contain venous blood, that the oxygen content of these vessels is less than in any other part of the circulatory system, and that the sickling of erythrocytes, increased blood viscosity, and hemostasis are maximal in pulmonary arterioles.

Fresh pulmonary emboli that are composed mainly of sickled cells, in fresh-cut sections of the lung, appear as dark, moderately firm, and unattached plugs in the lumens of pulmonary arteries. Emboli that contain only a few fibrin threads are fragile. When fixed lung tissues are thinly cut in order to prepare sections for microscopic examination, there are breaks or cracks that are caused by mechanical trauma induced by the microtome knife.

The second, and less frequently occurring, occlusions of the lumens of pulmonary arteries are thromboemboli which are fragments of white clots. These thromboemboli originate in the flowing blood of systemic veins. Thrombi are most likely to form in the leg veins of patients with stasis ulcers or in pelvic and uterine veins in association with pregnancy. The nonpigmented portions of thromboemboli are composed of platelets and leukocytes entrapped in fibrin

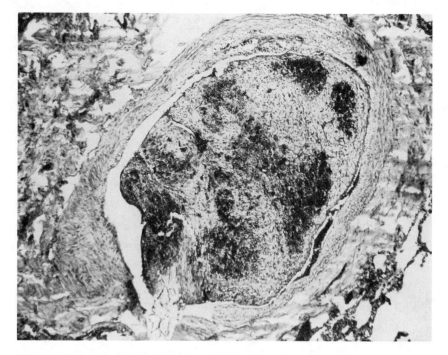

Figure 5.19.   Thromboembolic mass occluding the pulmonary artery.

webs. When sections of thromboemboli are microscopically examined, the fibrinous portions appear as colorless masses of varying shapes (Figure 5.19).
The shapes include linear structures (lines of Zahn).

The third and least frequently occurring pulmonary emboli consist of bits of
bone marrow that are dislodged from infarcted areas. Bone marrow emboli in
the lumens of pulmonary arterioles are identified by fragments of trabeculi (Figure
5.20), fat cells, megakaryocytes, and other morphologically identifiable marrow
structures. Some calcific spicules of bone contain Haversian canals (1) (see the
section on fat embolism).

When blood under arterial pressure is forcibly pushed through narrow fibrin
networks in pulmonary arteries, the membranes of elastic erythrocytes become
over-stretched, scuffed, and fragmented (26, 27). Manifestations of mechanical
trauma are revealed in peripheral blood smears by morphological erythrocyte
variants that include marginal achromia (blister cells), dome- and helmet-shaped
red cells, triangular cells, poikilospherocytes, and red cell fragments. These
morphological abnormalities are similar to those that occur in patients with other
types of microangiopathic hemolytic diseases. The presence, in peripheral blood
smears, of erythrocytes that have shape variations indicative of mechanical
trauma, is of value as a readily available, reliable, and inexpensive aid in the
differential diagnosis between pneumonia and pulmonary embolism (27).

Emboli that occlude the lumens of large pulmonary arteries and their major

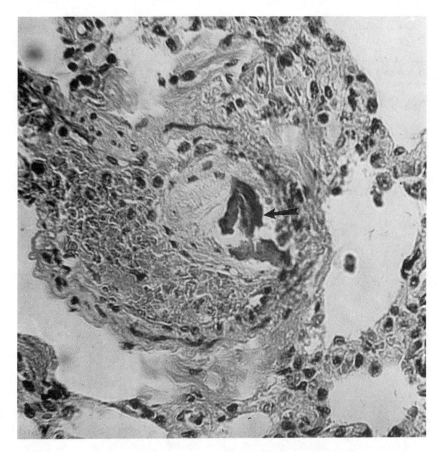

Figure 5.20.   Trabecular fragments in pulmonary artery (arrow) following ischemic
necrosis of the bone marrow.

branches cause the formation of cone-shaped infarcts. Sections of lung infarcts
that are cut in the vertical axis of the cone are wedge-shaped, with the widest
portion distal. Fibrous tissue adhesions form on the pleural surfaces of infarcted
areas. Infarcts occur most frequently in the lower lobes and in the right side.
Pulmonary infarcts, as a rule, reveal central pallor with hemorrhagic margins
(Figure 5.21). The alveolar capillaries of freshly infarcted areas usually are
packed with sickled erythrocytes. The alveolar spaces contain serum and networks of fibrin (Figure 5.22). There are relatively few leukocytes. Erythrocytes
usually are demonstrable in the sputum but gross hemoptysis seldom occurs.
Fibrocytes originating in the arterial walls proliferate and grow into embolic
masses, and new vascular channels may appear (recanalization, see Figure 5.23).
In some of the pulmonary arteries there is complete occlusion.

There is no anatomical evidence that thrombi originate in the lungs. The
margins of early emboli of all three types are not attached to intimal surfaces.

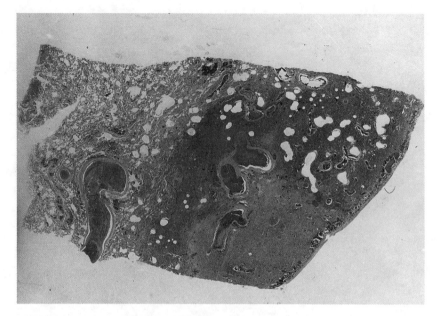

Figure 5.21.   Infarct of the lung due to red cell embolus.

The internal elastic lamellae are intact, and there are no signs of medial degenerative changes and no evidence of a perivascular inflammatory reaction. Collagen is not exposed, and there is an absence of platelet aggregates.

As the result of the progressive loss of lung tissue due to recurrent emboli, infarction, and fibrosis, the oxygen content of the arterial blood is decreased, and pulmonary function is progressively impaired. The occlusion of the lumens of pulmonary arteries results in chronic pulmonary hypertension. The impairment in blood flow in the arterial system of the lung is followed by dilatation and hypertrophy of right heart chambers (cor pulmonale; see the section on the heart).

HEART

Autopsies of children seldom reveal cardiac abnormalities other than the presence of sickled erythrocytes in vascular channels. As patients age there is abnormal cardiac enlargement. The hypertrophy involves all heart chambers. The heart is pale and flabby. The widths of the lumens of coronary arteries are normal, and arteriosclerotic changes, coronary thrombi, focal myocardial infarcts, and pericardial adhesions are seldom demonstrable. A recent discussion of this topic has been published by Falk and Hood (28).

The hearts of patients past the third decade of life usually reveal gross evidence of patchy fibrosis (6). Microscopic examination shows, in addition to fibrosis (Figure 5.24), degenerative changes in muscle cells manifested by loss of stria-

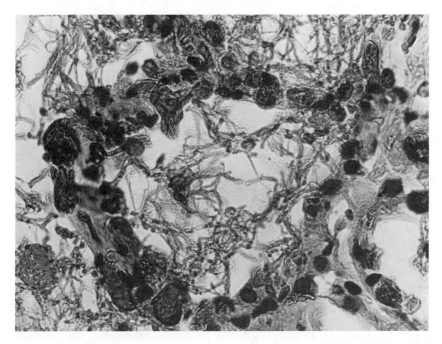

Figure 5.22.   Engorgement of aveolar blood vessels by sickled red cells, showing fibrin threads in alveoli.

tions, basophilic nuclei, and cytoplasmic vacuoles. In rare instances there is fibrosis of the distal portions of papillary muscles of the mitral valve (Figure 5.25) and nodularity and fusion of the cusps (6). Fibrotic lesions in hearts of patients with sickle cell diseases grossly resemble those that occur in individuals who have had symptoms and signs of rheumatic fever. Granulomatous lesions of the Ashoff body type are not microscopically demonstrable in patients with S-hemoglobinopathies who have no history of rheumatic fever (29, 30).

As the result of and following embolic occlusion of pulmonary arteries, pulmonary fibrosis, and chronic pulmonary hypertension, there is a dilatation and hypertrophy of the right heart chambers (cor pulmonale) (31). Manifestations of right-sided heart failure include passive congestion of the liver, hepatomegaly, and generalized edema.

KIDNEYS

The kidneys of young patients are slightly larger than normal. The surface is smooth and the capsule strips easily. The color is normal. With advancing years, there are cortical as well as medullary atrophic, vascular occlusive, degenerative, and fibrotic anatomical changes as well as a progressive loss of nephron units (32, 33).

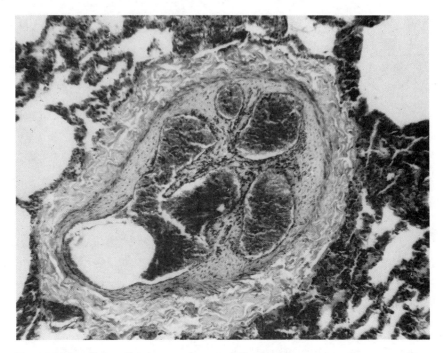

Figure 5.23.   Sicle cell aggregates in a recanalized pulmonary artery.

The pre-capillary arterioles of the glomeruli in patients of all ages are distended by sickled erythrocytes. The engorgement is of sufficient degree to make the glomeruli grossly visible on the surfaces of cut sections, where they appear as dark, pepper-like dots against a lighter and more brownish background. The engorgement of vascular channels is maximal in the cortico-medullary junctional areas.

Pale and yellowish infarcts that vary in size and in number may be demonstrable in the sub-capsular areas of the renal cortex (1). There is no anatomical evidence of emboli or primary arterial thrombi, and the infarcts are spherical rather than cone-shaped. It is thus evident that the ischemic infarcts are due to an impairment in blood flow in focal capillary areas rather than to arterial occlusions. When necrotic areas heal, they are replaced by fibrous tissue. Scars of old infarcts appear as surface depressions. The epithelial cells of renal tubules adjacent to glomeruli contain hemosiderin granules. Tests for hemosiderin in specimens of urinary sediment are positive.

The medullae of older patients may reveal degenerative changes in tubular epithelial cells. In some areas there is a loss of tubules, which are replaced by hyalinized fibrous tissue (Figure 5.26). The medullary arterioles (vasa recta) are distorted and tortuous (34), and their number is significantly decreased. In some medullary areas there are lakes of blood that contain sickled erythrocytes in endothelial-lined spaces. Hyaline casts may be demonstrable. Old proteinaceous

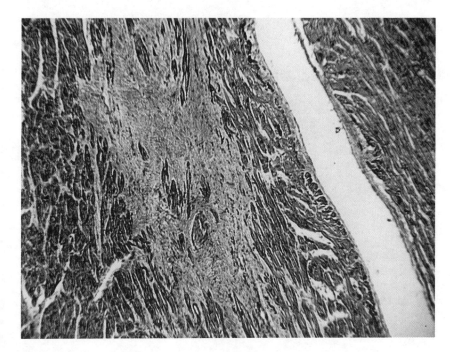

Figure 5.24.   Cardiac fibrosis.

urinary casts in fibrotic areas are infiltrated with calcium and iron. In microscopic sections, stained by the hematoxylin and eosin method, these residual casts are revealed as black, round or elongated, and fragmented amorphous structures.

Papillary Renal Necrosis

Individuals with all types of S-hemoglobinopathies, including those with the sickle cell trait, are subject to episodes of unilateral urinary tract bleeding due to a necrosis of the tips of renal papillae (Figure 5.27) (35). Papillary sickling of erythrocytes, hemostasis, necrosis, and hematuria are favored by hypoxemia, acidosis, hyperosmolarity, and inadequency of the collateral blood vessels. The pelvic epithelium is denuded. There is bleeding into interstitial tissues and tubules as well as into the renal pelvis. Clotting of blood is retarded by urokinase, which is an activator that catalyzes the conversion of plasminogen into plasmin. Papillary renal infarcts are most likely to occur in the left kidney and the upper calyces. Following the retrograde injection of radio-opaque substances into the renal pelvis, the sloughed-out papillary areas are revealed in X-ray plates as filled cavities. The abnormalities vary in size and shape.

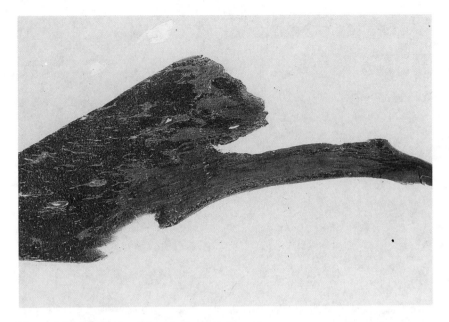

Figure 5.25.   Fibrosis of the papillary heart muscle.

Nephrotic Syndrome

The nephrotic syndrome, which is characterized by generalized edema, hyperproteinuria and hypoalbuminemia, develops as a superimposed anomaly in a small percentage of patients with sickle cell diseases (36–38). Theories differ concerning the explanation for the development of nephrosis in association with sickle cell hemoglobinopathies.

The anatomical lesions that have been observed by electron microscopy are an exaggeration of those that occur in patients without the nephrotic syndrome. These changes include the presence of sickled erythrocytes in vascular channels, glomerular sclerosis, loss of nephron units, a splitting and reduplication of basement membranes and dense bodies, and iron complexes within mesangial areas. There is fusion of the epithelial foot processes and changes in cytoplasmic organelles. Occasionally there are needle-like crystalline structures (39).

Patients who acquire the nephrotic syndrome are especially susceptible to bacterial, viral and other infectious agents. There is a decrease in plasma coagulation components with abnormal bleeding as a terminal manifestation in some patients. Death is due to combined factors.

Kidney Failure

Patients with sickle cell diseases, as well as all other individuals, are subject to pyelonephritis, glomerular nephritis, blood stream infections, and countless

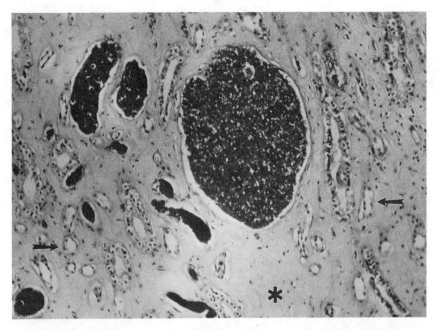

Figure 5.26. Medulla of the kidney, showing sickle cell aggregates in arterioles,
atrophic tubules (arrows), showing replacement of tubules by
hyalinized tissue (asterick).

other diseases and conditions that are characterized by renal anatomical abnormalities. It is difficult and often impossible, on the basis of tissue abnormalities,
to differentiate between sickle cell nephropathies and complicating diseases. It
is seldom that patients live long enough to develop kidney failure and uremia
due to the presence of Hb S as the sole etiologic agent. This may change as
better supportive care prolongs survival.

GENITAL ORGANS

Penis

Males of all ages with sickle cell diseases, and, in rare instances, those with
the sickle cell trait, may have episodes of sustained painful erections of the penis
(40, 41). At the time of priapism there is a firm engorgement of the sinusoids
of the corpus cavernosa by sickled erythrocytes. Aspirated specimens of blood
from the cavernous sinusoids are dark, thick, and noncoagulable. The erythrocytes are irreversibly sickled. Following recurrent episodes of priapism there is
a decrease in the number and width of vascular channels and an increase in the
thickness of intervascular structures. There is no evidence of thrombosis, hemosiderosis or calcification.

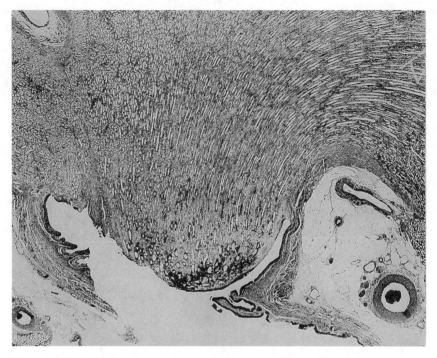

Figure 5.27.   Papillary renal necrosis.

Placenta

Sickled erythrocytes are demonstrable in the maternal sinusoids of the placenta. Due to the presence of Hb F as a major component, there is an absence of sickling in the circulatory system of the fetus. The majority of placentas reveal focal areas of necrosis, fibrosis and/or calcification. Spontaneous abortions are frequent. Aggregates composed mainly of sickled erythrocytes (Figure 5.2) with minimal amounts of fibrin as well as fragments of clots that form in intervillous spaces and in uterine veins may be dislodged and conveyed to the lungs. Pulmonary embolization is the main cause of maternal mortality. For further information, the author recommends Milner, Jones, and Dobler (42), Powars, Sandhu, Niland-Weiss, et al. (43), and Koshy, Burd, Wallace, et al. (44).

BRAIN

Infarcts

Infarcts of the brain cause serious disabilities and are a frequent cause of death (45). Focal areas of ischemic cerebral necrosis may occur at any age but are

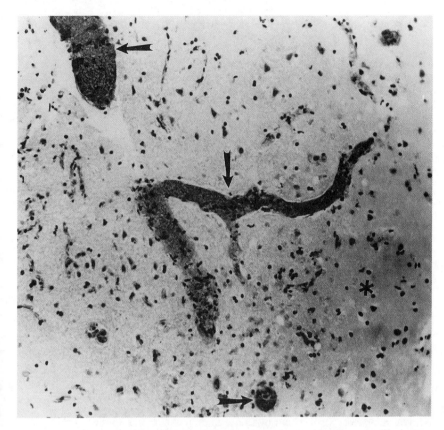

Figure 5.28. Small area of cerebral necrosis (asterisk) due to ischemia in a capillary
region. Pre-capillary arterioles (arrows).

most likely to develop in infants and in young children. Those who survive
initial cerebral vascular occlusive crises are prone to have recurrences involving
the same and/or additional areas. The infarcts often are bilateral, and vary in
size and in number. Small focal areas of degeneration are frequently observed
(Figure 5.28). Large necrotic and hemorrhagic lesions, as a rule, are confluent
(Figure 5.29).

Infarcts may occur in any portion of the cerebral hemisphere, cerebellum, or
hind brain. The most frequent infarcts are in the cerebral cortex in portions that
are supplied with blood by the anterior and middle cerebral arteries. Boundary
or watershed areas, as a rule, are included. The necrosis is primarily caused by
ischemia involving the cortical and subcortical capillaries. This is followed by
the engorgement of precapillary arterioles by sickled erythrocytes and the shunting of arterial blood into thin-walled venules. These changes are followed by
subarachnoid hemorrhages and by the development of thrombi in capillaries,
precapillary arterioles, arteriovenous shunts, and post capillary venous channels.

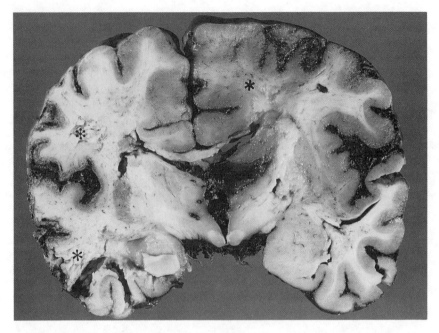

Figure 5.29. Multiple and confluent infarcts, showing ventricular and subarachnoid hemorrhage, encephalacia (asterisks).

Intravascular clots also extend in a retrograde manner back to the nearest patent arterial branches.

At the time of autopsy of a patient who dies within a few hours following the first cortical infarct, the surface of the brain of the involved side is swollen and cyanotic. The subarachnoid blood vessels are distended. The gray matter and subcortical white matter are soft and friable. The microscopic examination of sections of initial and recent infarcts reveals aggregates of sickled cells within dilated arterioles. Longitudinal sections of engorged precapillary arterioles have tapering (Figure 5.28) or ''tadpole'' shapes (46). Peri-arteriolar hemorrhages are demonstrable in some areas. In other areas there are accumulations of leukocytes and arterioles. Older lesions are characterized by degenerative changes in vessel walls and perivascular infiltration by macrophages, some of which contain in their cytoplasm hemosiderin and lipid granules. There is also injury to and loss of nerve cells, astrocytosis and evidences of demyelinization.

When cerebral infarcts heal and parenchymal structures are replaced by scar tissue, there is dilatation of the ventricles and a shift of central brain structures toward the involved side (Figure 5.30). If there have been infarcts in both hemispheres the shift is in the direction of maximal atrophy. Old fibrotic and atrophic lesions, as a rule, are pigmented.

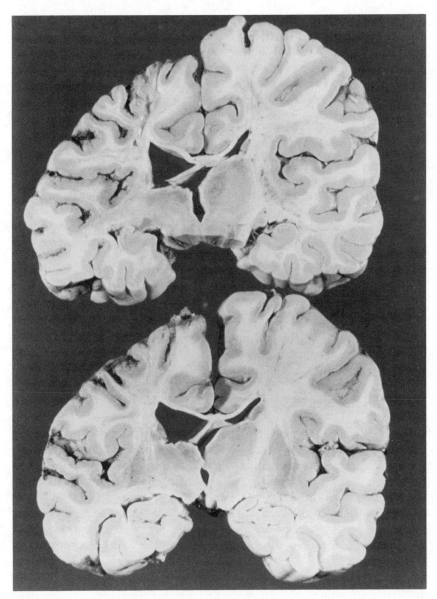

Figure 5.30. Dilation of ventricle on the side of a healed cortical infarct.

Subarachnoid and Ventricular Hemorrhages

Ruptures of dilated and thin-walled cortical venules result in escape of blood into subarachnoid spaces. Necrosis that occurs in the more central portions of cerebral hemispheres is followed by bleeding into ventricles (Figure 5.29). Another cause of cerebral hemorrhage is the rupture of an aneurysm (see below). In association with subarachnoid and ventricular hemorrhages the cerebrospinal fluid is xanthochromatic and contains sickled red cells. The pressure of the spinal fluid is increased. There also is an increase in proteins and a moderate increase in leukocytes, most of which are neutrophilic granulocytes. The concentration of glucose is normal.

Subdural Hematomas

Dilated venules that convey blood from the subarachnoid areas into dural sinuses may rupture as they pass between the arachnoid membrane and the dura, thus producing subdural hematomas. Subdural hematomas may be massive and cause a loss of consciousness and death without localizing clinical symptoms and signs.

Thrombi in Dural Veins

Clots that form in cerebral infarcts and in venules and veins in subarachnoid spaces may extend into dural veins (47).

Atrophic Changes

The oxygen uptake by the cells of the brain is high. Brain tissues are extremely sensitive to hypoxemia. In spite of a rapid flow of blood and numerous freely communicating blood vessels, hemostasis due to the presence of sickled cells in the microvasculature is a continuing process. No one has ever weighed the brains of a large number of patients of different ages with various types of sickle cell diseases in whom there was a negative history of ictus. There is, however, convincing evidence that the brain, like all other organs, in patients who never had clinical manifestations of cerebral infarcts nonetheless undergoes progressive atrophic changes.

Gross morphological proof of brain atrophy in the absence of infarctive lesions, manifested by a shrinkage of cortical gyri and a widening of sulci, has been observed by the author in a 17-year-old patient with Hb SS disease who was mentally retarded (Figure 5.31). He had no history of cerebral vascular occlusive crises. Death was caused by pneumonia. Parenchymal abnormalities are disclosed by computerized tomography (CT) scans, magnetic resonance imaging (MRI), and by electroencephalographic studies. Injury to brain tissues is manifested also by statistically significant low scores when standard psychometric (neuropsychological) assessment procedures are employed.

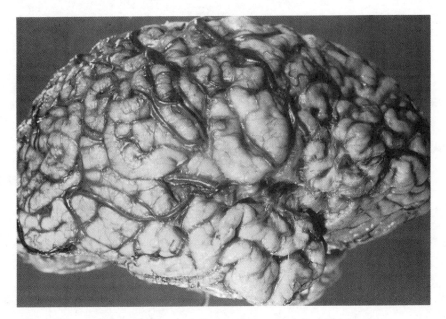

Figure 5.31.   Unevenly distributed cortical atrophic changes, with dilated
subarachnoid venules.

Fibrinous Thrombi in Cerebral Arteries

In addition to the atrophic, ischemic, necrotic, hemorrhagic, thrombotic and
fibrotic abnormalities described above in association with the blockade of capillaries and other small and terminal vascular channels by sickled erythrocytes,
there are in some, but not in all stroke cases, fibrinous thrombi in the internal
carotid, the basal arteries and their branches.

Awareness of cerebral arterial occlusions and speculations concerning the role
that focal obstructions may play in the production of infarcts were initiated by
Stockman, Nigro, Mishkin, et. al. in 1972 (48). These investigators employed
angiographic procedures. They reported stenotic lesions in the intracranial arteries
of six of seven Hb SS patients with stroke or other symptoms and signs of
neurological abnormalities. Two patients revealed progressive changes. Collateral circulation was a prominent feature in 3 patients. Two patients showed
evidence of neovascularization of the "moyamoya" type.

Since 1972 numerous angiographic studies have confirmed the presence of
partial or complete occlusions in focal areas (49–54). The stenotic lesions may
precede or follow the development of initial cerebral vascular occlusive crises.

Technological procedures, in addition to those that require the injection of
radio-opaque contrast agents into the blood include unenhanced and/or contrast-

enhanced computerized tomography (CT scans) (49, 51, 53, 55), magnetic resonance imaging (MRI) (49, 51, 53, 56), cerebral blood flow (57) and intracranial Doppler ultra-sonography (56).

Ingenious and expensive technical devices have been useful as research tools and have expanded greatly our knowledge concerning the location, number and degree of obstructed intracranial arteries, dilatated lumens above focal stenotic lesions, restoration of blood flow in some instances and parenchymal abnormalities. Technological procedures, however, are not capable of providing information concerning the morphological characteristics of arterial walls or the structure of the luminal occlusive masses.

Unfortunately, there is a paucity of anatomical information concerning the walls and the lumens of cerebral arteries and arterioles previous to the development of infarcts. Most of the reports of pathology relate to abnormalities that were demonstrated at the time of autopsies that were performed multiple hours or days, weeks, months, or years following the initial stroke or other clinical manifestations of intracranial vascular occlusive crises. Many of the stenotic arterial lesions that have been reported have been demonstrated in patients who had a history of multiple neurological crises. The most noteworthy anatomical descriptions and illustrations are by Bridgers (58), Hughes, Diggs, and Gillespie (47), Boros, Thomas, and Weiner (50), Merkel, Ginsberg, Parker, et al. (54), and Rothman, Fulling, and Nelson (59).

Based on the limited anatomical evidence that is now available, the initial arterial stenotic lesions are characterized by the deposition of a few fibrin strands on intimal surfaces. This is followed by a disappearance of endothelial cells below the fibrin cover. The internal elastic lamellae are intact (Figure 5.32). There is no evidence of primary degenerative changes involving the intima, media, adventitia, or perivascular tissues. Collagen is not exposed. There is an absence of aggregates of platelets intermingled with fibrin fibers. Sickled erythrocytes in vasa vasorum, clumps of sickled cells adherent to endothelial surfaces and/or atherosclerotic lesions have never been observed by the author or documented in the literature.

As new layers of fibrin are superimposed the arterial lumens become progressively narrowed. The thrombi have homogenous and hyalinized appearance. Partial occlusions, as a rule, are asymmetrical (Figure 5.33). The thickening of the inner walls is due to fibrin strands that are derived from the plasma and are not due to the proliferation of intimal cells. The term *intimal hyperplasia*, therefore, is inappropriate.

Fibrinous thrombi differ from clots that form in blood that has ceased flowing, such as occurs within and closely adjacent to infarcted areas. They do not contain red cells or heme pigments. Fibrinous thrombi differ from the so-called "white thrombi" or "mixed white and red thrombi" that form as the result of vessel wall injury in a blood stream that is rapidly flowing. Fibrinous thrombi do not contain irregularly shaped colorless structures that are surrounded by red cells, leukocytes and fibrin strands. Fibrinous thrombi do not reveal, at the time of

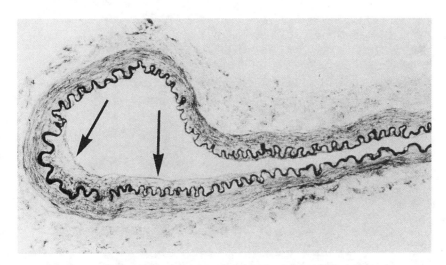

Figure 5.32.   Section of basal artery, showing narrowing of lumen due to deposits of fibrin on intimal surface (arrows).

Source: SM Rothman and JS Nelson, Spinal cord infarction in a patient with sickle cell anemia, *Neurology* 30 (1972): 1072–1076. Reproduced with permission.

the microscopic examinations of cut sections, linear structures (*stria of Zahn* or *lines of Zahn*).

Diffusely and fairly evenly distributed throughout older fibrinous thrombi, there are cells, the nuclei of which appear in stained sections as small, round and dark objects or as elongated, narrow structures with each end tapering. Opinions differ concerning the origin of these infiltrating cells. One theory is that they are derived from multipotent mononuclear blood cells. Another theory is that they are endothelial or smooth muscle cells or fibrocytes that migrate from the arterial walls into the fibrinous matrix. Whatever the origin of these cells, they have the ability to form new endothelial linings when the luminal occlusions are partial and new (recanalized) vascular channels when obstructions are complete.

The internal elastic lamellae of cerebral arteries that contain older fibrinous thrombi are distorted and may be thickened, reduplicated or fragmented but they remain as well defined and easily identifiable structures (Figure 5.33). This is irrefutable evidence that severe injury to the intima has not occurred.

The mediae of cerebral arteries of adults with sickle cell diseases are narrowed. This is a manifestation of the progressive atrophic process that occurs in all organs as the result of chronic anemia and stasis of blood in the microvasculature. It is possible and probable that the thinning and weakening of arterial walls, combined with stenotic lesions, are the cause of the development of aneurysms in older patients.

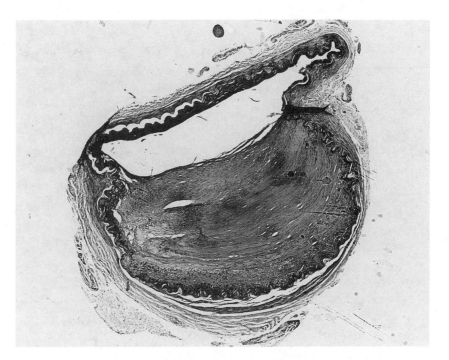

Figure 5.33.   Fibrinous thrombus in internal carotid artery, showing parallel layers of fibrin deposited in intimal surfaces, atrophic media. Prepared with PAS stain.

Courtesy Dr. J. J. Jenkins, St. Jude Children's Hospital, Tenn.

The demonstration of focal occlusions in cerebral arteries that are clinically silent and in cerebral hemispheres that are opposite (contra-lateral) to hemispheres which are infarcted is ample proof that the luminal obstructions, in some cases, may precede the development of ischemia and necrosis.

Fibrinous thrombi that develop in focal areas of cerebral arteries most frequently occur distal to bifurcation points. The deposition of fibrin in these areas probably is due to turbulence and hemostasis that occurs when blood in a proximal blood stream that is rapidly flowing meets with a stream in a branch that is slowly flowing due to upstream blockage of capillaries by sickled erythrocytes. A favorite site for focal stenosis of the internal carotid artery is distal to the point where the ophthalmic artery branches off. Other frequent sites are the lower portions of the anterior and middle cerebral arteries and major branches of basal arteries. Arteries of intermediate and small sizes also may be occluded.

Since the lumens of many cerebral arteries distal to focal occlusions are kept open by collateral arterioles and arteries, it is theoretically possible for an upper portion of a thrombus to break off and to be transported upstream as an artery to artery embolic mass. Insofar as the author is aware, no one has ever observed thromboemboli of this type. It is extremely unlikely that fibrinous thrombi in focal downstream areas will serve as sources of emboli because they are firm, tough, and tightly attached.

It is my opinion that fibrinous thrombi that develop in intracranial arteries are secondary to hemostasis and occlusions that are primary in capillaries, precapillary arterioles, arteriovenous shunts and venules. There is no anatomical evidence that the thrombotic lesions are associated with or due to degenerative lesions that are primary in arterial walls. The fibrinous obstructive lesions are best explained by the retarded rate of blood flow combined with the presence of multiple hypercoagulable factors.

One of the hypercoagulable factors is tissue thromboplastin which is released at the time of injury to parenchymal as well as hemic cells in association with hypoxemia, sickling of erythrocytes, and hemostasis. There are numerous normally functioning platelets. The concentrations of fibrinogen and Factor VIII are high. The concentrations of coagulation factors such as calcium, prothrombin, the fibrin stabilization factor (Factor XIII) as well as other clotting components, insofar as we now know, are within normal limits. There is a decrease in the delivery of the plasminogen activator factor into the blood stream. Defective conversion of plasminogen into plasmin retards the lysis of fibrin as well as fibrinogen.

The reduction in the speed of blood flow in intracranial arteries is due to the upstream blockage of the microvasculature by sickled erythrocytes. A decreased volume and rate of blood flow in a given artery favors the deposition of fibrin strands on intimal surfaces and a retention of tissue thromboplastin and other clot activating factors. Impairment of blood flow prevents the rapid escape of activator factors into the systemic circulation and their denaturation in the liver.

Periarterial Neovascularization (Moyamoya Syndrome)

The development of occlusions of intracranial arteries, in some cases, is followed by the formation of myriads of tiny perivascular arterioles (60). These telangiectatic vascular channels aid in the detour of blood around stenotic areas. When visualized by angiographic procedures they appear as opaque, hazy and dust-like areas or nebulous clouds that vary in density, size and shape. These newly formed small blood vessels are said to have a *moyamoya* pattern. (*Moyamoya* is a Japanese expression for a puff of cigarette smoke.) Periarterial neovascularization following stenotic lesions in arteries is not limited to the brain. Moyamoya-like patterns have been observed in the retina following arterial occlusions. New networks of arterioles also develop beneath the granulating base of chronic leg ulcers in areas surrounding arteries that are partially occluded by depositions of fibrin on intimal surfaces.

Aneurysms

Angiographic studies of older patients with sickle cell diseases sometimes reveal dilatation of cerebral arteries to a degree sufficient to be identified as aneurysms. The existence of thin-walled arterial sacs has been confirmed in a few cases at the time of craniotomies and autopsies. The aneurysms are often multiple. They usually involve the internal carotid or basal arteries and their communicating and/or major branches. The location of the aneurysm is proximal to focal stenotic lesions. It is probable that the weakening and bulbus dilatations are due to atrophic changes in the arterial walls combined with an increase in intravascular pressure below focal luminal obstructions. The rupture of intracranial aneurysms, in most cases, is followed by subarachnoid hemorrhage manifested by bleeding into the cerebrospinal fluid.

The clinical symptoms and signs vary depending on the size and location of the hemorrhage. The onset usually is sudden and is characterized by headache, nausea and vomiting, lethargy and signs of meningeal irritation. Intracranial bleeding may compress the optic nerve and cause blindness (61).

SPINAL CORD

The spinal cords of patients with sickle cell diseases have been inadequately studied. The few reports that are available indicate that lesions that are produced are anatomically similar to those produced in the brain by chronic and acute occlusions of the microcirculation by sickled erythrocytes.

EYE

Examination of the superficial vessels in the bulbar conjunctiva by means of a slit lamp or an ophthalmoscope with a $^+40$ diopter lens provides a readily available and inexpensive procedure for the study of terminal vascular channels. The most suitable area for visual examination is the lower temporal region at the junction of the bulbar and palpebral conjunctivae. In areas which are covered by the lower eyelid and thus protected from exposure to the oxygen in the air, the sickling of erythrocytes is maximal (62, 63).

The number of visible blood vessels in the conjunctiva of patients with sickle diseases is less than in normal individuals or in those with sickle cell trait. The circulatory abnormality is characterized by dark, isolated and dilated vascular loops (Figure 5.34). The segments vary in number, in length and in width. They may be fairly straight but usually they have comma, corkscrew or curlicue shapes. The blood in some of these superficial vessels has a sludged or beaded appearance due to sickle cell aggregates separated by plasma. Stasis of blood in superficial vessels is transient. Exposure of the surface of the conjunctiva to the air and to the warmth of a slit lamp causes the restoration of the continuity of superficial blood vessels. The use of drops that contain vasodilator drugs causes the isolated loops to disappear. Vasoconstrictor drugs, in contrast, favor an increase in the visibility of isolated loops. These phenomena furnish evidence that there is a vasoconstrictive factor.

The abnormalities revealed at the time of examination of the surface of the

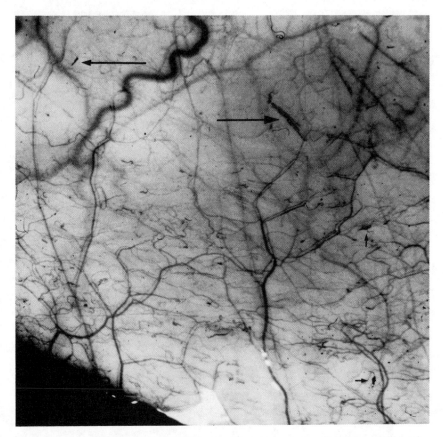

Figure 5.34.   Surface of bulbar conjunctiva, showing paucity of visible small blood
vessels, isolated vascular loops (arrows).

bulbar conjunctiva in hypoxic areas probably are due to the presence of sickled
erythrocytes that engorge precapillary arterioles and arteriovenous shunts combined with vasoconstriction at each end of the distended loops.

Retina

The peripheral areas of the retina are frequent sites of focal ischemic necrosis
because the circulation in these areas is terminal and anastomotic channels are
limited. Following the development of retinal infarcts and dilatation of precapillary arterioles and arteriovenous shunts, superficial hemorrhages may occur.
When these bleeding spots first appear they are red. Later they acquire a pink
or salmon color and are designated as "salmon patches" (Figure 5.35). As these
areas age there is replacement by fibrous tissue which is non-pigmented and
greyish-white. Hemorrhages and atrophic lesions involving deeper chorio-retinal

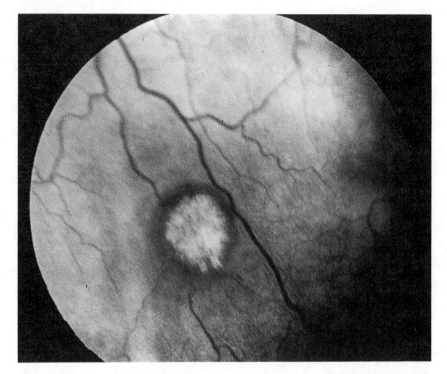

Figure 5.35. "Salmon patch" retina.

areas reveal black granules and spiculated pigments ("black sunbursts") (Figure 5.36). Older degenerative and atrophic areas that are depressed and non-pigmented are called "schisis cavities". Hemosiderin-laden macrophages and structures associated with tissue destruction appear as lustrous granules (iridescent deposits). The arborizing pattern of new blood vessels that develop in infarcted areas, when visualized by fluorescein angiography, resemble coral growths and are called "sea fans" (Figure 5.37).

Additional anatomical lesions include: retinal tears and detachments, vitreous hemorrhages (Figure 5.38), spoke-like angioid streaks, thrombosis of retinal arteries and veins, neovascularization of the optic nerve head and vascular occlusions in macular areas.

Uvea

Occlusions of the lumens of terminal vascular channels of the eye may, in rare instances, cause ischemia and atrophy of the iris and other structures in the anterior chamber of the eye. Edema and an inflammatory reaction in the region

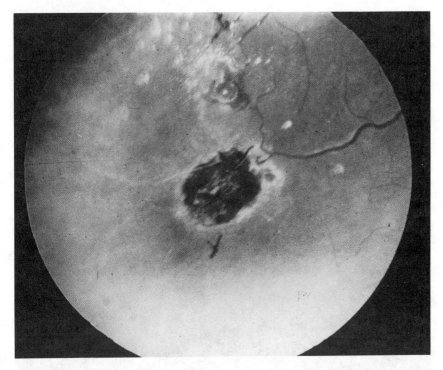

Figure 5.36. ''Black sunburst'' retina.

of drainage of the aqueous humor may cause an increase in intraocular pressure (glaucoma).

LEG ULCERS

Older children, adolescents and adults are prone to develop ulcers of the lower legs that are difficult to heal (64, 65). The ulcers usually are on the lateral sides. They are often bilateral (Figure 5.39) and may encircle the leg. The ulcers vary in shape. As a rule, they are roughly round or oval. The skin at the edge is thin and tapering. The marginal areas reveal pigmentation of differing degrees. The necrosis of the skin is due to the chronic anemia combined with the obstruction of small blood vessels by sickled erythrocytes in areas where there is venous stasis.

A common sign of impending ulceration is hyperpigmentation of the lower legs. Initial lesions may be caused by an insect bite or by a wound produced by mechanical trauma but in many instances the first manifestations include soft

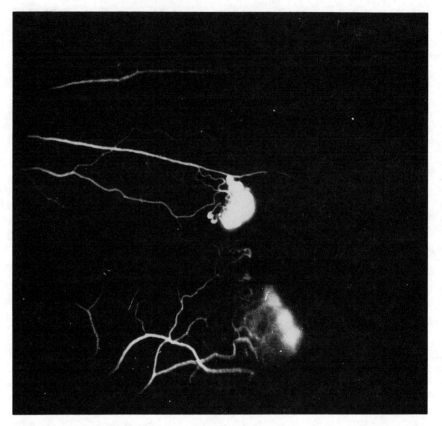

Figure 5.37. "Sea fans" Fluorescein angiography.

tissue swelling, itching and tenderness. This is followed by central necrosis in a small focal area. If improperly treated, the ulcer progressively enlarges. The base of untreated ulcers has a dull grey color and consists of fibrin, bacteria, fungi and amorphous debris. Following treatment the ulcer surface has a bright color due to exposed capillary loops which are filled with red cells in contact with the oxygen in the air which prevents sickling.

The lumens of arteries that supply blood to chronic leg ulcers are partially occluded by fibrous deposits (6). There is microscopic evidence of neo-vascularization in the form of peri-arterial arterioles (moyamoya syndrome). These new blood vessels aid in by-passing luminal arterial obstructions and in supplying blood to skin at the margins of ulcers.

Secondary anatomical lesions associated with large and chronic ulcers include thrombosis of leg veins, systemic infections and periosteal proliferation of bones beneath the ulcers.

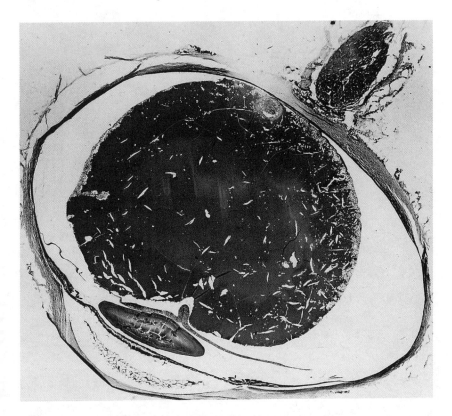

Figure 5.38. Hemorrhage into vitreous.

FAT EMBOLIZATION

Necrosis due to the blockage of sinusoids and reticular spaces of the bone marrow is followed by edema and an inflammatory reaction. Pressure in marrow spaces is increased by the inflow of arterial blood. The rigid cortical bone and trabeculae prevent the collapse of venous channels. Portions of partially necrotic marrow are dislodged and forced into efferent veins. Globules of fat released from necrotic areas are transported to the lungs and from the lungs to the brain, kidney, skin and all other organs (66–70).

The fat droplets are soluble in xylol and appear, in sections stained by standard methods, as colorless and structureless small circles of varying sizes (Figure 5.40). Their identity as globules of fat is confirmed in frozen sections by Oil-Red-O or other fat stains.

Some of the droplets of fat are large enough and firm enough to obstruct the lumens of arterioles and the production of perivascular hemorrhages. Petechiae in the skin are most numerous in the upper trunk. Petechial hemorrhages occur in all areas of the brain but are most numerous and most conspicuous in the

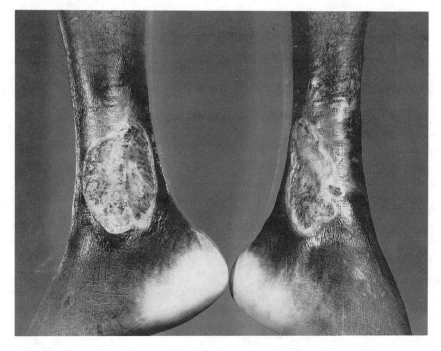

Figure 5.39.   Chronic leg ulcers.

white matter (Figure 5.41). Fat droplets are demonstrable in the sputum and the urine.

Fat embolization is more likely to occur in patients with Hb SC disease, S-thalassemia, or other heterozygous sickle cell diseases than in homozygous sickle cell anemias (Hb SS) because the bone marrow of those who inherit genes for the production of Hb S in combination with other types of abnormal hemoglobins contains many fat cells.

HETEROZYGOUS SICKLE CELL HEMOGLOBINOPATHIES

General

All of the erythrocytes of all individuals who inherit all types of sickle cell diseases and conditions contain sickle cell hemoglobin (Hb S). The frequency and severity of untoward clinical manifestations are in proportion to the concentration of Hb S within the cytoplasm of erythrocytes. If the oxygen content of the blood ever gets low enough and stays low enough in the body as a whole or in focal areas there will be a transformation of soluble Hb S to elongated polymers that distort the elastic membranes of erythrocytes. Blood that contains sickled cells is more viscous than blood with the same number of red cells that

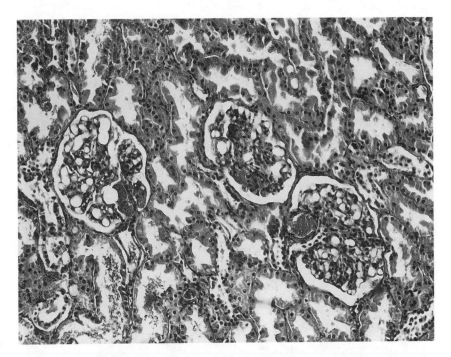

Figure 5.40.   Globules of fat in glomerular arterioles.

are not sickled. Blood that contains sickled cells flows less readily through small and terminal vascular channels, thus producing ischemic infarcts in focal areas.

The anatomical lesions that are produced in heterozygous sickle cell hemoglobinopathies, as a rule, appear later in life than in patients with homozygous sickle cell anemia (Hb SS). The degree of anemia and hemolytic jaundice is less marked in heterozygotes. Painful and febrile crises are less frequent in heterozygotic individuals but when they do occur they are equally as severe and disabling. The mechanisms that are involved and the anatomical characteristics are the same.

The spleens of patients with heterozygous sickle cell diseases are usually enlarged after the first year and remain enlarged throughout life. The degree of enlargement at any given age is highly variable. Splenic infarcts may develop when there is exposure to hypoxic environments and in association with strenuous and prolonged exertion, dehydration, hyperthermia, acidosis, febrile illness, and other situations of stress.

Infarcts may occur in any portion that still contains red pulp. They usually occur in spleens that are larger than normal. The infarcts vary in size, shape and in number. The smaller infarcts, as a rule, are roughly spherical or egg shaped. There is no evidence of primary arterial or venous thrombi. The color of infarcts varies depending on the age of the lesions. Early infarcts are dark due to entrapment of sickled erythrocytes. Old infarcts are pale and gray. The lumens of arteries supplying blood to infarcted areas are narrowed due to deposits of fibrin on intimal surfaces.

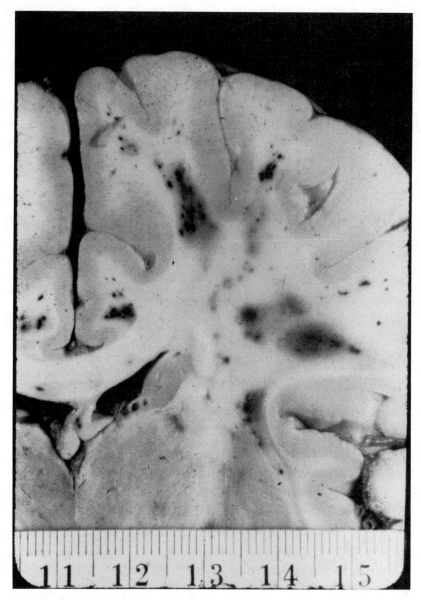

Figure 5.41.   Focal hemorrhages in white matter of brain, showing fat embolization.

Individuals with all types of heterozygous S disease have a longer survival rate than those with homozygous sickle cell anemia (Hb SS). As a rule, patients with heterozygous Hb S diseases do not develop leg ulcers or marked atrophic lesions.

Hemoglobin SC Disease

A distinctive characteristic of Hb SC disease is the presence of crystals of hemoglobin in the cytoplasm of erythrocytes (71). Most of the Hb SC crystals are elongated with parallel sides and with round or bluntly pointed ends. The shape resembles that of the Washington Monument. The narrow and elongated crystals may be condensed at both ends with the central portion achromic. Some red cells contain crystals that have pyramid shapes. When there are multiple crystals within a given cell they protrude in varying directions and in a finger-like manner from the same focal point. Some of the red cells that contain crystals are bent (Figure 5.41). The number of crystals in a given red cell is in the 1 to 4 range.

Hb SC crystals are demonstrable in small numbers in moist preparations and in dry smears of peripheral blood in approximately 75 percent of the cases. In some blood smears there may be several crystal-containing red cells in a single oil immersion field, but as a rule, it is necessary to search in multiple fields in order to find typical SC cells. The inability to demonstrate crystals does not exclude Hb SC disease, but the presence of these structures is diagnostic.

Sickle Cell Thalassemia

Thalassemia is an umbrella term for an extremely large and complex group of hereditary diseases and conditions that have in common the inherited inability to synthesize globin chains of hemoglobin molecules in normal amounts. The globins that are produced in relatively low concentrations are chemically normal. The percentage value for any given globin is highly variable depending on the genetic defect.

When Hb S is inherited from one parent and thalassemia from the other parent in a heterozygous manner, the result is a decrease in the hemoglobin content and the size of the red cells (hypochromia, microcytic anemia). The hereditary deficiency in hemoglobin is not corrected by iron therapy.

Sickle Cell Trait

Individuals with the sickle cell trait who inherit normal adult hemoglobin (Hb A) as a major component and Hb S as a minor component, as a rule, do not reveal any anatomical abnormalities due to Hb S until the last few gasping moments of life when respiration fails and the oxygen concentration of the blood decreases to a degree sufficient to cause systemic sickling of erythrocytes. Sickling continues in all organs following death and is microscopically demonstrable in sections of blocks of tissues that have been fixed in formaldehyde or gluter-aldehyde solutions.

Individuals with the sickle cell trait, however, are subject to the development of ischemic infarcts in any and all organs if there is severe and sustained hypoxemia in focal areas (72). When individuals with the sickle cell trait are exposed to hypoxic environments associated with flying in unpressurized air craft, climbing mountains, underwater swimming, anesthestic complications or other situations that cause systemic hypoxemia they may develop enlargement of the spleen and splenic infarcts (73, 74). Strenuous, prolonged and exhaustive muscular activities may result in systemic sickling of erythrocytes, collapse and sudden death or death within a few days (73, 75). Dehydration, hyperthermia, and acidosis are contributing factors. Anatomical manifestations of exertional syndromes include cerebral edema, splenomegaly, focal infarcts in the bone marrow and other organs, muscular degenerative changes (rhabdomyolysis), disseminated intravascular coagulation (DIC) and tubular renal necrosis (73, 75).

Other Heterozygous S-Hemoglobinopathies

When Hb S is combined in a heterozygous manner with the hereditary persistence of fetal hemoglobin (Hb S-HPFH) the benign condition that is produced is comparable to the sickle cell trait in its clinical and anatomical manifestations. The fetal hemoglobin (Hb F) usually is in the 20 to 30 percent range and Hb S is a major component. Polymerization of Hb S, however, does not occur unless there is a severe oxygen deficiency.

The mutant genes responsible for the production of Hb S, in addition to the genes for the production of hemoglobins C and HPFH, may be inherited in combination with several hundred other types of abnormal hemoglobins. The number of individuals with heterogenous hemoglobinopathies other than Hb SC, S-thal, and AS that have been studied and reported are too few to establish the natural history of each variant and to determine any specific anatomical lesions that may exist.

SUMMARY

Elongated, multipointed and rigid (sickled) erythrocytes continually impede the flow of blood in capillaries and in other small and terminal blood vessels. Continuing hemostasis combined with a chronic anemia cause progressive atrophic changes in patients with sickle cell anemia at a rate that is more rapid than normal. All organs are affected. In addition, there are focal areas of ischemic necrosis and replacement of parenchymal cells by fibrous tissue. Following the development of infarcts there is a release of tissue thromboplastin followed by intravascular coagulation. The organs that are most severely affected are the spleen, bone marrow, brain, kidney, lungs, heart and liver.

If the oxygen in the blood gets low enough and stays low long enough in the body as a whole or in focal areas of individuals with heterozygous S hemoglobinopathies, including the sickle cell trait (Hb AS), the lesions that are produced are similar to those that occur in patients with homozygous sickle cell anemia (Hb SS).

REFERENCES

1. Kimmelstiel P: Vascular occlusion and ischemic infarction in sickle cell disease. *Am J Med Sci* 216 (1948): 11–18.
2. Reynolds J: *The roentgenological factors of sickle cell disease and related hemoglobinopathies.* Springfield, IL: Charles C. Thomas, 1965.
3. Diggs LW: Sickle cell crisis. *Am J Clin Pathol* 44 (1965): 1–19.
4. Edington GM, and Gilles HM: *Pathology in the tropics,* pp. 362–396. Baltimore, MD: Williams and Wilkins, 1969.
5. Song YS: *Pathology of sickle cell disease.* Springfield, IL: Charles C. Thomas, 1971.
6. Diggs LW: Anatomic lesions in sickle cell disease. In M Abramson, D Wethers, and JF Bertles, eds.: *Sickle cell disease: Diagnosis, management, education and research,* pp. 199–229. St. Louis, MO: C. V. Mosby, 1973.
7. Konotey-Ahula FID: The sickle cell diseases. *Arch Intern Med* 133 (1974): 611–619.
8. Serjeant GR: *Sickle cell disease.* New York: Oxford University Press, 1985.
9. Embury SH: The clinical pathophysiology of sickle cell disease. *Ann Rev Med* 37 (1986): 361–376.
10. Bunn HF, and Forget BG: *Hemoglobin: Molecular, genetic and clinical aspects.* Philadelphia, PA: W. B. Saunders, 1986.
11. Lewkow L, and Shah I: Sickle cell anemia and epidural extramedullary hematopoiesis. *Am J Med* 76 (1984): 748–751.
12. Sebes JI, Massie JD, White TJ, et al.: Pelvic extramedullary hematopoiesis. *J Nucl Med* 25 (1984): 209–210.
13. Bohrer SP: *Bone ischemia and infarction in sickle cell disease.* St. Louis, MO: Warren H. Green, 1981.
14. Schumacher HR: Rheumatological manifestations of sickle cell disease and other hereditary hemoglobinopathies. *Clin Rheuma Dis* 1 (1975): 37–52.
15. Diggs LW: Bone and joint lesions in sickle cell disease. *Clin Orthop* 52 (1967): 119–143.
16. Sebes JI, and Diggs LW: Radiographic changes in skull in sickle cell anemia. *Am J Rad* 132 (1979): 373–377.
17. Konotey-Ahula FID: Mental nerve neuropathy: A complication of sickle cell crisis. *Lancet* no. 8 (1972): 388–389.
18. Pearson HA, Spencer RP, and Cornelius EA: Functional asplenia in sickle cell anemia. *N Engl J Med* 281 (1969): 923–926.
19. Edmond AM, Collis R, Darvill D, et al.: Acute splenic sequestration in homozygous sickle cell disease: Natural history and management. *J Peds* 107 (1985): 201–206.
20. Diggs LW: Siderofibrosis of the spleen in sickle cell anemia. *JAMA* 104 (1935): 538–541.
21. Diggs LW: Pathology of the spleen: Sickle cell disease. In A Blaustein, ed.: *The spleen,* pp. 89–109. New York: McGraw-Hill, 1963.
22. Bauer TW, Moore CW, and Hutchins GM: The liver in sickle cell disease: A clinicopathologic study of 70 patients. *Am J Med* 69 (1980): 833–837.
23. Rosenblate HJ, Eisentein R, and Holnes AW: The liver in sickle cell anemia: A clinical-pathologic study. *Arch Path* 90 (1970): 235–245.
24. Muirhead EE, Halden ER, and Wilson BJ: Recurrent crises in sickle cell anemia

responding to cholecystectomy: A syndrome apparently based on cholecysto- and choledocho-stasis. *Am J Med* 20 (1956): 953.

25. Diggs LW: Pulmonary lesions in sickle cell anemia. *Blood* 34 (1969): 734.
26. Barreras L, Diggs LW, and Bell A: Erythrocyte morphology in patients with sickle cell anemia and pulmonary emboli. *JAMA* 203 (1968): 569–573.
27. Diggs LW, and Barreras L: Pulmonary emboli vs. pneumonia in patients with sickle cell anemia. *Mid South Med J* 42 (1967) 375–378.
28. Falk RH, and Hood WB: The heart in sickle cell anemia. *Arch Intern Med* 143 (1984): 1680–1684.
29. Gerry JL, Bukley B, and Hutchins GM: Clinicopathologic analysis of cardiac dysfunction in 52 patients with sickle cell anemia. *Am J Cardiol* 42 (1978): 211–216.
30. McKusick VA: The diagnosis of organic mitral stenosis in the presence of sickle cell anemia. *Am Heart J* 46 (1953): 467–475.
31. Moser KM, and Shea JG: The relationship between pulmonary infarction, corpulmonale and sickle states. *Am J Med* 22 (1957): 561–579.
32. Addae SK: *The kidney in sickle cell disease.* Accra, Ghana: Universities Press, 1975.
33. Bernstein J, and Whitten CF: A histologic appraisal of the kidney in sickle cell anemia. *Arch Path* 70 (1960): 407–418.
34. Alleyne GAO, VanEps LWS, Addae SK, et al.: The kidney in sickle cell anemia. *Kidney Int* 133 (1975): 660–669.
35. McCoy RC: Ultrastructural alterations in the kidney of patients with sickle cell disease and the nephrotic syndrome. *Lab Invest* 212 (1969): 85–95.
36. Pardo V, Strauss J, Kramer H, et al.: Nephropathy associated with sickle cell anemia: An autologous immune complex nephritis. *Am J Med* 59 (1975): 650–659.
37. Walker BR, Alexander F, Birsall TR, et al.: Glomerular lesions in sickle cell nephropathy. *JAMA* 215 (1971): 437–440.
38. VanEps LWS, Pinedo-Veels C, DeVries GH, et al.: Nature of concentrating defects in sickle cell nephropathy: Micro-radio angiographic studies. *Lancet* no. 1 (1970): 450–452.
39. Pitcock JA, Hatch FE, Roy S, et al.: Renal changes in sickle cell disease. In EF Mannen, GF Anderson, and MI Barnhart, eds., *Sickle cell disease,* pp. 231–242. Stuttgart: S.K. Schattauer, 1973.
40. Campbell JH, and Cummins SD: Priapism in sickle cell anemia. *J Urol* 66 (1951): 697–703.
41. Hasen HB, and Raines SL: Priapism associated with sickle cell disease. *J Urol* 88 (1962): 71–76.
42. Milner PF, Jones BR, and Dobler J: Outcome of pregnancy in sickle cell anemia and sickle cell hemoglobin C disease: An analysis of 181 pregnancies in 98 patients and a review of the literature. *Am J Obstet Gynecol* 138 (1980): 239–245.
43. Powars DR, Sandhu M, Niland-Weiss J, et al.: Pregnancy in sickle cell disease. *Obstet Gynecol* 67 (1986): 217–218.
44. Koshy M, Burd L, Wallace D, et al.: Prophylactic red cell transfusions in pregnant patients with sickle cell disease. *N Engl J Med* 319 (1988): 1447–1452.
45. Powers D, Wilson B, Imbus C, et al.: The natural history of stroke in sickle cell disease. *Am J Med* 65 (1978): 461–467.
46. Baird RL, Weiss DL, Ferguson AD, et al.: Clinico-pathological aspects of neurological manifestations. *Pediatrics* 34 (1964): 92–100.

47. Hughes JG, Diggs LW, and Gillespie CE: The involvement of the nervous system in sickle cell anemia. *J Peds* 17 (1940): 166–184.

48. Stockman JA, Nigro MA, Mishkin MM, et al.: Occlusion of large cerebral vessels in sickle cell anemia. *N Engl J Med* 287 (1972): 846–849.

49. Adams RJ, Nichols FT, McKie V, et al.: Cerebral infarction in sickle cell anemia: Mechanism based on CT and MRI. *Neurology* 38 (1988): 1012–1017.

50. Boros L, Thomas C, and Weiner WJ: Large cerebral vessel disease in sickle cell anemia. *J Neur Neurosurg Psychiatry* 39 (1976): 1236–1239.

51. El Gammal T, Adams RJ, Nichols FT, et al.: MR and CT investigation of cerebrovascular disease in sickle cell patients. *Am J Neur Rad* 7 (1986): 1043–1049.

52. Gerald B, Sebes JI, and Langston JW: Cerebral infarction secondary to sickle cell disease: Angiographic findings. *Am J Rad* 134 (1980): 1209–1212.

53. Goldberg HI, and Zimmerman RA: Central nervous system (sickle cell anemia). *Semin Roentgenol* 22 (1987): 205–212.

54. Merkel KHH, Ginsberg PI, Parker JC, et al.: Cerebrovascular disease in sickle cell anemia: A clinical pathological and radiological correlation. *Stroke* 9 (1978): 45–52.

55. Jeffries BF, Lipper MH, and Kishore PRS: Major intracerebral arterial involvement in sickle cell disease. *Surg Neurol* 14 (1980): 291–295.

56. Adams RJ, Aaskid R, El Gammal T, et al.: Detection of cerebral vasculopathy in sickle cell disease using transcranial doppler ultrasonography and magnetic resonance imaging. *Stroke* 19 (1988): 518–520.

57. Huttenlocher PR, Moohr JW, and Johns L: Cerebral blood flow in sickle cell cerebrovascular disease. *Pediatrics* 73 (1984): 615–621.

58. Bridgers WH: Cerebral vascular disease accompanying sickle cell anemia. *Am J Pathol* 15 (1931): 353–361.

59. Rothman SM, Fulling KH, and Nelson JH: Sickle cell anemia and central nervous system infarction: A neuropathological study. *Ann Neurol* 30 (1986): 685–690.

60. Seeler RA, Royal JE, Powe L, et al.: Moyamoya in children with sickle cell anemia and cerebrovascular occlusion. *J Peds* 93 (1978): 808–810.

61. Caprioli JC, Fagadau W, and Lesser R: Acute monocular visual loss secondary to anterior communicating artery aneurysm in a patient with sickle cell disease. *Ann Ophthal* 15 (1983): 873–876.

62. Comer PB, and Fred HJ: Diagnosis of sickle cell disease by ophthalmoscopic inspection of the conjunctiva. *N Engl J Med* 271 (1964): 544–546.

63. Paton D: The conjunctival sign of sickle cell disease: Further observations. *Arch Ophthal* 68 (1962): 627–632.

64. Diggs LW: Sickle cell leg ulcers: Pathophysiology and treatment. *Sphere* 6 (1981): 5–6.

65. Serjeant GR: Leg ulceration in sickle cell anemia. *Arch Intern Med* 133 (1974): 690–694.

66. Wyatt JB, and Orrahood MD: Massive fat embolization following marrow infarction in sickle cell anemia. *Arch Path* 53 (1952): 233–238.

67. Shelley WM, and Curtis EM: Bone marrow and fat embolism in sickle cell anemia and sickle cell hemoglobin-C dislease. *Bull J Hopkins Hosp* 103 (1958): 8–25.

68. Graber S: Fat embolization associated with sickle cell anemia. *Southern Med J* 34 (1961): 1395–1398.

69. Charache S, and Page DL: Infarction of bone marrow in the sickle cell disorders. *Ann Intern Med* 67 (1967): 1085–1200.
70. Hutchinson RM, Merrick MV, and White JM: Fat embolism in sickle cell disease. *J Clin Pathol* 26 (1973): 620–622.
71. Diggs LW, and Bell A: Intraerythrocytic hemoglobin crystals in sickle cell hemoglobin-C disease. *Blood* 25 (1965): 218–223.
72. Sears DA: The morbidity of sickle cell trait. *Am J Med* 64 (1978): 1021–1026.
73. Jones SR, Binder RA, and Donowho EM: Sudden death in sickle cell trait. *N Engl J Med* 262 (1970): 323–325.
74. Diggs LW: The sickle cell trait in relation to the training and assignment of duties in the Armed Forces. II: Aseptic splenic necrosis. *Aviat Space Environ Med* 55 (1984): 271–276.
75. Diggs LW: The sickle cell trait in relation to the training and assignment of duties in the Armed Forces. III: Hyposthenuria, hematuria, sudden death, rhabdomyolysis and acute tubular necrosis. *Aviat Space Environ Med* 55 (1984): 358–364.
76. Felson B, and Wiot JF, eds.: *Seminars in roentgenology; sickle cell anemia.* Orlando, FL: Grune and Stratton, 1987.

Part II

CLINICAL DIAGNOSIS AND MANAGEMENT OF SICKLE CELL DISEASE

6

Diagnosis of Sickle Cell Disease and Its Related Hemoglobin Disorders

Yih-Ming Yang, Susan Brigham, and Paul I. Liu

Sickle cell anemia was first described in medical literature by James Herrick in 1910 when he observed large numbers of elongated, sickle-shaped red blood cells in the peripheral blood smear of a 20-year-old West Indian student with severe anemia (1). Herrick recognized the chronic nature of the disease and the diversity of clinical findings, including frequent infections, intermittent pain of the muscles of the legs and arms, chronic jaundice with occasional exacerbation of icterus, attacks of pain resembling liver or gall-bladder disease, prolonged leg ulcers, enlargement of the heart, and evidence of kidney damage while he followed the patient for 6 years. He suggested that the disease could not be explained by a lesion of any one organ and might be caused by some unrecognized pathology in the red blood cells.

The definitive laboratory diagnosis of sickle cell disease was not possible until 1949 when Linus Pauling analyzed hemolysate by moving boundary electrophoresis and found that the hemoglobin from a patient with sickle cell anemia had a different mobility from hemoglobin of a normal person (2). An individual with sickle cell trait had both hemoglobins in approximately equal amounts. The work originated the concept of molecular disease and provided a sound explanation of its inheritance pattern.

In 1957, Vernon Ingram demonstrated that sickle hemoglobin was the result of single amino acid substitution of glutamic acid with valine in the number six position of the beta-globin chain by peptide analysis, and thus introduced the science of molecular biology (3).

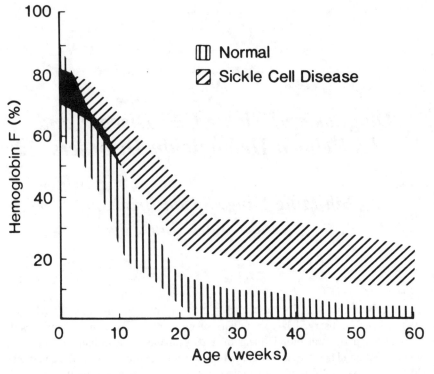

Figure 6.1.   Hemoglobin F decline in children with hemoglobn AA and SS.

Source: Redrawn, with permission, from DG Nathan and FA Oski, eds., *Hematology of Infancy and Childhood* (Philadelphia, W. B. Saunders, 1987). Data from RT O'Brien, S McIntosh; GT Aspnes, et al. (1976); and GR Serjeant, *Clin Hematol* 4 (1975): 109, Fig. 22.10.

GENERAL CONSIDERATIONS

Sickle cell disease may be identified by characteristic clinical manifestations of the disease, evidence of hemolytic anemia, abnormal morphological findings of red blood cells on a peripheral blood smear, or positive screening tests of populations or families.

The clinical syndromes of sickle cell disease are caused by chronic hemolytic anemia and vaso-occlusion due to the sickling process. Clinical manifestations usually occur after the first few months of life as hemoglobin F declines and hemoglobin S increases (see reference 4 and Figure 6.1). Pallor and jaundice due to chronic hemolysis are common after early infancy. Painful swelling of the hands and feet (hand-foot syndrome) due to sickle cell vaso-occlusion may be found in infancy. Recurrent episodes of vaso-occlusive pain crisis of the extremities, joints, and abdomen are common in all ages. Splenic sequestration crisis characterized by a suddenly enlarging spleen and profound anemia associated with cardiovascular collapse, although not common, typically occurs in early age. Aplastic crisis, a transient decrease in red cell production resulting in severe anemia, may occur at any age after infancy. Sickle cell patients are much more susceptible to infections, especially pneumococcal septicemia, mainly due to defective splenic function. Hemoglobin SC disease is a double heterozygous disorder characterized by mild to moderate anemia, enlarged spleen, and recurrent attacks of abdominal, bone, or joint pain. When compared to sickle cell anemia, persons with hemoglobin SC disease have a milder degree of anemia but have similar clinical manifestations with a greater variation in severity. Sickle thalassemia is another double heterozygous hemoglobinopathy. Patients with sickle-β° thalassemia have clinical presentations similar to those with homozygous sickle cell disease; those with sickle-β^+ thalassemia are usually milder clinically. These characteristic clinical manifestations in high risk populations often lead to further laboratory testing and diagnosis of the disease.

A chronic hemolytic anemia in individuals at risk, such as African-Americans, is often caused by sickle cell disease. Hemolytic anemia caused by sickle cell disease may occur early in life or may escape detection until late childhood or even adulthood. Abnormal morphological findings of red blood cells on a peripheral blood smear may be the first noted manifestation of a sickling disorder. The demonstration of irreversibly sickled cells (ISC), increased numbers of target cells or nucleated red cells may herald the diagnosis of a sickle cell disease in a minimally symptomatic patient (see Table 6.1).

Many individuals with sickle cell trait and some with sickle cell disease are diagnosed by screening tests used for populations or families. These include the screening of newborn infants and at-risk populations in schools and in the community. Prenatal diagnosis of sickle cell disease has recently become available for pregnant women who are known to have an increased risk of affected children.

It is important to emphasize that both clinical information and laboratory data are needed for the accurate diagnosis of sickle cell disease and other hemoglobinopathies. Several methods of laboratory testing are available. The necessity of the precise diagnosis of sickle cell disease may vary depending on its use in clinical management or academic research. In clinical practice, satisfactory diagnosis is made by characteristic clinical manifestations and laboratory findings, while in academic research, efforts for precise genotypic determination of hemoglobin variants are usually pursued.

LABORATORY FEATURES IN SICKLE CELL DISEASE

A patient with sickle cell anemia usually presents a moderately severe normocytic normochromic hemolytic anemia by the age of 4 months. Hemoglobin is in the range of 5.5–9.5 gm/dl with an average of 7.5 gm/dl and hematocrit is in the range of 17–29 percent with an average of 22 percent. The reticulocyte count is in the range of 3–25 percent with an average of 12 percent. Nucleated

Table 6.1
Diagnostic Guide for Common Sickle Cell Disease

Diagnosis	Hb/Hct (gm/dl)(%)	Retic (%)	MCV (fl)	Red Cells		Hb F Distribution	Hb Pattern (%)	Clinical Severity
				ISC	Target			
SS	5.5-9.5/17-29	3-25	80-98	4+	2+	uneven	S 80-98 F 2-20	severe
SC	9.5-12/30-36	1-7	65-95	1+	4+		S 45-55 C 45-55	mild to severe
S-β° Thal	6.5-10/20-30	3-18	63-88	3+	3+	uneven	S 70-95 F 2-20 A_2 3-6	moderate to severe
S-β^+ Thal	9.5-12/30-36	2-6	62-84	1+	3+	uneven	S 50-90 F 0-20 A 10-30 A_2 2-4	mild to moderate
SS-α Thal	8-10/25-30	5-15	59-79	2+	2+	uneven	S 65-95 F 2-30 A_2 2-4	mild to severe
SD Los Angeles or Punjab	7-10/20-30	4-14	81-120	3+	3+		S 45-55 D 45-55	moderate to severe
S-HPFH	12-16/38-48	0.5-3	75-88	-	±	even	S 60-80 F 15-35 A_2 0-2	asymptomatic

red blood cells are commonly observed with 1 to 20 per 100 white blood cells. Peripheral blood smear shows red blood cell morphologic abnormalities including irreversibly sickled cells, polychromatophilia, target cells, spherocytes, fragments, biconcave discs, nucleated red cells, and Howell-Jolly bodies. The presence of Howell-Jolly bodies suggests the state of functional hyposplenia.

Double heterozygous sickle cell disease, such as Hb SC disease, Hb $SD_{Los\ Angeles}$ or SD_{Punjab} disease, S-β° thalassemia, S-β^+ thalassemia, and SS α-thalassemia, all manifest chronic hemolysis and sickling complications with varieties of severity. It is important to differentiate sickle-hereditary persistence of fetal hemoglobin (S-HPFH) from clinically significant sickle cell disease since individuals with S-HPFH are asymptomatic. The representative hematological findings and clinical severity are summarized in Table 6.1 for diagnostic reference.

The white blood cell count is consistently increased with a range of $10-30 \times 10^9/L$ and an average of $12 \times 10^9/L$. This elevated white blood cell count in steady state is possibly due to a shift of neutrophils from the marginated pool to the circulating compartment and to loss of splenic function.

The bone marrow usually shows hypercellularity and marked erythroid hyperplasia reflecting the state of increased bone marrow activity caused by the chronic hemolysis. Iron metabolism and stores are usually normal, with normal ferritin, serum iron–binding capacity, and marrow iron stores unless repeated transfusions have been given. Levels of coagulation factor VIII and fibrinogen may be increased, along with elevated platelet count in steady state.

SIMPLIFIED TESTS FOR IDENTIFICATION OF SICKLE HEMOGLOBINS

Solubility Tests

The solubility test is based on the fact that solubility is markedly decreased in deoxygenated hemoglobin S (Hb S). Insoluable and precipitating polymers called tactoids are formed when Hb S is deoxygenated with a reducing substance and is exposed to concentrated salt solutions. Tactoids refract and deflect light rays, producing a visual turbidity (5). This test quickly identifies blood that contains Hb S. Although the solubility test confirms the presence of sickling hemoglobins, it is not specific for Hb S. Positive sickling tests should be substantiated by hemoglobin electrophoresis or other diagnostic laboratory tests since other sickling hemoglobins, such as C_{Harlem}, $C_{Georgetown}$, S_{Travis}, and $C_{Zinguincher}$, will also give positive tests.

The solubility test is primarily used to distinguish Hb S from the similar electrophoretically migrating Hb variants D, G, and Lepore, and is also used in clinical laboratories as the rapid test for screening potential sickle cell patients in the emergency room or hospital. This method can not be used as a testing technique for screening programs where the results will be used for genetic counseling.

The reagents in most commercialized methods include: (1) saponin—a detergent that lyses red blood cells and conveniently allows the use of whole blood, (2) sodium hydrosulfite (or sodium dithionite) to deoxygenate oxyhemoglobin, and (3) a high-molarity phosphate buffer to induce the insolubility of deoxyhemoglobin. A specimen of anticoagulated whole blood is added to the prepared reagents. Five minutes later, the mixture is held in front of a black-lined white card. A positive test for Hb S is indicated by a very turbid solution in which black lines on the white card cannot be distinguished through the solution. A negative solubility test is indicated when the black lines are clearly visible through the solution (see Figure 6.2). False positive tests can occur due to hyperlipidemia, dysglobulinemia, and polycythemia. In many such cases, it is useful to prepare a hemolysate or to wash the red blood cells in 0.9 percent saline. False negative tests are often attributed to anemia (Hb < 7gm/dl) and newborn infants with sickle cell disease or trait who express low percentages (< 15% of total) of sickling hemoglobins. The solubility test is the most commonly used method for quick identification of sickle hemoglobin because of its simplicity and quickness and the minimal equipment involved.

Mechanical Instability Test

The mechanical instability test is a qualitative and semiquantitative assay for Hb S. It is based on the observation that vigorous shaking of oxygenated Hb S in solution results in denaturation and precipitation of the hemoglobin. Turbidity of the solution implies the presence of Hb S or other mechanically unstable hemoglobins. There are many variations of the mechanical instability test. The basic method is performed by adding a concentrated solution of red blood cells to a tube containing 0.01 M sodium phosphate buffer, pH 8.0 (6). The solution is then shaken or vortexed for a short period of time. Next, the tube is inspected for turbidity, which indicates the presence of Hb S. Quantitation of the percentage of Hb S can be measured by spectrophotometer before and after shaking.

In a study of 599 blood samples, including 55 persons with sickling disorders and 47 others with unusual hemoglobin patterns, the shake test accurately identified patients with Hbs AS, SA, or SS as confirmed by the solubility and electrophoretic tests (7). There were no false negative results. The clinical implication of this technique is similar to that of the solubility test. However, several rare hemoglobin variants, such as Hb C_{Harlem}, Hb $M_{Saskatoon}$, Hb Leiden, Hb Gun Hill, Hb Shepherds Bush, Hb Zürich and Hb H can also form precipitation by vigorous shaking.

Slide Sickling Test

Red blood cells may form crescentic shapes when red cells containing 20 percent Hb S are deoxygenated. The sickling phenomenon can be observed by simply sealing blood between glass slides for 24 hours. A rapid and reliable test

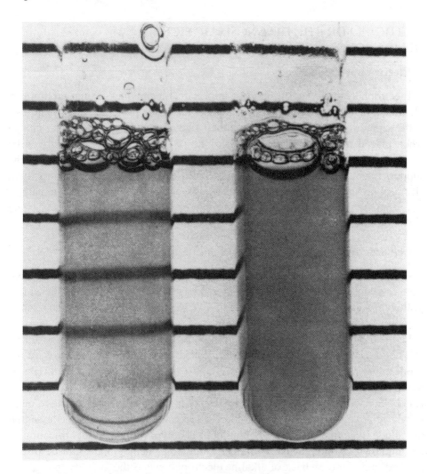

Figure 6.2. Positive (right) and negative (left) solubility tests.

Source: Dade^R Sickle-Sol^{TM} product package insert, Dade Division, Baxter Healthcare Corporation. Reproduced with permission.

for sickling formation is accomplished by mixing blood to be tested with a freshly prepared solution of 2 percent sodium metabisulphite, a reducing agent, and then sealing it under a glass coverslip (8). Sickling usually occurs within a few minutes in cells of individuals with sickle cell disease containing greater than 50 percent Hb S. In red blood cells of sickle cell trait patients containing 40 percent or less Hb S, sickling occurs slowly and usually assume a ''holly leaf'' shape.

METHODS FOR THE DIAGNOSIS OF SICKLE
HEMOGLOBIN AND ABNORMAL HEMOGLOBINS

Electrophoretic Methods

Electrophoresis is one of the most informative techniques for the preliminary identification of normal and abnormal hemoglobins. In principle, electrophoresis is the separation of proteins based on their size, structure, and molecular charge when placed in an electrical field. The rate of separation or migration can be manipulated by altering the pH and ionic strength of the buffer system, the support medium, and the voltage applied. Based on the results of hemoglobin electrophoresis, the diagnosis of sickle cell disease and other hemoglobinopathies can be made. Hemoglobin patterns of common forms of sickle cell disease and thalassemia are shown in Table 6.2 (9).

Cellulose Acetate Electrophoresis

Cellulose acetate membranes can discriminate many of the major hemoglobin bands within a short time period, and vendors have made this medium widely available. At a pH of 8.4–8.6 with a Tris-EDTA borate (TEB) buffer, the relative mobilities of hemoglobins on cellulose acetate from anode to cathode are depicted in Figure 6.3 (10). Abnormal hemoglobins with amino acid substitutions resulting in a net negative charge such as Hbs H, I, N, Bart's, J, and K move toward the anode more rapidly than Hb A. Hbs H and I are the most anodal with Hbs J, K, N, and Bart's, having mobilities intermediate between those of H and A. Hbs F, S, C and A_2, with varying degrees of a net positive charge, move more slowly relative to Hb A. When a clinical specimen is evaluated, it is essential to include a sample of known hemoglobin genotypes to aid in identification of the unknown. Although many clinically important hemoglobins can be distinguished, a major drawback of alkaline electrophoresis is the inability to discriminate different abnormal hemoglobins that migrate together. For instance, over 20 hemoglobin variants have electrophoretic mobilities similar to Hb S; with Hbs D, $G_{Philadelphia}$, and Lepore being the more frequently encountered. Likewise, Hbs A_2, C, O_{Arab}, and E cannot be differentiated on the basis of electrophoretic mobility on cellulose acetate alone. In addition, hemoglobin F may be poorly resolved from Hb A. A major limitation in the analysis of cord blood with alkaline electrophoresis is the distinction of homozygous Hb S disease from Hb AS heterozygote or S-β^+ thalassemia, since acetylated Hb F and Hb A migrate closely together. Many of these difficulties of interpretation can be overcome by an additional electrophoretic separation on citrate agar.

Citrate Agar Electrophoresis

Hemoglobin electrophoresis on citrate agar provides a greater degree of discrimination between Hbs F, A, S, and C and essential confirmation of other variants. This method employs a citrate buffer at pH 6.0–6.2 and an agar base as the

Table 6.2

Hemoglobin Patterns and Red Blood Cell Morphology in Sickle Cell Disease and Thalassemia

Hemoglobin Pattern	A(%)	A₂(%)	F(%)	Abnormal Hb(%)	RBC Morphology
Normal	97	0-2	0-2		Normal
Sickle Cell Anemia	0	2-4	2-20	S 80-98	Sickle Cell 4+
Sickle Cell Trait	48-60	0-2	0-2	S 38-48	Normal
Sickle-β° Thalassemia	0	3-6	2-20	S 70-95	Sickle Cell 2+ Target Cell 2+
Sickle-β⁺ Thalassemia	10-30	3-6	0-20	S 50-87	Sickle Cell 1+ Target Cell 3+
Sickle-HPFH	0	0-2	15-35	S 60-80	Target Cell 2+
Hb SS α Thalassemia	0	2-4	2-30	S 65-95	Sickle Cell 2+ Target Cell 2+
Hb SC Disease	0	0-2	0-8	S 45-55 C 45-55	Sickle Cell 1+ Target Cell 4+
Hb CC Disease	0		0-3	C 97-100	Target Cell 4+
Hb SE Disease	0		0-2	S 60-64 E 34-40	Sickle Cell ± Target Cell 2+
β Thalassemia Major	0-30	1-6	70-90		Target Cell 4+
β Thalassemia Minor	90	3-9	0-10		Target Cell 2+
Hb H Disease	0-85	0-2	0-4	H 15-40	Target Cell 2+
Hb SO_Arab Disease	0		2-28	S 40-56 O 41-46	Sickle Cell 3+ Target Cell 1+
Hb SS-G Disease	0		1-3	S 62-63 G 34-37	Sickle Cell 3+ Target Cell 1+
Hb SD Disease	0	0-3	2-20	S 45-55 D 45-55	Sickle Cell 3+ Target Cell 1+

Source: Adapted from PI Liu, Erythrocyte disorders, in PI Liu, ed., *Diagnostic Tests* (Philadelphia: W. B. Saunders, Blue Book Series, 1986), p. 23.

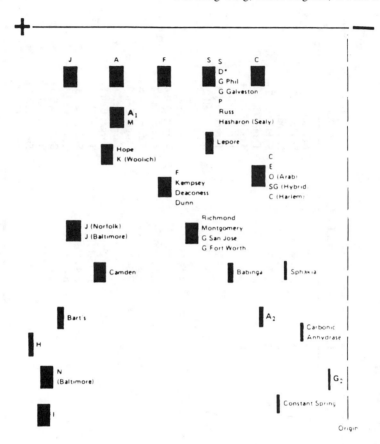

Figure 6.3. Relative mobilities of hemoglobins on cellulose acetate at pH 8.4.

Source: U.S. Department of Health Services, *Laboratory Methods for Detecting Hemoglobinopathies*. (Atlanta: Centers for Disease Control, 1984), p. 84. Reproduced with permission.

support medium (10). Agaropectin, a major component of purified agar, has the ability to bind reversibly with a small number of amino acids of hemoglobin at the surface, within heme pockets or at the 2,3 DPG binding sites of the β-globin chains. Complexed hemoglobin-agaropectin migrates through the gel matrix toward the anode, whereas noncomplexed hemoglobin is carried toward the cathode. Hbs D_{Punjab} and $G_{Philadelphia}$, with similar substitutions deeper in the molecule, have low affinities for agaropectin. Likewise, Hb C has a high affinity for agaropectin, while Hb E does not. Thus, migration of the hemoglobins is influenced not only by molecular charge but also by the relative solubility and affinity for agaropectin in the agar medium. Electrophoretically, Hbs C and F show the most anodal and cathodal migration patterns respectively. Hbs A, D, G, and Lepore co-migrate

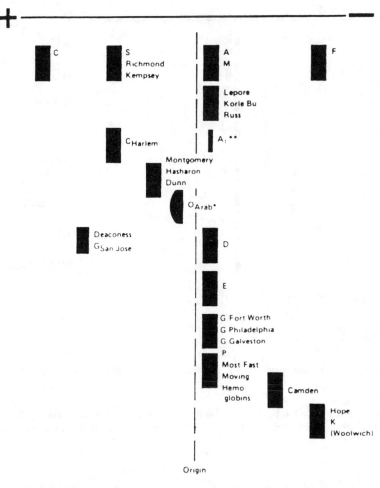

Figure 6.4.   Relative mobilities of some hemoglobins on citrate agar at pH 6.0–6.2.

Source: U.S. Department of Health Services, *Laboratory Methods for Detecting Hemoglobinopathies* (Atlanta: Centers for Disease Control, 1984), p. 87. Reproduced with permission.

slightly toward the cathode and are thus easily differentiated from the anodal migration of Hb S. Hb E, which also migrates with A, is readily discriminated from C. Hb O$_{Arab}$ is slightly more cathodal than A and thus serves to delineate it from C, in addition to Hbs A, D, G, and E. Hb A$_2$ co-migrates with Hb A. The relative mobilities of hemoglobins in citrate agar are depicted in Figure 6.4 (10).

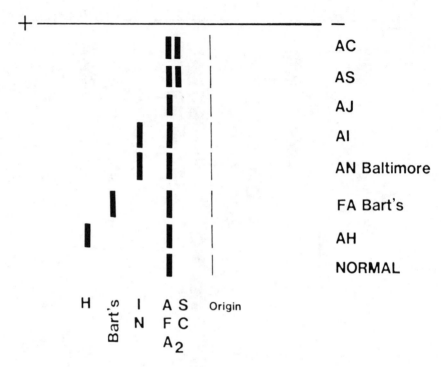

Figure 6.5.   Comparison of some fast-moving hemoglobins on cellulose acetate at pH 7.0.

Source: Redrawn from U.S. Department of Health Services, *Laboratory Methods for Detecting Hemoglobinopathies* (Atlanta: Center for Disease Control, 1984), p. 76. Used with permission.

Neutral pH Electrophoresis

For many of the fast-moving Hbs, N, I, Bart's and H, their exact identification on alkaline cellulose acetate is a definite challenge. Verification is complicated by their potentially low concentration and rapid diffusion of these fast-moving bands (10). However, a sharper demarcation of these fast-moving hemoglobins can be obtained when electrophoresis is performed at a neutral pH. This method employs a sodium phosphate buffer at pH 6.9–7.1 with migration on cellulose acetate of Hbs H and Bart's toward the anode, causing them to separate from Hb A and other fast-migrating hemoglobins (Figure 6.5).

Globin Chain Electrophoresis

In instances where a combination of cellulose acetate and citrate agar electrophoresis alone are not sufficient to differentiate abnormal hemoglobin variants, disassociation of the hemoglobin tetramer with urea and mercaptoethanol can aid in its identification. Specifically, the hemoglobin molecule is disassociated into heme and globin moieties upon treatment with urea and mercaptoethanol. Mercaptoethanol removes heme, whereas globin chains are disassociated from each other by treatment with urea and are separated by electrophoresis. A combination of acid TEB buffers (pH 6.0) or alkaline TEB buffers (pH 8.9) are most useful in differentiating abnormal variants (10). In either type of electrophoresis, α-chains migrate toward the cathode, and β-chains toward the anode. Acid globin electrophoresis will differentiate Hbs O and β^D, which migrates anodaly from Hb E.

In addition, acid electrophoresis can distinguish the globin chains β^D from β^S and G from Hasharon, thus helping to discriminate between Hbs D_{Punjab}, $G_{Philadelphia}$, and Hasharon. Alkaline globin electrophoresis is most useful in differentiating Hbs I and N.

Isoelectric Focusing Electrophoresis

Another form of electrophoresis referred to as isoelectric focusing (IEF) has been developed to detect and quantitate hemoglobins. Isoelectric focusing utilizes the concept that proteins have a sharply defined isoelectric point (PI) within a narrow pH range. A pH gradient is created by the use of carrier ampholytes which, under electrophoretic conditions, form a natural pH gradient. By varying the pH of the medium and applying an electric field, proteins migrate until the pH of the agarose medium equals the isoelectric point of the protein. Proteins that differ in their isoelectric point values by only 0.02 pH unit have been identified. Hemoglobins can best be separated with a pH gradient between pH 6 and 8 on 4 percent polyacrylamide gels developed with carrier ampholyte (7). The separated hemoglobins can be quantitated by use of a densitometer with or without a general protein stain. The relative migration of hemoglobins after IEF from anode to cathode is in the order: Hbs A, F, S, and C and is shown in Figure 6.6. Isoelectric focusing clearly separates Hbs A and F, in addition to D and S.

Isoelectric focusing can often obtain results that are more sensitive and resolving for abnormal Hb variants than conventional alkaline electrophoresis. For instance, many hemoglobin variants migrate closely with Hbs A, S, and C on cellulose acetate, and additional methods are often necessary for identification. In contrast, IEF has been shown to clearly distinguish as many as 70 variants in a one-step procedure (11). Only one variant, Hb $G_{Galveston}$, was indistinguishable from other Hb S–like variants in this study. Acid electrophoresis can clarify these migration patterns in the majority of cases but IEF offers an alternative possibility. In a large-scale cord blood screening program for sickle cell disease and related thalassemias utilizing 835 cord blood samples, IEF correctly identified 100 percent of normal and abnormal hemoglobins, whereas 22 samples were misdiagnosed by a combined alkaline and acid electrophoresis interpretation (12). This combination failed to detect 20 samples containing Bart's hemoglobin and gave incorrect results in two FAS samples. In contrast, IEF clearly separated

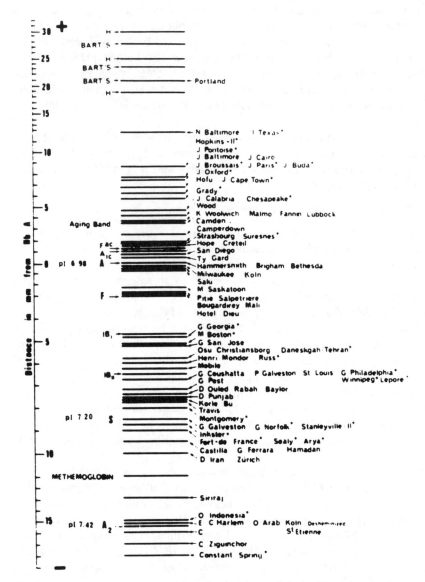

Figure 6.6. Characterization of 70 mutations of human hemoglobin by isoelectric focusing.

Source: P Basset, F Braconnier, and J Rosa: An update on electrophoretic and chromatographic methods in the diagnosis of hemoglobinopathies. *J Chromatogra Biomed Appl* 227, (1982): 284, Fig. 10.

Hb Bart's, acetylated Hb F, Hb A, nonacetylated Hb F, and Hb S, in addition to accurately identifying Hbs C, D, and E variants.

In the past, isoelectric focusing for hemoglobin used to be a time-consuming, bulky, and expensive technique that restricted its use in most clinical laboratories. However, the advent of commercial precast thin-layer gels containing ampholytes and the application of high voltages have streamlined this method into a convenient, rapid, and economical alternative. The primary disadvantage of IEF is the rather significant degree of technical acumen required to discriminate the variant hemoglobins scattered over numerous focusing positions.

Chromatography

For a better preparative isolation, quantitative identification, and quantitative analysis of hemoglobin variants, chromatographic techniques are currently a useful and popular method. In these techniques, a hemoglobin solution is layered on the top of a column filled with support particles and allowed to flow through this bed. The physical characteristics of the hemoglobin variant result in different degrees of retention in the support particle matrix and subsequently, under appropriate conditions, permits separation. The amphoteric property of hemoglobin molecule and the availability of both anion and cation exchanges make ion exchange chromatography, which separates proteins based on differing electrical charges, the most powerful and widely used method of all types of chromatography.

Macrochromatography

Macrochromatography, employing a large-size column and handling up to 150 mg of hemoglobin, is primarily used to separate and quantitate normal and abnormal hemoglobin fractions. Up to seven hemoglobin fractions have been separated from normal and cord red blood cell hemolysates. Similar separations can also be obtained for sickle cell and Hb C homozygote patients. Use of the ion exchanges DEAE-cellulose, DEAE-Sephadex, or CM-cellulose thus far offers the best separation of Hbs S, F, A_0 and A_1. Although macrochromatography techniques as reproducible and quantitative data are reliable, their lengthy procedures (2–3 days) do not easily lend to self-automation in which several chromatographic profiles can be obtained.

Microchromatography

Microchromatography is an inexpensive and rapid means for the detection and quantitative determination of primarily Hb A_2, as well as the hemoglobin variants S, D, C, J, and N. In addition, it is becoming a method of choice for large-scale cord blood screening programs for hemoglobinopathies, especially sickle cell anemia. Microchromatography quantitation of A_2 typically employs the use of pasture pipets, 5 ml serological pipets, or small disposable commercial columns. The column is usually packed with DEAE-cellulose, and then either whole blood or red cell hemolysate are added to the gel bed. With the appropriate developers, Hb A_2 and remaining hemoglobins are eluted separately and the optical densities at 415 nm are determined. Within a 30-minute time span, an accurate quantitation of Hb A_2 can be obtained. Hb A_2 level is often helpful in the differentiation between sickle cell anemia and sickle-$\beta°$ thalassemia and in the diagnosis of β thalassemia minor. The rapid diagnosis of sickle cell anemia at birth has recently been approached through microchromatography (13). Using the cation exchange, CM-Sephadex, and appropriate developers, Hb F is quickly washed from the columns while Hbs A, S, and C remain fixed. At the end of development, a presumptive diagnosis of sickle cell anemia, sickle cell trait, and C trait can be obtained. In all, microchromatography techniques offer a rapid and accurate identification of the most common hemoglobin variants.

High-Performance Liquid Chromatography

The use of high-performance liquid chromatography (HPLC) for the identification and quantitation of hemoglobin variants is a rather new and exciting phase emerging from progressive improvements in chromatographic techniques. The HPLC system consists of a rigid microparticulate support medium, a high-pressure continuous-flow gradient pumping system, and a variety of highly sensitive detectors. This system results in a rapid, sensitive, and highly resolved technique. Several types of ion exchangers have been prepared for HPLC application. In general, HPLC of human hemoglobin molecules with anion exchanges has been able to resolve many of the major hemoglobins with improved separation over electrophoresis of Hb A and Hb F in the neonate (14). In addition, an anion exchanger prepared by the cross-linking of low-molecular-weight polyethylenimine has successfully diagnosed hemoglobin disorders such as AS, AC, SS, CC, SC, and S(C)-β^+ thalassemia (see Figure 6.7; and reference 15). However, the limitation of anion exchangers is their inability to detect fast-moving variants such as Hbs J, N, or Bart's, and their lack of ability to resolve rare hemoglobin variants. Major advances in resolving hemoglobin variants rapidly and accurately have been achieved through the use of cation exchangers. The most successful material thus far is a weak cation exchanger prepared by coating silica with poly-aspartic acid (16, 17). The resolution and sensitivity of this method is excellent, providing chromatographic patterns and identifying infants and children with various hemoglobinopathies that standard electrophoretic techniques would have failed to detect. In addition, a complete resolution of A_2 as compared to the reference method, DEAE-cellulose, can also be obtained. The high resolution of this technique makes it possible to identify hemoglobin variants such as Bart's, AC, AD, AE, AG, AS, ASG, CC, SC, SS, Camden, Lepore, Koln, Osu Christianberg, $Q_{Thailand}$, O_{Arab}, Winnipeg, and Sealy. The sensitivity and accuracy of the method make it also possible to diagnose the variants of thalassemia. The system can be fully automated and requires minimal technician time. Moreover, the column gel material is stable for at least 300 analyses without compromising resolution and efficiency. This new achieve-

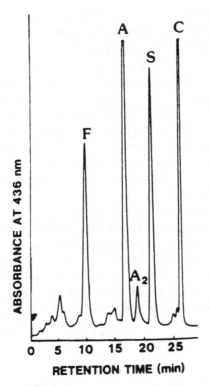

Figure 6.7. Cation-exchange high-performance liquid chromatography pattern of control containing hemoglobin F, A, A$_2$, S, and C.

Source: BB Rogers; RA Wessels, CN Ou, et al.: High performance liquid chromatography in the diagnosis of hemoglobinopathies and thalasemias, *Am J Clin Path* 84 (1985): 672.

ment in HPLC technology should provide an efficient and accurate diagnosis of common and rare hemoglobinopathies in the adult and high-risk newborn populations.

Immunoassays

Several immunoassays have recently been developed for the detection of hemoglobin variants. These assays are based on the exquisite sensitivity and specificity of the immune system for recognizing single amino acid substitutions. Both radioimmunoassays (RIA) and enzyme-linked immunosorbant assays (ELISA) employing monospecific polyclonal antisera or monoclonal antibodies have been shown to be useful for the identification and quantification of variants (18, 19). Hemoglobin variants with a structural alteration on the surface of the molecule are more antigenic, and these include the most frequently encountered variants.

The monospecific antibody recognizes only the single amino acid substitution in the variant hemoglobin polypeptide chain, with no cross-reactivity for normal hemoglobins or other hemoglobin variants containing a different amino acid substitution at the same position.

Recent advances in hybridoma technologies have produced monoclonal antibodies to the major hemoglobin variants. The innate restricted specificity of a monoclonal antibody for the variant hemoglobin makes it even more ideal for most immunoassays as compared to the conventional polyclonal antisera. Radioimmunoassays have been developed employing monospecific antisera capable of recognizing and quantifying approximately 40 hemoglobin variants in red cell hemolysates of adults and newborns (20). The advantages of these assays are that only a very small amount of the sample is needed (nanograms of abnormal hemoglobin can be detected in micrograms of sample) and no purification of the hemoglobin variant is required. The major limitations of this method include the time-consuming production and screening of the antisera and the ever-present hazards of radioactive material. Thus, RIAs for the detection of variant hemoglobins have primarily remained a research tool. A new commercial ELISA kit has been developed for rapid screening of newborn and adult. It employs a Hb S-specific monoclonal antibody and may be used for large-scale screening programs (19).

Peptide Analysis

Peptide analysis has remained the major method used to precisely identify the exact amino acid substitution of hemoglobin variants since Vernon Ingram first applied it to characterize the molecular defect of sickle hemoglobin (3).

The globin chain is purified after being separated from heme and is then digested by a proteolytic enzyme, trypsin. Trypsin specifically cleaves the polypeptide on the carboxyl side of its lysine and arginine residues, leading to the formation of different small peptides. Separation of these peptides is accomplished by using high-voltage electrophoresis followed by cross-dimentional paper chromatography based on their degree of polarity and net charge. The pattern of peptide spots is visualized by staining with ninhydrin and is called fingerprinting or peptide mapping. Amino acid analysis and sequencing is then performed on the abnormal peptide to determine the amino acid substitution of the hemoglobin variant.

Most hemoglobin variants have had their amino acid substitution identified by peptide analysis and amino acid sequencing. Because of the complexity of these techniques, they are only performed in some well-equipped research laboratories and are only used when a precise analysis of abnormal hemoglobin is indicated or when a possible new variant is anticipated.

DNA Analysis

Recombinant DNA technology has rapidly expanded our knowledge of the organization and structure of human globin genes. Established gene maps of globin DNA have been prepared and are now used to detect the presence or absence of a specific gene. At present, DNA analysis can precisely identify almost all the sickle cell disease and clinically significant hemoglobinopathies. Moreover, fetal DNA obtained by amniocentesis or chorionic villus sampling can be analyzed making prenatal diagnosis of the hemoglobinopathies possible. (The technical aspect and clinical application of DNA analysis are discussed in the "Prenatal Diagnosis" section in Chapter 7.)

REFERENCES

1. Herrick JB: Peculiar elongated and sickle-shaped red blood corpuscles in a case of severe anemia. *Arch Intern Med* 6 (1910): 517–521.
2. Pauling L, Itano HA, Singer SJ, et al.: Sickle cell anemia: A molecular disease. *Science* 110 (1949): 543–548.
3. Ingram VM: Gene mutation in human haemoglobin: The clinical difference between normal and sickle cell haemoglobin. *Nature* 180 (1957): 326–328.
4. O'Brien RT, McIntosh S, Aspnes GT, et al.: Prospective study of sickle cell anemia in infancy. *J Peds* 89 (1976): 205–210.
5. Nalbandian RM, Nichols BM, Camp FR, et al.: Dithionite tube test—A rapid, inexpensive technique for detection of hemoglobin S and non-S sickling hemoglobin. *Clin Chem* 17 (1971): 1028–1032.
6. Asakura T, Agarwal PL, Relman DA, et al.: Mechanical instability of the oxy form of sickle hemoglobin. *Nature* 244 (1973): 437–438.
7. Asakura T, Segal M, Friedman S, et al.: A rapid test for sickle hemoglobin. *JAMA* 233 (1975): 156–157.
8. Daland GA and Castle WB: A simple and rapid method for demonstrating sickling of the red cells: The use of reducing agents. *J Lab Clin Med* 33 (1948): 1082–1088.
9. Liu PI: Erythrocytic disorders. In PI Liu, ed.: *Blue book of diagnostic tests*, pp. 22–23. Philadelphia: W. B. Saunders, 1986.
10. U.S. Dept. of Health Services/Public Health Service Center for Disease Control/ Division of Host Factors: *Laboratory methods for detecting hemoglobinopathies*, pp. 45–76. Atlanta: Centers for Disease Control, 1984.
11. Basset P, Beozard Y, Garcel MD, et al.: Isoelectric focusing of human hemoglobin: Its application to screening to the characterization of 70 variants, and to the study of modified fractions of normal hemoglobins. *Blood* 51 (1978): 971–982.
12. Galacteros F, Kleman K, Caburi-Martin J, et al.: Blood screening of hemoglobin abnormalities by thin layer isoelectric focusing. *Blood* 56 (1980): 1068–1071.
13. Powers D, Schroeder W, and White L: Rapid diagnosis of sickle cell disease at birth by microcolumn chromatography. *Pediatrics* 55 (1975): 630–635.
14. Huisman JHH, Gardner MB, and Wilson JB: Experiences with the quantitation of

human hemoglobin types by high pressure liquid chromatography. In SM Hanash and GJ Brewer, eds.: *Advances in hemoglobin analysis, Progress in clinical and biological research,* Vol. 60, pp. 69–82. New York: Alan R. Liss, 1981.

15. Hanash SM and Shapiro DN: Separation of human hemoglobins by ion exchange high performance liquid chromatography. *Hemoglobin* 5 (1981): 165–175.

16. Ou CN, Buffone GJ, and Reimer GL: High performance liquid chromatography of human hemoglobins on a new cation exchanger. *J Chromatogra* 266 (1983): 197–205.

17. Rogers BB, Wessels RA, Ou CN, et al.: High performance liquid chromatography in the diagnosis of hemoglobinopathies and thalassemias. *Am J Clin Pathol* 84 (1985): 671–674.

18. Garver FA, Baker MB, Jones CS, et al.: Radioimmunoassay for abnormal hemo-globins. *Science* 196 (1977): 1334–1336.

19. Grenett HE and Garver FA: Identification and quantitation of sickle cell hemoglobin with an enzyme-linked immunosorbent assay (ELISA). *J Lab Clin Med* 96 (1980): 597–605.

20. Garver FA, Baker MB, Jones CS, et al.: Immunochemical identification and quan-titation of variant hemoglobins. *Tex Rep Biol Med* 40 (1980–1981): 167–178.

7

Screening for Sickle Cell Disease

Yih-Ming Yang and Paul I. Liu

Genetic screening is a search for individuals in a population who possess certain genotypes associated with existing disease or are predisposed to future disease that may lead to disease in their offspring or that produce other variants that are of interest but not known to be associated with disease (1). It is a process by which a large population of individuals are separated into a much smaller population of high-risk individuals. Diagnoses are made from this smaller population so that disease can be treated or prevented. Screening for sickle cell disease and other hemoglobinopathies is a selected genetic screening for newborns and other age groups for this inherited disorder.

Absolute prevention is not yet available for sickle cell disease; however, the implementation of a sickle cell screening program can help reduce the mortality and morbidity of the disease by providing optimum medical care to individuals with sickle cell disease and prevent the disease through genetic counseling and education to patients, parents, and relatives. Sickle cell screening, like other genetic screening, should be offered to everyone, although economy may favor limiting the search to high-risk groups. In the United States, high-risk populations for sickle cell genes are African-Americans and some Spanish-speaking groups.

THE NEED FOR SICKLE CELL SCREENING

Ten percent of the population in the United States is of Afro-American origin. Approximately 1 in every 10 Afro-Americans carries genes for hemoglobin S, hemoglobin C, or β-thalassemia, which produce sickle cell disease or its related hemoglobin disorders. One of every 500 black infants born in the United States suffers from sickle cell disease (2).

It has been shown that bacterial infections, especially pneumococcal septicemia, are the main cause of death during infancy and early childhood (3–12). A life-threatening infection like sepsis, meningitis, or pneumonia may be the first manifestation of sickle cell disease. This serious infection may occur early in the first few months of age or even in the neonatal period (9). It is estimated that the susceptibility to pneumococcal infection in individuals with sickle cell disease is 600 times that for the normal population, with 85 percent of all episodes occurring before five years of age (3, 4). The mortality rate may be as high as 35 percent (3, 10, 11).

Gaston and colleagues of the Prophylactic Penicillin Study Group of the Sickle Cell Disease Branch, National Institutes of Health, reported the result of a randomized trial of oral penicillin prophylaxis in children with sickle cell disease in 1986. They concluded that prophylactic oral penicillin significantly reduced the frequency of pneumococcal infection and also prevented the mortality of pneumococcal infection during the study period (13). They recommended that children should be screened at birth for sickle cell disease and that those with sickle cell disease should receive prophylactic therapy with oral penicillin by four months of age in order to decrease the morbidity and mortality associated with pneumococcal septicemia. An earlier report by John, Ramial, Jackson, et al. in 1984 (14) supported these findings and conclusions. Recently, Vichinsky, Hurst, Earles, et al. reported that newborn screening for sickle cell disease, when combined with adequate follow-up care and education, greatly reduced patient mortality (15). It is apparent that practical prophylactic measures could virtually eliminate the most common fatal complication of sickle cell disease.

Acute splenic sequestration crisis is a life-threatening complication in young sickle cell patients which may contribute to early death (9, 16). Aplastic crisis may lead to severe anemia and result in congestive heart failure. Both conditions must be recognized and treated promptly to prevent irreversible consequences. It has been suggested that mortality can be decreased by educating parents about the clinical manifestations of these crises, which should lead to early recognition and management of episodes (17, 18).

When there is early identification of infants with sickle cell disease by screening newborns, morbidity and mortality can be decreased by the provision of early penicillin prophylaxis, and comprehensive medical care and follow-up as well as education of the parents and family. Early diagnosis of the disease may provide an opportunity to study the natural history of the disease and allow the research and testing of potential interventions.

Screening for the sickle cell gene in other age groups of the high-risk population can lead to the genetic counseling of prospective parents who carry heterozygous sickle cell or other hemoglobinopathy genes. Adequate genetic counseling and education will provide information for parental reproductive decision-making, which may prevent the birth of individuals with the disease.

Some milder forms of sickle cell disease may escape detection until late childhood or even adulthood. The screening for and identification of sickle cell disease in pregnant women and other patients in the at-risk population before they undergo anesthesia or other potentially hypoxic experiences will allow the provision of proper medical care and prevent complications.

Specific goals of sickle cell screening are to: (1) reduce the mortality and morbidity of affected individuals by comprehensive medical care, prophylactic measures such as the administration of oral prophylactic penicillin, education, and supportive service; (2) prevent the disease by providing genetic counseling to patients, parents, and to individuals with the sickle cell trait, disease, or other hemoglobinopathies, through which offspring with homozygous disease may be avoided by reproduction options; and (3) provide information by appropriate follow-up studies that ultimately will be helpful to patients, families, and health care providers in acquiring a better understanding about the heterogeneity, pathological effects, and diverse clinical aspects of this disease.

NEONATAL SCREENING

In early 1970, Robert Scott drew attention to sickle cell disease in the United States by pointing out its high prevalence and relatively low priority in research programs and funding compared to less common childhood diseases (19). Comprehensive sickle cell disease centers and screening programs were subsequently proposed and developed. The passage of the National Sickle Cell Anemia Control Act by the U.S. Congress in 1972 provided appropriated funds for increased research in the pathophysiology and treatment of the disease and for the education, screening, and counseling of individuals with sickle cell trait.

Neonatal testing for sickle cell disease was first done by Howard Pearson and colleagues at Yale–New Haven Hospital in 1972, where they conducted a comprehensive umbilical cord screening for the neonatal diagnosis of hemoglobinopathies (20). This screening program was implemented in a comprehensive sickle cell program, including a clinic for infants with sickle cell disease, extensive education of families regarding the disease, social assistance, and continuing comprehensive medical care. There were no deaths over a 3-year period (21).

Unfortunately, some early mass newborn sickle cell screening efforts created social, ethical, political, and legal problems. These were caused by the failure to distinguish the sickle cell trait from the disease, the compulsory preschool and premarital screening mandated by state laws, the inadequacy in administering community programs, and the confusion resulting from improper testing methods or incorrect screening results (22). These problems raised controversies and created difficulties in screening for sickle cell disease.

With the efforts of many institutions, as well as local, state, and federal groups, to improve the quality of sickle cell screening programs, examples of successful endeavors have been established. A good newborn screening program for sickle cell disease should inform parents properly; use reliable laboratory methods; protect confidentiality; provide adequate education, counseling, and psychosocial support; and ensure optimal medical care and follow-up.

Provision for Mandating Screening

A recent consensus development conference on newborn screening for sickle cell disease and other hemoglobinopathies sponsored by the National Institutes of Health suggested that screening be provided for all newborns as a part of standard health care (23). It is suggested that the implementation of the planning and organization should be required by state law.

The New York Experience

Screening for sickle cell disease was included in New York State's newborn screening program in 1974, 10 years after the program was first established. In the early phase of the sickle cell screening program, of 110,000 initial blood samples tested in the newborn screening laboratory, 440 required repeat testing for definitive diagnosis. Only 227 (52%) of requested samples were received in the screening laboratory to verify the original diagnosis. The failure was caused by a lack of funds and facilities for outreach services and the follow-up of presumptive positive cases (24). Insufficiencies were also experienced by physicians involved in the screening program and by the parents of affected children. They suggested several areas for improvement: (1) maintaining communication among the screening laboratory, the hospitals and the physicians; (2) encouraging physicians to educate parents thoroughly; (3) providing genetic counseling and testing for families of the neonates identified as possessing Hb S; and (4) providing a well-delineated follow-up system for every infant with sickle cell disease (25). In 1979, with funds available from the New York State Genetics Grant, a follow-up program was set up and effective communication established between the initial screening program and the follow-up program. This allowed the screening program to obtain repeat blood samples for definitive diagnosis and referral of diagnosed patients for ongoing medical care. Of the 106,565 blood samples tested over a one-year period; 141 infants were identified on repeat blood testing as having various forms of sickle cell disease. There were no deaths reported among the 131 study patients followed for the period of 8–20 months (26). This experience demonstrated the importance of a well-planned, well-organized screening and follow-up program in newborn sickle cell screening.

The ultimate goal of newborn sickle cell testing is to include the screening procedure as an integral part of standard health care. Implementation of the neonatal screening program can be best achieved by implanting into, or coordinating with, an ongoing comprehensive sickle cell program or an existing newborn screening follow-up program. Adequate funding should be sought and secured from appropriate local, state, or federal agencies.

A successful newborn sickle cell screening program needs a well-structured program that should not only establish a proper testing and follow-up procedure as well as adequate communication between the participating services but also should monitor the efficiency and quality of screening and follow-up programs. A steering committee formed by the representatives of all major services or

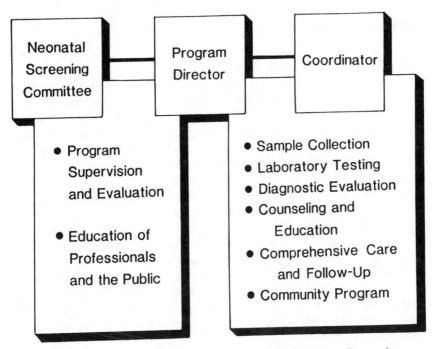

Figure 7.1. Suggested structure of organization in neonatal sickle cell screening
programs.

departments of the screening program, along with an executive director and
coordinator, can enhance the program by overall planning, supervision, and
coordination of participating personnel and services (27). A suggested structure
of organization is shown in Figure 7.1.

Informing Mother/Parents

The health care provider should inform expectant mothers about the reason
for and availability of newborn sickle cell screening along with other newborn
screening tests as part of prenatal education. Thorough information on sickle
cell screening should be provided in understandable language and should explain
that: (1) sickle cell disease and other hemoglobinopathies are diseases of the
blood that primarily affect black Americans, people of Mediterranian and South-
east Asian descent, and some Spanish-speaking groups; (2) by obtaining either
cord blood or heel-stick blood sample screening for sickle cell disease will
produce no side effects for the newborn baby; and (3) individuals have the right
to withdraw from the screening program and are assured of confidentiality of
testing results; and it should describe (4) the difference between sickle cell disease
and sickle cell trait; and (5) how sickle cell disease is manifested.

Laboratory Methods

Either cord blood specimen or filter paper specimen taken by heel-stick of the newborn is adequate for laboratory analysis of hemoglobins. Both methods have advantages and disadvantages. The advantages of using cord blood samples for screening are that the various types of hemoglobins within the samples (e.g., Hb Bart's) are more stable, a sufficiently large sample can be collected at one time for repeated and further analysis when necessary, contamination by transfusion is avoided, and there is no pain to the baby. The disadvantages are that cord blood sample is more cumbersome to transport, and maternal blood contamination can occur.

Blood collected in filter paper by heel-stick is advantageous because it is the commonly used method of sample collection for screening newborns for inborn metabolic errors such as phenylketunuria and hypothyroidism, and the system for sample collection and transport already exists. The disadvantages are that the sample is more susceptible to deterioration and could be contaminated by neonatal blood transfusion, sample collection may be missed when infants are in intensive care nurseries or are discharged early, and the fact that additional sample collection may be difficult when further hemoglobin analysis is required. Most of the sickle cell neonatal screening programs are currently using blood collected in filter paper.

Laboratory methods for newborn screening for sickle cell disease and other hemoglobinopathies should be reliable, standardizable, simple, economical, and adaptable for mass screening (20, 23). The screening method should be specifically able to identify Hb S; to detect when Hb A is absent, thus suggesting an SS homozygote or a double heterozygote for S and another globin variant; and to screen for other potentially pathological hemoglobin states. Tests that detect sickle hemoglobin on the basis of its insolubility in deoxy state or mechanical instability are not suitable in the neonatal period because fetal hemoglobin will render a false negative. Such tests are not suitable even at older ages because traits for C hemoglobin and thalassemias are not detected. There are several reliable laboratory methods that are being applied in newborn screening programs, and they are presented briefly here.

Electrophoresis is presently the most popular procedure used for neonatal and other mass screening. Electrophoresis of hemoglobin at alkaline pH on cellulose acetate, followed by further analysis of abnormal samples by acid electrophoresis on citrate agar, allows reliable detection of Hb S, C, and A in the presence of high concentration of fetal hemoglobin in newborn sample. Some screening programs use both alkaline and acid electrophoreses simultaneously. This is an established standardized method and is simple to perform at low cost. Disadvantages are the requirement of two different electrophoretic procedures to detect certain abnormal hemoglobins, limited resolution in some hemoglobin variants, and possibly lower sensitivity and specificity compared to other methods such as thin layer isoelectric focusing and high-performance liquid chromatography.

The standard laboratory method for detecting hemoglobinopathies established by the U.S. Department of Health and Human Services, Center for Disease Control (28), should be followed.

Thin layer isoelectric focusing has been employed in several newborn screening programs. This analysis gives better resolution of Hb A, S, and C from Hb F and can detect many other abnormal hemoglobins (29). This method requires high technical skill and is used less commonly.

High-performance liquid chromatography (HPLC) is a very sensitive and specific method for hemoglobin analysis (30). With its recently improved high resolution, HPLC is capable of diagnosing and distinguishing many abnormal hemoglobins (31). This method is also highly reproducible. With complete automation, this procedure is simple, rapid, and feasible for use in mass screening (31).

Until a satisfactory method for one-time screening and confirmatory diagnosis of hemoglobinopathies is available, abnormal screening results should be confirmed by a followup repeat testing. Every screening laboratory should have a quality-control program. New methodologies for the precise diagnosis of hemoglobinopathies in the newborn are still developing. The application of DNA analysis can lead to the precise determination of the α and β genotype of the patient in the neonatal period.

Results of Neonatal Screening for Sickle Cell Disease

The incidence of abnormal hemoglobins in neonatal screening programs for the black population is about 12 percent, of which Hb FAS is 6–8 percent; FAC, 2 percent; FA Bart's, 2–4 percent; FS, 0.12–0.30 percent; and FSC, 0.1 percent.*
In screening programs for mixed ethnic groups in the United States and England, the incidence of abnormal hemoglobins is 0.5–2 percent. The incidence of sickle cell disease varies greatly with the population and area screened in the United States and England (Table 7.1).

Notification and Interpretation of the Results

Screening results should be centralized in the screening program in order to assure the proper notification of each client result. All results with normal hemoglobin patterns are sent directly to the parent—usually the mother—and the health care provider by mail. If parents and the general public are well informed about the screening, results with abnormal hemoglobins may be reported to the parent

---

*Conventionally, hemoglobins are abbreviated in symbols in order of decreasing proportion. Therefore, FAS in newborns usually suggests sickle cell trait (Hb AS); FAC suggests C trait (Hb AC); FS suggests homozygous sickle cell anemia (Hb SS), sickle-β° thalassemia, or sickle-HPFH (hereditary persistence of fetal hemoglobin); FA Bart's suggests increased Bart's hemoglobin seen in α-thalassemia traits; and FSC suggests Hb SC disease.

Table 7.1
Incidences of Sickle Cell Disease in the Newborn

| Location | Total No. | Black % | Abnormal Hemoglobin %[*] | | | |
			AS	AC	SS	SC	CC
New York	106,223	35	3.26	0.83	0.18	0.12	0.002
Buffalo	2,435	5-10	0.58	0.12			
Galveston	9,224	100	6.10	1.60	0.13	0.07	
New Haven	3,976	100	7.30	0.13	0.50	0.20	0.001
Birmingham (Eng.)	43,500	10	1.19	0.46	0.006	0.006	
Jamaica	8,000	>95	8.60	2.89	0.30	0.20	0.003

*Percent of all newborns screened.

and the health care provider expeditiously and confidentially. An explanatory letter on the significance of the test result and an appointment with a health care provider or a health worker/counselor of the screening program is offered so that the result can be explained fully and further confirmatory tests or genetic counseling can be arranged. Some screening programs prefer to mail a statement that the test has been completed and a counselor is available to discuss the results. The results with abnormal hemoglobins are not indicated in the notification letter so that people may be less anxious and may benefit more from counseling when the counselor informs them directly.

Interpretation of the test results should include appropriate information on sickle cell trait, sickle cell disease, or other hemoglobinopathies. Further discussion and counseling are also provided in a formal clinic setting. Brief genetic information on the inherited nature of the disease is presented and sickle cell testing is recommended to the parents or other family members. Printed materials with information on sickle cell disease, sickle cell trait, and other hemoglobinopathies may be helpful to parents and relatives.

Follow-Up and Outreach

Results of sickle cell disease or other major hemoglobinopathies may fail to reach the parent of the affected infant or the parent may fail to bring the affected infant back for interpretation of the results, counseling, and follow-up. Therefore, a mechanism of outreach and follow-up is required to assure that adequate medical surveillance and care are provided. This service should be set up and coordinated by the screening program and can be incorporated with a community program or the existing public health system.

Community Aspect

Community participation and support are essential to a successful sickle cell screening program. Community members should be informed and educated to the significance and purpose of sickle cell screening as well as the medical and technical aspects of the program. Screening program members should understand the community need. The administrators of the screening program and the community should work together to discuss the ethical, legal, educational, and socioeconomic aspects of sickle cell screening. Objectives and guidelines of the screening program can be developed by a joint effort of both groups.

Many sickle cell community programs in the United States are actively participating in screening and provide services which are usually integrated into the comprehensive care program, such as education and supplying reference information to the public; medical care referral; counseling services for individuals with the trait, the disease, or at risk; outreach service; supportive service; peer groups; tutoring; vocational training and job placement; and intracommunity referrals and advocacy.

Education

Education of professionals and health care providers is important to the overall, ultimate care of sickle cell patients. Continuing education and training should provide medical professionals and allied health personnel with the knowledge and skills of etiology, pathophysiology, genetics, diagnosis, management, and psychosocial aspects of this disease to assure the comprehensive care of patients with sickle cell disease. This education should also be included within the curricula of schools of medicine, nursing, allied health, and social work.

Public education is also vital to an effective newborn screening program. Misconceptions and lack of knowledge about sickle cell disease and sickle cell trait in the general population have been reported and have been of concern. Education of the general public should include a clear understanding of the disease, the difference between the sickle cell trait and disease, hereditary pattern of the sickle cell gene, the complications and treatment, the purpose of the screening, and the benefits and potential risks of participation in such screening programs. Education should be directed to students at all levels, individuals of childbearing age in the population at risk, and mass media personnel.

Education on the inheritance pattern, clinical manifestations, early complications, and life-threatening symptoms, such as sudden onset of high fever, pallor, or collapse, and available treatment, as well as prophylactic measures, should be emphasized to parents, affected individuals when they are older, and other family members. The primary health care provider should assume this responsibility.

Counseling

Counseling in the areas of general health concerns, genetic significance, and socioeconomic problems should be made available to the general population and especially to individuals with sickle cell trait and disease. Supportive service and other social services should also be provided when needed. Screening programs should work with community program and health care providers to assure the availability of such services.

Genetic counseling should be provided to all individuals who are identified as having sickle cell disease or trait or other hemoglobinopathies. General genetic counseling may be sufficient for individuals who are carriers and can be provided by counselors at the screening or community program. Genetic counseling should be provided to parents of infants with sickle cell disease or other major hemoglobinopathies by a genetic counselor, and the counseling service should be arranged by the screening program or health care provider.

A thorough understanding of the genetic ramifications of sickle cell disease is of practical importance in families of a newborn with sickle cell disease. When an affected newborn is diagnosed, primary functions of the genetic counselor include collecting the family history and pertinent medical, developmental and social histories; identifying and responding to the family's immediate genetic concerns; and briefly introducing the most basic genetic principles. Two to 3 months later, as the family has begun to adjust to their newborn, they are usually much more receptive to a detailed discussion of the inheritance of sickle cell disease and the necessity of carrier detection among relatives. About 6 months after this meeting it is important to assess the family's needs and understanding of sickle cell disease as well as its impact on the family unit, to reinforce prior counseling, and to introduce the issues of planned future pregnancies and options for prenatal diagnosis. Thereafter, a yearly follow-up will allow for updates in areas such as reproductive intentions, carrier testing, and risk counseling for relatives, as well as explanations to the child, siblings, and others.

The genetic counselor can be an integral part of team functions such as assessment and planning in the neonatal screening program. Interface with genetic services is also critical when implementing prenatal diagnosis in families which choose the option in subsequent pregnancies.

Although the major purpose of neonatal screening is to identify infants with sickle cell disease, neonates with the heterozygous state are also identified. It is important to understand that sickle cell trait is invariably a benign state. The key implication of this heterozygous state is a genetic one, for the individual may pass a sickle cell gene to his or her offspring.

When a neonate with sickle cell trait is identified, the screening program should inform a health care provider or designated counseling service to contact the family with the screening result. Counseling and education on the significance of sickle cell trait and the inheritance pattern, as well as family testing, should be offered. Parents and individuals with the trait should be assured that the condition is benign and that it is not necessary to alter their regular activity. They should also be informed about the preventive health implication of this condition. Persons with the trait should avoid extreme altitudes or circumstances in which hypoxia may be experienced. The health care provider and counselor need to be aware that this information could disturb family well-being because it may raise fears of the disease, doubts regarding paternity, and worries about affecting future children. Therefore, sensitivity and prudence should be applied when individual family members are counseled.

Comprehensive Care

Every child who is identified as having sickle cell disease or a clinically significant hemoglobin disorder should have comprehensive care and follow-up (20–23). Continuous, consistent, and comprehensive care should be provided for the physical and psychosocial needs of sickle cell patients and their families. This follow-up program can be placed in a sickle cell center or provided by local health care services and health professionals. This comprehensive program requires good communication and mutual respect between all disciplines and between medical facilities and community organizations.

Components of the comprehensive care program should include sickle cell specialists, knowledgeable nurses, genetic counselors, social workers, and consultant specialists of various disciplines who are familiar with sickle cell problems. Services should include:

1. Laboratory testing to confirm or make the definitive diagnosis of the type of sickle cell disease.
2. Health surveillance
   a. Infection prophylaxis with oral penicillin starting by 4 months of age.
   b. Routine immunization and special vaccinations with hemophilus influenzae B and streptococcus pneumoniae vaccines.
   c. Periodic health maintenance check-up with necessary laboratory tests and growth and development monitoring.
   d. Nutritional advice.
3. Education and counseling
   a. Knowledge of common symptoms and early recognition of manifestations impending serious complications (i.e., fever, pallor, lethargy, enlarging abdomen, weakness of the extremities on one side of the body, and shortness of breath).
   b. Health care management advice.
4. Supportive services and social service
   a. Assistance and counseling on socioeconomic problems.
   b. Peer groups.
   c. Vocational training and job placement and retention.
5. Medical care
   a. Medical service for emergency care and comprehensive medical care.
   b. Transfusion therapy support.
   c. Medical referral system.

SCREENING OF OTHER AGE GROUPS

Sickle cell screening is also recommended for populations at risk other than newborns. The aims of this screening are either to detect the carrier state or to identify homozygous disease in the high-risk population.

Carrier Testing

The primary goal of identifying the carrier state for sickle hemoglobin or an abnormal hemoglobin is to provide accurate genetic information for counseling carriers on reproduction decisions. The health implication of carrier screening is that individuals with sickle cell trait may avoid exposing themselves to reduced oxygen environments. Carrier testing should be coupled with genetic counseling and education.

Carrier testing is best offered to people at risk during, or just prior to, their reproductive years. This carrier screening program may be implemented in target populations, such as communities with high percentages of people at risk, family planning clinics, factories with young workers, and secondary schools and colleges. People at risk for the sickle cell genes need to be screened before they experience hypoxic states, such as occur when climbing high mountains, flying in unpressurized aircraft, and possibly undergoing general anesthesia. Laboratory method for carrier testing should be capable of detecting many β-chain abnormalities such as Hb S, Hb C, and β-thalassemia traits, as any of these traits, when inherited in combination with the sickle cell trait, will result in sickle cell disease.

Screening during Pregnancy

Screening for sickle hemoglobin and other abnormal hemoglobins during pregnancy may serve special purposes or goals. Screening in early pregnancy may serve to detect pregnant women with milder forms of sickle cell disease to whom medical care can be provided to reduce morbidity and mortality during pregnancy and may detect couples who are both carriers of abnormal hemoglobin and to whom genetic counseling and prenatal diagnosis should be offered. Carrier testing for all pregnant women of the population at risk may also serve as the initial screening test for further testing of newborns for the detection of sickle cell disease. This is a more selective approach in which only pregnant women at risk for sickle cell gene or other abnormal hemoglobin gene are screened and only the newborns of mothers who have any of the abnormal hemoglobins will be tested for sickle cell disease.

Screening before Anesthetic Procedures and Experiencing Potentially Hypoxic States

Some patients with sickle cell anemia and double heterozygous sickle cell disease, such as hemoglobin SC disease and sickle β-thalassemia, may have milder clinical manifestation and may escape detection until late childhood or adulthood. Patients or individuals in the high-risk population need to be screened to identify previously unrecognized sickle cell disease before they undergo anesthesia or other potentially hypoxic experiences such as flying in high altitude in nonpressurized aircraft. Proper medical care and precautions can then be undertaken to prevent hypoxia and untoward complications.

RISKS AND BURDENS OF SCREENING

There are risks and burdens of neonatal sickle cell screening (22, 32), but it is clear that the benefits of screening outweigh the risks. Potential risks and burdens include misdiagnosis; interference with parent–child bonding or over-protection of the child; stigmatization; diminished self-esteem; discrimination, especially in employment opportunities; anxiety and guilt of parents and family; family disruption; discovery of nonpaternity; and cost to the public.

These risks or burdens can be minimized or avoided by careful programmatic design and monitoring. Anxiety to the family or individual from the discovery of sickle disease can be reduced through emotional support and appropriate education regarding the nature of the disease and its management. Anxiety resulting from the identification of an individual with sickle cell trait may be minimized by careful counseling that emphasizes that the condition will not affect the health of the individual and that serious complications can be prevented by observing certain precautions. If retesting a child to confirm an uncertain screening result is required, the parent(s) should be approached with sensitivity and caring. Direct patient or parent contact by providers in a screening program rather than indirect methods such as mailed information can reduce the anxiety and potential family disruption. Legal safeguards against discrimination in employment opportunities and insurance eligibility are also necessary. Great care should be taken to ensure the confidentiality of screening results and to maintain the privacy of the family.

PRENATAL DIAGNOSIS

Despite the fact that a reduction of morbidity and mortality of sickle cell disease has been made possible by early detection through newborn screening and early comprehensive care, unpreventable complications with serious or fatal outcomes still exist. Before a cure of sickle cell disease is available, the development of reliable methods for prenatal diagnosis and the availability and safety of early termination of the pregnancy provide an opportunity to prevent the disease.

With the sickle cell screening of the population at risk, couples who are at risk can be identified. Prenatal diagnosis can be discussed and offered to couples who are both carriers of sickle cell or other abnormal hemoglobins. It is important to recognize that prenatal diagnosis is not simply a laboratory exercise. It is a process that requires the identification of pregnancies at risk, genetic counseling, prenatal education about sickle cell disease and trait, procedures involved and potential risks of prenatal diagnosis, and emotional support at a time when difficult and sensitive issues are being discussed and decided. Prenatal diagnosis also needs a well-planned follow-up, both for verification of the diagnosis and for continued interaction with the parents, who frequently have guilt feelings and may feel uncertain about their decision. Good communication between the geneticist, obstetrician and referring physician is essential. Supportive services, including community programs, social services, and the clergy, may be required.

Methods

There are two general ways to establish sickle cell disease and its related hemoglobin disorders. One is to demonstrate the abnormal globin chains by using fetal blood sampling and the other is to analyze globin DNA by using fetal DNA obtained either from amniotic fluid cells or by chorionic villus sampling.

Globin Chain Synthesis Studies

Fetal blood sampling is performed during the second trimester by either fetoscopy or placental aspiration. The fetal blood sample is incubated in a culture medium containing ^{3}H-leucine, which is incorporated into the newly synthesized globin chain. Globin chains are then separated by chromatography and the proportion of radioactivity contained in each chain is calculated (33).

The overall results of prenatal diagnosis of sickle cell disease and other hemoglobin disorders by this method have been very successful. An analysis of 3,959 diagnostic studies (34) showed a diagnostic error of 0.8 percent and had 6.2 percent fetal loss and 1.6 percent maternal complications. This data suggests that this diagnostic approach is reliable and safe in centers performing these procedures regularly.

The major disadvantage is that fetal blood sampling cannot be carried out until late in the second trimester. The parents may therefore have a great deal of anxiety because of the long period of waiting and uncertainty. Therapeutic abortion, if indicated, at 20 weeks gestation or later may be difficult.

DNA Analysis

Fetal DNA can be obtained either from cells in amniotic fluid or chorionic villus sampling. Amniotic fluid cells are usually obtained by transabdominal amniocentesis under guidance of ultra-sonography at 14 to 16 weeks of gestation. About 10 to 30 ml of amniotic fluid is aspirated and transported to a laboratory for processing and subsequent analysis. The yield of DNA from amniotic fluid is usually low and it is usually necessary to culture the fluid for several weeks to obtain sufficient DNA. This process makes the diagnosis unavailable until late in the second trimester (35, 36). Recently, chorionic villus sampling has been used to obtain fetal DNA during the first trimester of pregnancy or at 8 to 12 weeks of gestation. It is possible to obtain a sufficient amount of fetal DNA for analysis by chorionic villus biopsy (37, 38). Fetal loss following amniocentesis is 3.5 percent, and is slightly increased, compared to 3.2 percent, on control subjects. Fetal loss induced by chorionic villus biopsy is about 4 percent.

The technique of DNA analysis for prenatal diagnosis has been greatly advanced over the past 10 years and is still evolving. Gene mapping by restriction enzymes or by oligonucleotide probes have been applied to the prenatal diagnosis of sickle cell anemia and other hemoglonopathies.

Gene Mapping by Restriction Enzyme.   Several restriction endonucleases are known to cut specifically in the region around the sixth codon of the β-globin gene, and this cleavage is prevented by the substitution of T for A in the β^S-mutation. Mst II is the most reliable restriction enzyme to identify the A to T change (39). Prenatal diagnosis of sickle cell disease is accomplished by using Mst II to cleave the total DNA. DNA fragments are detected by electrophoresis and then transferred to filter paper and probed with cDNA probes for the β-globin gene (Southern Blotting).

Oligonucleotide Probes   Short synthetic DNA fragments (i.e., oligonucleotide or oligomers) can be constructed that will hybridize to homologous, but not to heterologous, sequences. Short probes consisting of 19 nucleotides (19-mers), which contain the sequences of the normal β-globin gene in the region of β^S-mutation, hybridize specifically with the normal gene (β^A) but not with β^S-gene (40, 41). Normal and sickle cell DNA sequences can be distinguished after hybridization of restricted total fetal DNA by using highly specific labelling of these synthetic probes. Recently, new enzymatic amplification procedures by using polymerase chain reaction (PCR) have been developed that are much more sensitive and rapid. The β-globin genotype can be determined within 24 hours on minute amounts (less than 1 μg) of genomic DNA (42).

These new reliable and rapid methods make the early prenatal diagnosis of sickle cell disease more feasible and acceptable. The application and utilization of these diagnostic procedures will depend on the perception of the severity of disease by the medical profession, the community, and prospective parents, and by the availability of medical facilities in the area.

REFERENCES

1. Committee for the Study of Inborn Errors of Metabolism, Division of Medical Science, Assembly of Life Science, National Research Council. *Genetic screening: Programs, principles and research.* National Academy of Sciences, Washington, D.C., 1975

2. Motulsky AG: Frequency of sickling disorders in U.S. blacks. *N Engl J Med* 288, no. 1 (1973): 31–33.

3. Overturf GD, Powars D, and Baraff LJ: Bacterial meningitis and septicemia in sickle cell disease. *Am J Dis Child* 131 (1977): 784–787.

4. Robinson MG, and Watson RJ: Pneumococcal meningitis in sickle cell anemia. *N Engl J Med* 274 (1966): 1006–1008

5. Ecckels R, Gatu F, and Kenaurie AM: Abnormal distribution of hemoglobin genotypes in Negro children with severe bacterial infections. *Nature* 216 (1967): 382.

6. Seeler RA, Metzger W, and Mufson MA: Diplococcus pneumoniae infections in children with sickle cell anemia. *Am J Dis Child* 123 (1972): 8–10.

7. Pearson HA: Sickle cell anemia and serious infections due to encapsulated bacteria. *J Infect Dis* 126 (1977): S25–S30.

8. Barrett CF: Bacterial infection and sickle cell anemia: An analysis of 250 infections in 166 patients and a review of the literature. *Medicine (Baltimore)* 50 (1974): 97–112.

9. Roger DW, Clarke JM, Cupidore L, et al.: Early deaths in Jamaican chilu. sickle cell disease. *Br Med J* 1 (1978): 1515–1516.
10. Powers D, Overturf G, Weiss J, et al.: Pneumococcal septisemia in children with sickle cell anemia: Changing trend of survival. *JAMA* 345 (1981): 1839–1842.
11. Kabins SA, and Lerrer C: Fulminant pneumonecemia and sickle cell anemia. *JAMA* 211 (1978): 467–471.
12. Zarkowsky HS, Gallagher D, Gill FM, et al.: Bacteremia in sickle hemoglobino-pathies. *J Pediatr* 109 (1986): 579–585
13. Gaston MH, Verter JI, Woods G, et al. for the Prophylactic Pencillin Study Group: Prophylaxis with oral penicillin in children with sickle cell anemia. *N Engl J Med* 314 (1986): 1593–1599.
14. John AB, Ramial A, Jackson J, et al.: Prevention of pneumococcal infection in children with homozygous sickle cell disease. *Br Med J* 288 (1984): 1567–1570.
15. Vichinsky E, Hurst D, Earles A, et al.: Newborn screening for sickle cell disease: Effect on mortality. *Pediatrics* 81 (1988): 749–755.
16. Powars, D. Natural history of sickle cell disease, The first ten years. *Semin Hematol* 12; no. 3 (1975): 267–285.
17. Emond AM, Collis R, Maude GH, et al.: Acute splenic sequestiation in homozygous sickle cell disease: Natural history and management. *J Peds* 107 (1985): 201–206.
18. Emond AM, Morais P, Venugopal S, Carpenter RG, Serjeant GR: Role of sple-nectomy in homozygous sickle cell disease in childhood. Lancet 8368, no. 1 (1984): 88–91.
19. Scott RB. Health care priority and sickle cell anemia. *JAMA* 214 (1970): 731–734.
20. Pearson HA, O'Brian RT, McIntosh S, et al.: Routine screening of umbilical cord blood for sickle cell disease. *JAMA* 227 (1974): 420–421.
21. Kramer MS, Rooks Y, and Pearson HA. Cord blood screening for sickle hemo-globins. *J Peds* 93 (1978): 998–1000.
22. Miller, DR. Pitfalls of newborn screening for sickle cell anemia. *Am J Dis Child* 133 (1979): 1235–1236.
23. U.S. National Institutes of Health; Office of Medical Applications of Research, Concensus Conference: Newborn screening for sickle cell disease and other hem-oglobinopathies. *JAMA* 258 (1987): 1205–1209.
24. Grover R, Wethers D, Shahidi S, et al.: Evaluation of the expanded newborn screening program in New York City. *Pediatrics* 61 (1978): 740–749.
25. Warren NS, Carter TP, Humbert JR, et al.: Newborn screening for hemoglobino-pathies in New York State: Experience of physicians and parents of affected children. *J Peds* 100 (1982): 373–377.
26. Grover R, Shahidi S, Fisher B, et al.: Current sickle cell screening program for newborns in New York City. *Am J Publ Health* 73 (1983): 249–252.
27. Scott RB, and Harrison DL. Screening of the umbilical cord blood for sickle cell disease. *Am J Pediatr Hemat/Oncol* 4 (1982): 202–205.
28. U.S. Department of Health and Human Services, Public Health Services, Centers for Disease Control, *Laboratory methods for detecting hemoglobinopathies*. Atlanta: Centers for Disease Control, 1984.
29. Huisman THJ, and Jonxis JHD. *The hemoglobinopathies, Techniques of identifi-cation*. New York: Marcel Dekker, 1977.
30. Wilson JB, Headlee ME, and Huisman THJ. A new high performance liquid chro-

matographic procedure for the separation and quantitation of various hemoglobin variants in adults and newborn babies. *J Lab Clin Med* 104 (1984): 1027–1034.

31. Ou CN, Breffone RA, and Reimer GL. High performance liquid chromatography of human hemoglobins on a new cation exchanger. *J Chromatogr* 266 (1983): 197–205.

32. Rowley, PT. Newborn screening for sickle cell disease, benefits and burdens; New York State. *J Med* 78 (1978): 42–44.

33. Alter BP, Mondell CB, Fairweather D, et al.: Prenatal diagnosis of hemoglobinopathies: A review of 15 cases. *N Engl J Med* 295 (1976): 1437–1443.

34. Alter BP. Advances in the prenatal diagnosis of hematologic diseases. *Blood* 64 (1984): 329–349.

35. Jones JR, McCormack M, Dietzel C, et al.: Antenatal diagnosis of sickle cell disease: Amniotic fluid cell DNA analysis. *Obstet Gynecol* 59 (1982): 484.

36. Chang JC, Golburs MS, and Kan, YW. Antenatal diagnosis of sickle cell anemia by sensitive DNA assay. *Lancet* no. 1 (1982): 1463.

37. Old J, Ward RHT, Petrou M, et al.: First trimester diagnosis of haemoglobinopathies: A report of 3 cases. *Lancet* no. 2 (1982): 1413–1416.

38. Grossens M, Dumez Y, Kaplan L, et al.: Prenatal diagnosis of sickle cell anemia in the first trimester of pregnancy. *N Engl J Med* 309 (1983): 831–834.

39. Orkin SH, Little PFR, Kozazian HH, et al.: Improved detection of sickle mutation by DNA analysis. *N Engl J Med* 307 (1982): 32–36.

40. Wallace RB, Schold M, Johnson MJ, et al.: Oligonucleotide directed mutagenesis of the human β-globin gene, A general method for producing specific point mutations in cloned DNA. *Nucleic Acid Res* 9 (1981): 3647–3653.

41. Conner BJ, Reyes AA, Morin C, et al.: Detection of sickle β-globin allele by hybridigation with synthetic oligonucleotides. *Proc Natl Acad Sci USA* 80 (1983): 278–282.

42. Saiki RK, Scharf S, Faloona F, et al.: Enzymatic amplification of β-globin genomic sequences and restriction site analysis for diagnosis of sickle cell anemia. *Science* 230 (1985): 1350–1354.

8

Hematological Manifestations of Sickle Cell Disease

Vipul N. Mankad

Blood and blood-forming organs are significantly affected in major sickling disorders. Abnormal hemoglobin electrophoresis and other tests that differentiate sickle hemoglobin from normal hemoglobin and hemolytic anemia are hallmarks of sickle cell disease. In addition, leucocytosis and thrombocytosis are also commonly found. Furthermore, there are acute changes in the hematological status (e.g., anemic crises may be superimposed on the chronic hemolytic anemia). This chapter will review the hematological manifestations of sickle cell disease. (Hemoglobin electrophoresis findings are discussed in Chapters 6 and 7.)

ABNORMALITIES OF BLOOD COUNTS

The majority of patients with homozygous sickle cell anemia (SS) develop hemolytic anemia within the first 6 months of age (1). Their hemoglobin and red blood cell counts continue to decrease around 8–10 weeks of age, when babies with normal hemoglobin phenotype (AA) recover from physiologic anemia. The hemoglobin levels decrease further during the second year, after which they reach stable levels. The mean and standard deviations of the blood counts for patients with homozygous sickle cell anemia at the sickle cell clinic in Mobile, Alabama, are described in Table 8.1. Hemoglobin usually ranges between 6.5 gm and 8.5 gm percent. Reticulocyte counts are elevated and are usually in the range of 10–15 percent. The mean cell volume (MCV) is usually between 75 and 95 fl. but must be interpreted with respect to age of the patient. Beyond 5 years of age, MCV under 75 fl. should be considered microcytic. The mean corpuscular hemoglobin concentration (MCHC) is usually within normal limits unless iron deficiency or thalassemia coexists.

Table 8.1
Blood Counts in Patients with Homozygous Sickle Cell Anemia (N = 62)

	Mean	Standard Deviation	Range
White Blood Cell Count (x1000/cmm)	11.76	4.40	4.1-30.2
Red Blood Cell Count (millions/cmm)	2.72	0.53	1.74-4.37
Hemoglobin (gm/dl)	8.71	0.94	6.0-10.6
Hematocrit (%)	24.89	3.52	17.2-33.2
Platelet Count (x1000/cmm)	311.24	148.08	49.0-937.0

Leucocytosis is associated with sickle cell anemia, as shown in Table 8.1. The neutrophil count is elevated, with an average of 59 percent (2). While a shift to the left has been reported previously (3), band forms are usually not increased. Platelet counts are markedly increased during pain-free states in sickle cell anemia.

MORPHOLOGICAL ABNORMALITIES OF THE PERIPHERAL BLOOD SMEAR

Red cells vary in morphology in steady states of sickle cell patients (2). The number of sickled forms of erythrocytes varies among individuals and usually represent the irreversibly sickled cells (ISC). Strictly speaking, ISCs are defined as cells that retain a sickled shape upon reoxygenation under standard conditions in the laboratory. In the process of making the peripheral smear, the red cells are usually oxygenated. While this may not be the optimum oxygenation to precisely determine ISC counts, the sickled cells in the peripheral smear approximate the number of ISCs. More detailed studies of the morphological abnormalities of red cells have been performed, and the classification of these changes into six categories has been suggested (4). Dense red cells without central pallor, red cell fragments, target cells, and nucleated red cells may be seen. Dense red cells can be separated from light cells by density gradient fractionation (5). Howell-Jolly bodies and pitted red cells (in Nomarski optics) are increased in direct relationship to functional hyposplenia, which develops in early infancy (6).

ANEMIC CRISES

Aplastic crisis and acute splenic sequestration crisis are serious problems in patients with sickle cell anemia. Hyperhemolytic crisis is less well defined, but acute exacerbation of hemolysis is known to occur from mechanical stress during febrile and vaso-occlusive states and may contribute to worsening of the anemia. In addition, other causes of lower than usual hemoglobin, such as iron deficiency and thalassemia, need to be considered under appropriate circumstances in patients with sickle cell anemia.

APLASTIC CRISIS

Aplastic crisis is characterized by a sudden onset of anemia and a very low reticulocyte count. Prodromal symptoms include fever, chills, headache, abdominal pain, and occasionally respiratory illness (7–8). The hemoglobin may drop precipitously at a rate of over 50 percent in 3 days to levels below 2 gm/dl. This complication occurs predominantly in children between the ages of 4 and 10 years (7), but many cases have been reported in adults. The incidence of aplastic pathology is probably higher than recognized by overt clinical cases.

Multiple cases of aplastic crisis among sickle cell patients in the same family as well as the clustering of nonfamilial cases had been reported many years ago (9–10). This led to the hypothesis that infectious agents caused aplastic crises in patients with hemolytic anemias. A variety of microbial agents have been implicated in the causation of aplastic crises, including Strep. pneumoniae, Mycoplasma pneumoniae, Salmonella species, Epstein-Barr, and influenza viruses, and, most recently, parvovirus-like agents (7, 11). A deficiency of folic acid had been suggested in a study performed 25 years ago but has recently been questioned (12). Bone marrow necrosis and toxins have been suggested as other causes.

A human parvovirus–like agent has been shown to be the most common cause of aplastic crisis in sickle cell patients and in other hemolytic anemias (7, 10, 13, 14). Viremia occurs very early in the course of illness, as evidenced by the presence of an antigen in the serum, and may have cleared before the detection of the crisis. The virus has been shown to infect the erythroid stem cells (11), and plasma from patients with aplastic crises inhibits the formation of erythroid colonies in bone marrow cultures (CFU-E and BFU-E) in vitro.

Bone marrow in early stages of aplastic crisis shows decreased erythroid precursors which soon manifests as reticulocytopenia. Since the survival of sickle erythrocytes is short, shutdown of red cell production results in severe anemia, usually under 5 gm/dl of hemoglobin. Tachycardia, tachypnea, gallop rhythm, hepatosplenomegaly, and respiratory distress may follow. Recovery is heralded by the development of the IgM antibody to parvovirus, erythroid hyperplasia in the marrow, the appearance of nucleated precursors in the peripheral blood smear, and, finally, reticulocytosis. This usually takes approximately 1 week after clinical presentation of anemia.

Severe anemia and an extremely low reticulocyte count are sufficient for a diagnosis of aplastic crisis. Although the aplastic process usually involves erythroid cells, occasionally other myeloid cells are involved, resulting in leucopenia and thrombocytopenia. An examination of the bone marrow aspirate is usually not necessary but may be helpful in understanding the disease process. A transfusion of red cells may be necessary to prevent or treat cardiac failure. In the severely anemic patient who has maintained the blood volume by a shift of interstitial fluids into the intravascular space, transfused red cells may increase the blood volume as an immediate consequence of transfusion and, therefore, may aggravate pulmonary and systemic congestion. Pulmonary edema may ensue, which may compromize oxygenation. Therefore, partial exchange transfusion should be considered in such circumstances. It is difficult to recommend the level of hemoglobin at which exchange transfusion is preferred over simple transfusion. Instead, the decision should be individualized on the basis of the presence or absence of venous congestion, the severity of the anemia, and the rapidity with which the hemoglobin has declined.

ACUTE SPLENIC SEQUESTRATION CRISIS

Acute splenic sequestration crisis is a serious complication of sickle cell disease. In typical episodes, the spleen undergoes enlargement, trapping red cells and causing a precipitous fall in hemoglobin and possibly death. Prior to penicillin prophylaxis studies, splenic sequestration was second only to infections as a cause of death in children with sickle cell anemia (15, 16). As pneumococcal infections are controlled with penicillin prophylaxis, the splenic sequestration would remain the major cause of death in children. In many instances, sequestration may be minor (e.g., a fall in hemoglobin by 2 gm/dl associated with enlargement of spleen) (17). Since such episodes may be missed and early mortality from other causes may alter the statistics, the actual incidence of splenic sequestration may be higher than is generally recognized.

In a series in Chicago, 20 episodes were observed in 14 children between the ages of 6 months and 4.5 years (18). Anemia, enlarged spleen, high reticulocyte counts, high white counts, and thrombocytopenia were noted in these patients. The mortality rate was 29 percent. In a study of newborn cohort (216 children) in Jamaica, 71 episodes were recorded in 52 children with sickle cell disease in the first 5 years (17). The recurrence rate for the second episode was 26 percent, and of those, 35 percent had a third episode of sequestration. The mortality during the first, second, and third episodes of sequestration crises was 12 percent, 21 percent, and 20 percent, respectively.

The etiology of splenic sequestration is unknown. There is no evidence of infection as a precipitating cause of sequestration crisis. Symptoms associated with splenic sequestration include fever, cough, diarrhoea and vomiting, pallor, anorexia and drowsiness, and bone pain. An acute enlargement of the spleen (3–4 cm) is noted in all patients; however, comparison with splenic size in days immediately preceding the episode is rarely available. The spleen size may decrease during the follow-up, especially after the transfusion.

The hemoglobin declines by 3–4 gm below the basal levels, and often below 2 gm/dl. The reticulocyte count increases. The white blood cell counts are usually high but a high count is not specifically helpful. Since the platelet counts in steady state sickle cell patients are usually high, a decrease in platelet counts does not always exhibit thrombocytopenic range, but platelet counts are lower than in basal state. Death may occur within 24 hours in patients with severe sequestration crisis.

Treatment of the acute episode is transfusion of the appropriate blood products. In milder episodes without cardiovascular compromise, a transfusion of red cells should be administered. In more severe episodes, a simple transfusion or exchange transfusion with whole blood would be appropriate depending on the presence or absence of shock. Following the first severe attack, recurrences and mortality from sequestration crisis can be prevented by splenectomy. Since the enlarged spleen is usually not functional (18), the risk of sepsis is not likely to increase with splenectomy. If the first attack is mild, the decision to postpone splenectomy should be individualized on the basis of the ability of the physician and the parents to follow the course and provide adequate support in the event of a major recurrence.

Although splenectomy can prevent recurrences, mortality from the first attack of sequestration crisis remains a problem. It is prudent to educate the parents to palpate the spleen daily and to report any major changes in the spleen size for immediate medical attention.

MEGALOBLASTIC ANEMIA

Increased requirements for folic acid due to the rapid turnover of red cells have been recognized for a variety of hemolytic anemias including sickle cell disease (19, 20). Usually, folic acid in the diet is sufficient to meet the increased need for erythropoiesis. However, in special circumstances such as periods of rapid growth, diarrhoea or other intestinal conditions interfering with absorption, malaria causing additional hemolysis, treatment with folic acid antagonists, and pregnancy, the patient with sickle cell disease is prone to develop megaloblastic anemia (20–24). Several cases have been reported where megaloblastic anemia was reversed by folic acid supplementation (25, 26).

Since reticulocytes are larger than mature red cells and reticulocyte counts are usually higher in sickle cell patients, the range of MCV in patients with sickle cell disease is usually higher than in the normal population. A diagnosis of megaloblastic anemia can be suspected in a patient with a significant decrease in hemoglobin from the steady state, a low reticulocyte count, and MCV greater than 100 fl. Hypersegmentation of neutrophils on a peripheral smear is an additional hematological finding suggestive of folic acid deficiency. The measurement of the red cell folate level is the most sensitive biochemical test to confirm a deficiency of the vitamin. The most practical method is to conduct a therapeutic trial of folic acid.

Supplementation with folic acid (1 mg daily) is recommended during growth periods and pregnancy because (1) the vitamin is inexpensive and harmless; (2) megaloblastic anemia, when it occurs, can be reversed by folic acid and, therefore, probably prevented by routine supplementation; and (3) biochemical deficiency in nonsupplemented patients is common and may be associated with nonhematological consequences. Although the theoretical rationale for routine supplementation with folic acid exists, large-scale, double-blind, randomized controlled trials to demonstrate its effects are not available.

MICROCYTIC ANEMIA

Iron deficiency and thalassemia associated with sickle cell disease may cause microcytic anemia. Therefore, if the MCV is less than 75 fl., the patient should be investigated for the cause of microcytosis.

IRON DEFICIENCY

Iron deficiency as defined by decreased iron stores is not uncommon in sickle cell patients. Microcytic, hypochromic anemia due to iron deficiency occurs less frequently. However, the association of thalassemia genes is difficult to rule out as a cause of microcytosis and hypochromia. The etiology, diagnostic criteria, and treatment of iron deficiency states in sickle cell anemia are controversial. Low serum iron, high iron-binding capacity, and low serum ferritin are the usual laboratory parameters indicating iron deficiency. However, altered iron metabolism makes it difficult to assess the iron status of a sickle cell patient. In spite of diagnostic difficulties, it is important to establish the diagnosis of iron deficiency and to consider therapeutic options carefully.

Serum ferritin is usually elevated in sickle cell patients either due to intravascular hemolysis or due to increased absorption of iron (27, 28). Peterson, Graziano, deCurtis, et al. found elevated serum ferritin in sickle cell patients with absent bone marrow iron stores (27). However, in another study there was a good correlation between serum ferritin in sickle cell patients with absent bone marrow iron stores (29). In that study, serum ferritin less than 30 ng/ml was diagnostic of iron deficiency with 98 percent specificity. Increased excretion of iron in the urine rather than blood loss is thought to be the cause of iron deficiency in these individuals (29). While determination of occult blood in the stools would be a reasonable test in patients with suspected iron deficiency, extensive investigations of the gastrointestinal tract by endoscopy and radiography are usually unproductive (29).

Bone marrow aspirates show absent iron stores in about 28–34 percent of adults with sickle cell anemia in the United States (29). There is a significantly higher proportion of nontransfused patients among this group. However, there are reports of patients with absent bone marrow iron who had hemosiderosis of the liver and other organs (27). A very small number of sickle cell patients with low iron stores develop hypochromic, mirocytic indices with worsening of their anemia. Although treatment with iron can increase hemoglobin levels in these patients (30), such treatment is controversial. The opposing reasons are as follows:

First, iron deficiency can worsen the anemia in sickle cell patients and also place the patient at risk of developing nonhematological complications which have been reported in populations with an iron deficiency (31). It may cause growth retardation in children, behavioral changes and developmental delays, pica, gastrointestinal dysfunction, and skin and mucous membrane lesions. The role of iron deficiency in infection is controversial. However, a case can be made for administering iron to iron-deficient children who have sickle cell anemia.

Second, a low concentration of sickle cell hemoglobin in the red cells due to iron deficiency is an advantage to the patient from the point of view of manifestations of hemoglobin polymerization. There is a time delay before the appearance of the hemoglobin polymer. The delay in gelation is inversely proportional to the 30th power of deoxyhemoglobin S concentration (32). Therefore, a decrease in MCHC as a result of iron deficiency would result in a decreased sickling of the red cells. Indeed, there are reports of sickle cell patients with iron deficiency whose crisis history worsened as a result of treatment with iron (33, 34). Rao, Patel, Honig, et al. showed increased oxygen affinity and decreased *in vitro* sickling associated with iron-deficient, hypochromic anemia (34). Until further studies document the deleterious effects of iron deficiency in sickle cell patients specifically, it is prudent to withhold iron treatments.

HEMATOLOGICAL MANIFESTATIONS OF OTHER VARIANTS

Sickle-hemoglobin C (SC) disease patients have higher hemoglobin levels (9–11 gm %) than SS patients. Lower MCV and higher MCHC, a high percentage of dense cells, and a lower hemolytic rate are also characteristic of SC disease. Peripheral smear examination of erythrocytes shows sickle cells as well as target cells. Splenomegaly may persist in adult life and may be detected in as many as 50 percent of SC patients. Although the hemolytic manifestations are generally milder in SC disease patients, there is a higher incidence of retinal lesions, avascular necrosis of hip joint, and acute chest syndrome. The severity of SC disease varies among patients with this variant as it does in patients with SS disease. Although the hemoglobin levels are higher and a few asymptomatic individuals are found among SC disease patients, it is not accurate to state that SC disease is milder than SS disease.

REFERENCES

1. Platt OS, and Nathan DG: *Sickle cell disease in Hematology of Infancy and Childhood*. In DG Nathan and FA Oski, eds.: *Hematology of Infancy and Childhood*, p. 668. Philadelphia: WB. Saunders, 1987.
2. Diggs LW: Blood picture in sickle cell anemia. *Southern Med J* 25 (1932): 615–620.
3. Buchanan GR, and Glader BE: Leucocyte counts in children with sickle cell disease. Comparative values in the steady state, vaso-occlusive crisis, and bacterial infection. *Am J Dis Child* 132 (1978): 396–398.
4. Warth JA, and Rucknagel DL: Density ultracentrifugation of sickle cells during and after crisis; increased dense echinocyates in crisis. *Blood* 64, no. 2 (1984): 507–515.
5. Ohnishi ST: Inhibition of the *in vitro* formation of irreversibly sickled cells by cepharanthine. *Br J Haematol* 55 (1983): 665–671.
6. Pearson HA, Gallapher D, Chilcote R, et al.: Developmental patterns of splenic dysfunction in sickle cell disorders. *Pediatrics* 76, no. 3 (1985): 392–397.
7. Serjeant GR, Topley JM, Mason K, et al.: Outbreak of aplastic crisis in sickle cell anemia associated with parvovirus-like agent. *Lancet* no. 2 (1981): 595–598.
8. Kelleher JF Jr., Luban NLC, Cohen BJ, et al.: Human serum parvovirus as the cause of aplastic crisis in sickle cell disease. *Am J Dis Child* 138 (1984): 401–403.
9. Leikin SL: The aplastic crisis of sickle cell disease: Occurrence in several members of families within a short period of time *Am J Dis Child* 93 (1957): 128–139.
10. MacIver JE, and Parker-Williams EJ: Aplastic crisis in sickle cell anemia. *Lancet* no. 1 (1961): 1086–1088.
11. Mann JR, Cotter KP, Walker RA, et al.: Anemic crisis in sickle cell disease. *J Clin Pathol* 28 (1975): 341.
12. Purugganan G, Leikin S, and Gautier G: Folate metabolism in erythroid hyperplastic and hypoplastic states. *Am J Dis Child* 122 (1971): 48–52.
13. Rao KRP, Patel AR, Anderson MJ, et al.: Infection with parvovirus-like virus and aplastic crisis in chronic hemolytic anemia. *Ann Intern Med* 98 (1983): 930–932.
14. Bownell AI, McSwiggan DA, Cubitt WD, et al.: Aplastic and hypoplastic episodes in sickle cell disease and thalassemia intermedia. *J Clin Pathol* 39 (1986): 121–124.
15. Seeler RA: Death in children with sickle cell anemia. *Clin Pediatr* 11, no. 11 (1972): 634–637.
16. Powars DR: Natural history of sickle cell disease—The first ten years. *Semin Hematol* 12, no. 3 (1975): 267–285.
17. Topley JM, Rogers DW, Stevens MCG, et al.: Acute splenic sequestration and hypersplenism in the first five years in homozygous sickle cell disease. *Arch Dis Child* 56 (1981): 765–769.
18. Seeler RA, and Shwiaki MZ: Acute splenic sequestration crises in young children with sickle cell anemia. *Clin Pediatr* 11 (1972): 701–704.
19. Chanarin I, Dacie JV, and Mollin DL: Folic acid deficiency in haemolytic anaemia. *Br J Haematol* 5 (1959): 245–246.
20. Zuelzer WW, and Rutzky J: Megaloblastic anemia of infancy. In SZ Levine; ed.: *Advances in Pediatrics*, Vol. 6, pp. 243–306. New York: Year Book Publishers, 1953.

21. MacIver JE, and Went LN: Sickle cell anemia complicated by megaloblastic anaemia of infancy. *Br Med J* 1 (1960): 775–779.
22. Jonsson U, Roath OS, and Kirkpatrick CIF: Nutritional megaloblastic anaemia associated with sickle cell states. *Blood* 15 (1959): 535–547.
23. Fullerton WT, and Watson-Williams EJ: Haemoglobin SC disease and megaloblastic anaemia in pregnancy. *J Obstet Gynecol Brit Comm* 69 (1962): 729–735.
24. Shaldon S: Megaloblastic erythropoiesis associated with sickle cell anaemia. *Br Med J* 1 (1961): 640–641.
25. Pierce LE, and Rath CE: Evidence of folic acid deficiency in the genesis of anemic sickle cell crisis. *Blood* 20 (1962): 19–32.
26. Lindenbaum J, and Klipstein FA: Folic acid deficiency in sickle cell anemia. *N Engl J Med* 269 (1963): 875–882.
27. Peterson CM, Graziano JH, deCurtis A, et al.: Iron metabolism, sickle cell disease, and response to cyanate. *Blood* 46 (1975): 583–590.
28. Hussain MAM, Davis LR, Lauticht M, et al.: Value of serum ferritin estimation in sickle cell anemia. *Arch Dis Child* 53 (1978): 319–321.
29. Rao KRP, Patel AR, McGinnis P, et al.: Iron stores in adults with sickle cell anemia. *J Lab Clin Med* 103, no. 5 (1984): 792–797.
30. Vichinsky E, Kleman E, Embury S, et al.: The diagnosis of iron deficiency anemia in sickle cell disease. *Blood* 58 (1981): 963–968.
31. Oski VA: The nonhematologic manifestations of iron deficiency. *Am J Dis Child* 133 (1979): 315–322.
32. Hofrichter J, Ross PD, and Eaton WA: Kinetics and mechanism of deoxyhemoglobin S gelation. *Proc Natl Acad Sci USA* 71 (1974): 4864–4868.
33. Hardy TB, and Castro O: Overt iron deficiency in sickle cell disease. *Arch Intern Med* 142 (1982): 1621–1624.
34. Rao KRP, Patel AR, Honig GR, et al.: Iron deficiency and sickle cell anemia. *Arch Intern Med* 143 (1983): 1030–1032.

9

Conventional and Experimental Approaches to the Management of Acute Vaso-Occlusive Pain (Painful Crises)

Lennette J. Benjamin

Acute vaso-occlusive pain, or so-called painful crisis, is a devastating event that causes patients to seek hospital-based emergent or urgent care more than any other manifestation of sickle cell disease. The management of the acute painful event is generally suboptimal and fraught with obstacles. Optimal management of the pain involves the elimination or control of the cause. There is no specific treatment for the painful crises. Attempts to develop therapies are hampered by many problems. Some of the problems in drug development in sickle cell disease are:

Enormous heterogeneity in manifestations of disease;

No *in vitro* measures that predict *in vivo* response;

No animal model;

No objective measures of disease activity;

No uniform criteria for efficacy; and

Few controlled studies.

While many studies have been performed either in the prevention or the treatment of painful crises, these numbers are few in comparison to other disease states (1–5). Only 12 of these agents have progressed to controlled clinical trials. Moreover, 2 of these agents have shown modest efficacy but none has progressed to general clinical usage (6–8). The difficulty in developing a treatment for the acute vaso-occlusive event has been explained in part because when the patient presents in crisis, tissue ischemia sufficient to cause moderate to severe pain has already occurred and the circulation to the painful sites is either nonexistent or so severely compromised that the therapeutic agent cannot reach the affected areas (9). This does not explain why prophylaxis studies have also been unsuccessful. To some extent, a limited view of the pathophysiology of vaso-occlusive painful crises has also served as an obstacle in formulating therapies. It is understandable that many investigators have tended to approach treatment from a single, mechanistic perspective since the basic defect leading to the polymerization of hemoglobin S under deoxy conditions is central to any pathophysiologic event in sickle cell disease. However, in the patient, this single defect translates into multifaceted responses to multiple stimuli which can contribute to the pathophysiology.

The goal of any therapy for sickle cell disorders should be to intervene effectively in the pathophysiology of the disease. While curing the disease through genetic manipulation or controlling the disease by prevention and treatment of crises and other sequelae constitute the order of priority, neither of these has been accomplished. Hence, symptomatic treatment remains the mainstay of therapy. It is generally recognized that dehydration, hypoxia, or acidosis are precipitating events that can lead to polymerization *in vitro*. Thus, preventing or intervening *in vivo* in their occurrence should lessen the likelihood of vaso-occlusion. Polymer formation decreases hemoglobin S solubility and can lead to changes in cellular cation and water content (10, 11). The result is an increase in the concentration of hemoglobin within the red cell which further enhances polymerization (12). These abnormalities can lead to cells of varying density, adhesivity, and rigidity which can become entrapped in the microvasculature. This blockage of blood vessels thereby prevents the delivery of oxygen to tissues and results in ischemic pain.

A myriad of reactions accompany the initial vaso-occlusion and tissue injury secondarily which might contribute to the acute pain (13, 14). Some of these include vasospasm, inflammation at the site of injury, and elaboration of certain chemicals, including histamines, bradykinins, serotonin, prostaglandins, and potassium ions, all of which can influence vessel geometry, cellular functions, and/or pain at the acute vaso-occlusive sites. Thus, acute vaso-occlusive pain may well be mediated by different mechanisms, making single-agent therapy a misdirected goal. Accordingly, while some agents have shown promise, not one drug has come to general clinical use. Hence, the treatment of painful events is still dependent on symptomatic and conventional therapies and awaits more creative and successful experimental approaches with multipotent and combination methodologies.

The following chapter reviews the conventional ways of treating painful crises with the emphasis on pain management. It also reviews experimental efforts to prevent or treat painful crises as reported in controlled clinical trials. Reviews that include reports of uncontrolled studies may be found elsewhere (3, 4). Pitfalls in drug development in sickle cell disease and promising agents or approaches currently under investigation will be discussed, as well as the need for the establishment of better assessment tools and efficacy criteria.

CONVENTIONAL APPROACHES TO THE TREATMENT OF PAINFUL CRISES

The conventional therapy of acute vaso-occlusive painful events is supportive in nature and generally addresses the precipitating factors of dehydration, hypoxia, and infection. The most troublesome sequelae, pain, will be discussed under a separate heading.

Hydration

Hydration is required in individuals with sickle cell disease experiencing painful crisis primarily as a result of hyposthenuria, the inability of the kidney to maximally concentrate the urine (15). The condition results in a urinary output of > 2,000 cc per day, rendering the patient much more susceptible to dehydration than normal individuals. These fluid requirements are further exacerbated because painful crises are often accompanied by reduced fluid intake and increased insensible water losses. For uncomplicated painful crises, 5 percent dextrose in water (D5W) and ¼ to ½ normal saline can be used for initial fluid replacement. The total fluid intake should be approximately 3–5 liters/day in adults and 100–150 ml/kg/24 hrs in children to provide for both the obligatory urinary water loss and normal daily fluid requirements (16, 17). Hydration should be monitored closely, according to clinical state, to avoid iatrogenic congestive heart failure or electrolyte imbalance.

Oxygenation

Although deoxygenation induces sickling *in vitro,* there are no controlled clinical studies that indicate a general association of painful crisis and hypoxia. Studies involving the use of varying concentrations of oxygen and hyperbaric oxygen during sickle cell crisis have been performed with mixed reports regarding efficacy (3). Undesirable effects, such as possible toxicities related to oxygen therapy (18) as well as the depression of erythropoiesis during prolonged usage (19), have also been reported. Nevertheless, the practice of indiscriminately placing patients on oxygen without taking into account the state of oxygenation apparently still persists. Until such time as controlled studies provide evidence to the contrary, oxygen therapy should be reserved for those patients who are hypoxic.

Infection

A detailed description of infections and their management are detailed in Chapter 10. Infection should be identified and treated early (16). In particular, prophylactic penicillin should be given to children up to the age of at least 5 years (20). In addition to infections with pneumococcal, salmonella, staphylococcal, mycoplasma, chlamydia, and influenza organisms, infections associated with blood transfusions should be considered in those with appropriate histories.

Alkali Therapy

It is well documented that acidity enhances polymerization of hemoglobin S and decreases oxygen affinity *in vitro*. There are also reports of acidosis as a precipitating event in painful crises (21, 22). When acidosis is present, it should be managed appropriately. However, double-blind studies utilizing alkali to abort or ameliorate crises have not substantiated this approach in the general treatment of crises (23, 24).

Transfusion Therapy

Blood transfusions are rarely indicated in the treatment of painful crises (16). Patients adjust very well to the lowered hemoglobin that is representative of their steady state. Moreover, in most cases they do not experience a progression of anemia during painful crises that is sufficient to alter the hemodynamic balance. Transfusions are indicated when this stability is either threatened or disrupted by events such as aplastic crises and splenic sequestration or when complications ensue such as priapism, acute chest syndrome, and refractory painful crisis which have progressed or persisted beyond usual therapeutic measures. These approaches are based on clinical experience as there are no studies that evaluate the efficacy of transfusions in painful crises.

PAIN MANAGEMENT

Drug Therapy

Hampered by the absence of specific therapies for sickle cell disease, the treatment of pain takes on greater significance. To the patient, relief of pain is of paramount importance, while in medicine, pain control is a neglected area of symptomatic treatment. Since there is no treatment for the underlying disease, many physicians erroneously conclude that all one can do is prescribe narcotics. No effort is made to apply principles of clinical pharmacology of these drugs or to engage in studies centered around issues of understanding and controlling acute and chronic pain in this disorder. The paucity of literature on pain research in sickle cell disease is a reflection of this neglect. Management is generally hindered most by a lack of knowledge of the clinical pharmacology of the drugs or by attitudes that preclude application of this knowledge such as mistrust of the complaint of pain or fear of causing addiction, respiratory depression, or other side effects. Consequently, patients experiencing acute pain are often undermedicated, resulting in needless suffering, while being often overmedicated for chronic pain, leading to needless problems. Until appropriate studies are

Table 9.1

Oral Nonnarcotic and Narcotic Analgesics for Mild to Moderate Pain

	Dose (mg)	Duration (hrs)	Plasma Half-life (hrs)
Aspirin	650	4-6	3-5
Acetaminophen	650	4-6	1-4
Propoxyphene	65	4-6	12
Codeine	32	4-6	3
Meperidine	50	4-6	3-4
Pentazocine	30	4-6	2-3

performed, we must rely on guidelines for the use of analgesics derived from research primarily in cancer and post-operative pain.

The mainstay of medical treatment in managing pain in this disorder is analgesic drug therapy that includes nonnarcotic, narcotic, and adjuvant analgesic agents. The nonopioid agents most frequently used are acetaminophen and the nonsteroidal antiinflammatory agents (NSAIDs). Narcotic analgesics provide the basic framework for the treatment of acute painful episodes. These drugs are classified as agonist, antagonist, and mixed agonist-antagonist agents. The effective use of these agents requires an understanding of their clinical pharmacology, with the selection of a particular drug and dose geared to the needs of the individual. NSAID drugs work peripherally at the painful site; narcotic analgesics work primarily on the central nervous system.

The majority of patients with sickle cell disease experience pain of mild to moderate intensity, which can be controlled with nonnarcotic analgesics, of which aspirin (ASA) is the prototypic drug (Table 9.1). So-called "weak" narcotics are also used alone or in combination with nonnarcotics, and have been compared to ASA regarding equianalgesia. It is noteworthy that one 50 mg tablet of meperidine (demerol) is equivalent to two aspirin (650 mg). For severe pain, morphine is the prototypic narcotic agonist and is the standard by which all other drugs are evaluated for equianalgesia (Table 9.2). The potency of narcotic analgesics varies from one drug to another and from one route of administration to another. There seems to be no correlation between the half-lives of narcotics and their analgesic time course. Morphine, meperidine, and hydromorphone have a duration of action, according to most analgesic tables, of approximately 4–6 hrs and a plasma half-life of 2–3½ hrs. However, it should be noted that in clinical experience, the duration of action must be assessed in each individual and depends on the dose, pain intensity, prior narcotic experience, and individual pharmacokinetic differences. In sickle cell patients, pain medication might be required as frequently as every 1½–2 hrs. The hepatic and renal dysfunction and/or changes in various serum proteins that occur during acute vaso-occlusive painful episodes may alter the individual response to drugs (13, 14, 16). Drugs

Table 9.2
Oral and Parenteral Narcotic Analgesics for Severe Pain

Type of Drug	Route	Equianalgesic Dose (mg)	Duration (hrs)	Plasma Half-life (hrs)
Narcotic Agonists				
Morphine	IM	10	4-6	2-3.5
Meperidine (Demerol)	IM	75	4-5	3-4
	PO*	300	4-6	3-4
Normeperidine				
Levorphanol (Levodromoran)	IM	2	4-6	12-16
	PO	4	4-7	12-16
Hydromorphone (Dilaudid)	IM	1.5	4-5	2-3
	PO	7.5	4-6	2-3
Methadone (Dolophine)	IM	10	4-6	15-30
	PO	20	4-7	15-30
Mixed Agonist-antagonists				
Nalbuphine (Nubain)	IM	10	4-6	5
Butorphanol (Stadol)	IM	2	4-6	2.5-3.5

*Do not recommend.

such as levorphanol and methadone, which produce analgesia of a duration comparable to morphine and meperidine but have longer half-lives, can accumulate in the plasma with repeated doses and can result in excessive sedation and respiratory depression.

The clinical heterogeneity of sickle cell disease suggests a graded approach to treatment. There is no single drug that is appropriate or best for every sickle cell patient or for each painful event experienced by a given patient. Where one begins depends on the patient's previous analgesic experiences as well as on the current history and physical assessment of pain. Most clinicians use meperidine rather than morphine as a first-line drug in painful vaso-occlusive crises. The reasons for this are unclear but seem to be based on tradition derived from the empirical use of these drugs in clinical practice. Controlled studies regarding equianalgesia and pharmacokinetics of these drugs have not been performed in individuals with sickle cell disease. It is clear that there is a need for pharmacokinetic studies and relative potency assays in this patient population. Until these studies are performed, basic pharmacologic principles should be employed using available information and guidelines regarding peak effect, duration of action, and analgesic equivalence (25–29). Our approach to applying these principles in the management of pain in sickle cell disease has been reported and is summarized below (13).

In the case of mild to moderate sickle cell pain, begin with aspirin or one of the other NSAIDs to treat the pain peripherally. These drugs are not associated with dependence or tolerance but they do have a therapeutic dosage ceiling above which there is no added advantage. If the pain breaks from the peripheral site to the central nervous system, a mild narcotic analgesic is added to the nonopioid drug. Patients who present to emergency care facilities have usually exhausted these measures and are experiencing pain that supersedes control by these agents alone or in combination with mild narcotics. When the pain becomes more severe or relief is no longer achieved, the narcotic analgesic can be switched to a more potent opioid such as morphine or meperidine.

Combinations for Increased Analgesia and Reduced Side Effects

If needed, NSAIDs or antihistamines may be added to enhance the efficacy of morphine or meperidine. NSAIDs and acetaminophen have been determined to work additively with narcotic analgesics, thus permitting the simultaneous use of drugs that act on pain peripherally and centrally, as noted above. Moreover, meperidine or morphine can be administered in combination with hydroxyzine, not only to increase the analgesic efficacy but also to prevent or eliminate side effects such as nausea and vomiting. However, hydroxyzine should not be used routinely, and care must be taken to make certain that the patients are not oversedated. Thus, hydroxyzine is not given with every dose of narcotic when the narcotic dosing is at frequent intervals, such as every 2 hours. Phenergan can lower the seizure threshold of meperidine and is not recommended.

The mixed agonist-antagonist, nalbuphine and butorphanol, has been found to be particularly useful as an alternative therapy to narcotics in patients who develop side effects such as urinary retention or respiratory depression. One drawback to their use is the possibility of precipitating withdrawal, and they should not be administered to individuals who are receiving chronic agonist treatment (26). As noted previously, although probably not present in concentrations of any clinical consequence, the preservatives used in these preparations—sodium metabisulfite and sodium dithionite—are reducing agents that are used to induce sickling in the laboratory (13). Since constipation is also a common adverse reaction to narcotic analgesia, a bowel regimen consisting of stool softeners should be given routinely.

Dosing and Tapering of Drugs

Factors involved in determining the starting dose include the intensity of the pain and the prior analgesic history. For example, if a patient presents with severe pain and a negative history for treatment with narcotic analgesics, 10 mg of morphine or 75 mg of meperidine intramuscularly would be an appropriate starting dose for the level of pain. In children, the starting dose would be 0.1

to 0.15 mg/kg of morphine or 0.75–1.0 mg/kg of meperidine (16, 25). In a patient who has been managed with narcotics previously, the starting dose would be based on the dosage generally required by the patient for pain of similar intensity.

Once started, dose scheduling is crucial to the effectiveness of a given analgesic. The medication dose and intervals should be determined by a dose titration. Therefore, after the initial dose, medication (half the starting dose) should be given following each assessment at intervals as frequent as every 30 minutes to titrate to good pain relief and to determine the time for pain reappearance. During this time the vital signs should be monitored closely and the patient should be observed for signs of sedation. In most cases the dose titration is accomplished within 2 hours. After determining the appropriate dose and dosing intervals, an around-the-clock schedule should be instituted. A rescue dose should be written as needed (PRN) for breakthrough pain. Clinical judgment should be employed in determining whether to arouse a sleeping patient. Because the pharmacologic objective is to maintain the plasma level of the drug above a minimal effective level, it is probably unwise to bypass the scheduled administration of medication while the patient is asleep. On the other hand, because of the sequelae of oversedation, a patient should be awakened and assessed before being medicated.

If one chooses to switch from one narcotic drug to another for reasons of toxicity or lack of efficacy, decrease the equianalgesic starting dose of the new drug by one-half (because of cross-tolerance) and titrate the dose to the patient's need for relief. When switching from the parenteral to the oral route, use the exact equianalgesic dose because it increases the likelihood of providing pain relief. When intramuscular meperidine is used for severe pain, the practice of prescribing oral meperidine for acute and chronic pain is discouraged. This eliminates several problems: large oral equianalgesic doses (75 mg intramuscularly = 300 mg orally) place the patient in jeopardy for side effects related to the accumulation of the toxic metabolite normeperidine. On the other hand, prescription of less drug than the equianalgesic dose because of a fear of toxicity compromises the adequate relief of pain.

As soon as the patient shows sustained improvement, the opioid drug should be tapered slowly. Most often, patients experiencing acute, moderate to severe, and severe pain are treated with a narcotic by the parenteral route. The route and intervals of administration that have brought about improvement should not be changed. This is less anxiety-provoking for the patient, it permits the tapering process to proceed with greater confidence in predicting and assessing the response to medication; and it does not introduce confounding factors such as wide variations in the bioavailability of oral drugs.

Employ graded tapering as detailed elsewhere (13). Decrease the dose by 25 percent, alternating with the original dose at the onset of tapering. If the patient is receiving 100 mg of meperidine every 2 hours, give 100 mg alternatively with 75 mg every 2 hours. If both control pain equally, proceed to 75 mg and 75 mg, 75 mg and 50 mg, and so on. During this process, each dose must be adequate for maintaining pain control with a reduction in dosing as above until the patient is both pain-free and drug-free.

Following observation of this drug-free and pain-free period for at least 12, but preferably 24, hours, the patient is discharged. A nonnarcotic analgesic alone and a weak narcotic analgesic in combination with a nonnarcotic analgesic are prescribed for home use in managing mild to moderate pain, as outlined above. In the exceptional cases in which potent narcotics are also required for home use, the drug should not be the same as that utilized for acute severe pain. We do not prescribe oral meperidine as discussed above. Moreover, the routine use of oral meperidine for indiscriminate home management of any type of pain contributes unnecessarily to the development of tolerance and dependency while failing to provide adequate analgesia. It has been shown that 50 mg meperidine administered orally has the analgesic equivalent of two aspirin tablets (650 mg) (27).

Studies Needed to Increase the Efficacy of Pain Management

The efficacy of pain management should be enhanced considerably by therapy directed to the type of pain. Epidemiological studies that categorize and determine the prevalence and incidence of the types of pain that occur in sickle cell disease are needed. Pharmacokinetic studies on the major drugs that are used should be performed during crisis and steady state. The performance of relative potency assays are needed to ascertain whether the equianalgesic dosages from other pain studies are applicable in the sickle cell patient population. In addition, more creative ways of drug delivery are now becoming available, and efforts should be made to evaluate some of the modalities as to their potential usefulness during sickle cell painful crisis. These include:

Continuous infusions (30),

Sublingual, sustained-release, or epidural morphine,

Patient-controlled analgesia (31, 32),

Transdermal patches (33), and

Parenteral preparations of nonnarcotics such as the lysine derivative of aspirin (34) and ketorolac (35).

In addition, more attention should be given to the suffering or psychosocial components of pain and to therapeutic modalities such as behavior modification, hypnosis, and other modalities that address stress issues (13, 14, 25–29). Efforts should be made to determine the incidence and prevalence of physical dependency and addiction and properly define them. We must dissect out the subtle and/or unrecognized physical sequelae of pain management which might erroneously be attributed to sickle cell vaso-occlusive pain, and we must eliminate those components that are preventable through management modification.

Unlike therapy for the underlying disease, pain management need not await a major breakthrough. From a judicious use of the array of agents that are available and by varying drug combinations according to the pattern of pain and its severity, therapy can be adjusted to individual patient needs.

THE NEED FOR OBJECTIVE MEASURES IN EVALUATING PAINFUL CRISES

Whether therapy is in the context of clinical management (see the previous section) or research protocols (see the section that follows), the effect of the intervention on pain is central to any outcome measure. Accordingly, this section is positioned here because assessment is basic and pivotal for any intervention. The use of these analgesic agents as well as the investigation of experimental drugs in the treatment of painful crises will be facilitated by the application of better assessment tools that measure pain and the development of objective measures in evaluating painful crisis.

Thus, decisions about therapies depend on the patient's report of pain and assessment of the patient. In general, measures utilizing category scales, pain descriptors, and visual analogue scales address factors such as pain, relief, and some behavioral or psychosocial parameter such as mood. The pain assessment tools that are utilized have been validated in adults with cancer or post-operative pain and have been extrapolated to usage in sickle cell patients. The issue of pain assessment in children is less well studied in other pain states; thus, the clinical utility of these tools in children with sickle cell disease is even less clear.

Attempts to uncover objective correlates of crises utilizing improved cellular and biochemical assays and high-technology methods have identified some changes that occur during painful vaso-occlusive events. Alterations have been noted in the number of dense red blood cells (36); α-hydroxybutyrate dehydrogenase, or αHBD (37); red blood cell deformability (38); acute phase reactants (39); hemostatic parameters, including fibrinopeptide A (40, 41); high molecular fibrin-fibrinogen complexes (42); D-dimer fragments (41, 43); prostanoids (44); magnetic resonance imaging (45); and laser doppler velocimetry (46) provide a sampling of these measures. While to date the above evaluations are probably of more pathophysiologic significance, it is possible that selected combinations of some of these methodologies might provide surrogate end points of beneficial effects that might otherwise be undetected if pain reports remain the only evidence of efficacy. However, until the clinical utility of objective measures is established, the most successful methods of measuring pain and evaluating analgesics remain those that accept the patient's report of pain.

EXPERIMENTAL APPROACHES TO THE PREVENTION OR TREATMENT OF PAINFUL CRISES

Attempts at the prevention or attenuation of painful crises have resulted in many failures. However, an increase in the understanding of the basic mechanisms involved in sickling and sickling-related phenomena have permitted several approaches to the development of therapies designed to impact on events of pathophysiologic significance (3, 47, 48). Only 12 agents have been evaluated in controlled double-blind studies (Table 9.3). Their mechanisms of action as determined by *in vitro* studies include agents that affect (1) polymerization, either directly or indirectly by noncovalent or covalent interactions; (2) cellular rigidity and dehydration by altering cation permeability and by maintaining or increasing cellular hydration; (3) microvascular entrapment by impacting on sludging or vasoconstriction; (4) modifying factors such as fibrin formation by lysing fibrin; and (5) possible precipitating factors such as acidosis by using alkalinizing agents.

INHIBITORS OF HEMOGLOBIN POLYMERIZATION

Urea was thought to be potentially useful as a therapy in sickle cell disease because of its ability to interfere with the polymerization of hemoglobin S *in vitro* by disrupting hydrophobic bonds. Its evaluation led to the first clinical application of polymerization inhibitors to the treatment of painful vaso-occlusive crises. Early uncontrolled studies of urea reported a beneficial effect in painful crisis (49, 50); however, five controlled double-blind studies (the largest number of controlled studies performed with any agent) failed to substantiate these claims (51–55). Not only was there no beneficial effect of urea on painful crisis, controlled prophylactic studies also failed to demonstrate efficacy.

Sodium cyanate, an offspring of the urea studies, is the only other polymerization inhibitor that has been investigated in a controlled clinical trial. *In vitro,* cyanate exerts its antisickling effect primarily indirectly by carbamylation of the N-terminal valine residue of the α-globin chain (Val-l[α]) with a resultant increase in oxygen affinity of hemoglobin S (56). In open-label studies, the oral administration of cyanate to patients was reported to result in the reduction in the mean frequency of painful crises (57). However, the failure to document efficacy in a controlled double-blind study (58), coupled with reported toxicities (59), brought about the discontinuation of therapy with the oral form of the medication. Subsequent efforts to avoid toxicities by extracorporal carbamylation (60, 61) seemingly have been abandoned. While the clinical evaluation of cyanate was disappointing, it occupies an important place in drug development in general in that it was the first demonstration of the ability to chemically modify an abnormal gene product and it gave impetus for searching for other more specific chemical modifiers of sickle hemoglobin.

Increasing the Clinical Potential for Polymerization Inhibitors

A major problem in the use of drugs that react chemically with the hemoglobin molecule is that they also react with other proteins of the body, thereby increasing the potential for toxicity. The problem is further compounded because hemo-

Table 9.3
Double-blind Controlled Clinical Trials of the Prevention and Treatment of Painful Crisis

Action	Drug	Study Type	Number	Route	Efficacy
Polymerization Inhibitors	Urea	P	8	Oral	-
		P	5	Oral	-
		P	11	Oral	-
		T	19	IV	-
		T	23	IV	-
	Cyanate	P	22	Oral	-
Erythroactive	Promazine HCl Desmethyl	P	14	Oral	-
	Chlorpromazine	P	29	Oral	-
Vasoactive	Dihydroergotoxine	T	34	IV	+
Vasoerythroactive	Cetiedil	T	67	IV	+
		T	18	IV	+
		T	30	IV	+
Alkalinizing	NaHCO$_3$	T	18	IV	-
	Na lactate	T	21	IV	-
	Na citrate	T	10	Oral	
Antisludging	Rheomacrodex	T	11	IV	-
	Rheomacrodex	T	24	IV	-
Hemostatic	Ancrod	T	10	IV	-

Notes:

P = prophylactic.
T = treatment.

globin is present in such a large quantity that with some agents, the levels required for efficacy are prohibitive.

While polymerization agents to date have been discouraging clinically, *in vitro* studies have continued in search of compounds that have greater specificity for hemoglobin (62). Attempts at increased specificity utilizing acetylating agents serve to illustrate these efforts. Aspirin, for example, has long been known to acetylate hemoglobin and has been evaluated as a potential therapy in sickle cell disease but with disappointing results (63). Aspirin not only did not inhibit the polymerization process, but its lack of specificity resulted in the acetylation of lysine groups all along the globin chains. Derivatives of aspirin were synthesized in an effort to increase the specificity for reacting with the lysine residues in the 2,3-DPG pocket (64). Most notably, the bifunctional ASA derivatives cross-linked the two Lys-82 residues of the DPG binding site (65).

Methyl acetyl phosphate (MAP) is a nonaspirin acetylating compound that also shows considerably more specificity for hemoglobin than other acetylating agents that have been tested. Its degree of specificity is similar to that found for the bifunctional aspirin derivatives in that it reacts with Lys-82 (66). The fact that so few of the amino groups of the β-chain (Val-1, Lys-82, and Lys-143) and that none of the amino groups of the α-chain are acetylated by MAP under aerobic or anaerobic conditions is also indicative of the selectivity of this reagent (67). Moreover, while the bifunctional ASA derivatives crosslink proteins, with MAP there is no cross-linking and monoacetylation of the protein is achieved. MAP readily traverses the membrane of the sickle cell and reacts with intra-molecular Hb S to inhibit gelation of the protein (68). The presence of acetylated Hb S within the erythrocyte interferes with the aggregation process such that the density profile of the treated cells is nearly the same as that of oxygenated cells, indicating that the inhibition of gelation within the cell must be quite efficient.

At present it is unclear whether the increased specificity of MAP for hemo-globin will translate into nontoxic interactions with other proteins in the body. If so, its efficacy data warrants attempting other ways that circumvent this problem. In addition to the possibility of extracorporeal treatment, the problem of interactions with other proteins might be avoided by introducing the drug into cells via a vector of some type. Studies of MAP and other compounds continue as investigators attempt to selectively modify hemoglobin in a manner conducive for clinical usage.

DRUGS THAT ACT ON THE ERYTHROCYTE

The phenothiazines were perhaps the first agents reported to have membrane-related antisickling properties (69). Chlorpromazine was especially intriguing because of its ability to induce the formation of stomatocytes in normal cells, possibly by intercalating among the lipids of the erythrocyte membrane (70). Promazine HCl, the first agent evaluated in a double-blind controlled clinical trial in sickle cell disease, failed to prevent or decrease the number of painful crises. Before embarking on another clinical trial, *in vitro* studies were performed to identify the most potent of the available phenothiazines. Spin label studies of these compounds by Jones and Woodbury demonstrated a probable correlation between antisickling potency and the induction of membrane conformational changes (71). A double-blind clinical trial of desmethyl chlorpromazine, the most potent of the drugs in the spin label studies, failed to demonstrate therapeutic efficacy during painful crises (72).

Vaso-Active Drugs

Abnormal erythrocytes are entrapped and occlude blood vessels in the microcirculation, setting off a number of reactions which include vasospasm, vasoconstriction, and endothelial damage. It stands to reason, therefore, that agents that interfere with these vascular effects might impact favorably on painful vaso-occlusion. While uncontrolled studies have been performed with other agents (73, 74), only intravenous dihydroergotoxine has been evaluated in a double-blind clinical trial (6). In a multicenter study performed in West Africa, it was shown to shorten the duration of crises while having minimal side effects.

VASOACTIVE DRUGS THAT ALSO ACT ON THE ERYTHROCYTE

Agents in this category exert membrane effects on both the vasculature and erythrocytes and thus match well with an important aspect of the pathophysiology, blockage of blood vessels by red blood cells.

Cetiedil Citrate Monohydrate (Cetiedil)

Cetiedil (an *imindoester* developed from 3-thienyl acetic acid) is the only agent that has been shown in at least two double-blind controlled studies to bring about a measurable improvement in crises in adults and children (7, 8). It is representative of those drugs that have been determined by a circuitous route to alter membrane permeability and has become the protyptic agent for this class of compounds (75). Cetiedil was first evaluated in sickle cell disease by R. Cabannes and colleagues in the Ivory Coast because of its reported ability to cause an improvement in microvascular circulation. Cabannes noted clinical improvement in an uncontrolled trial which led to the investigation of antisickling properties of the drug (76).

Our laboratory (C.M. Peterson, L. Benjamin, et al.), and that of T. Asakura and his coworkers, began evaluating this agent in the United States. Both laboratories reported antisickling properties, the results of which led to the postulate that the compound exerted its antisickling effect by action on the red cell membrane (77, 78). Asakura and colleagues proposed that the observed swelling of the cells provided a possible explanation for the antisickling effect of cetiedil and in subsequent studies reported that cetiedil increases cellular hydration by passive sodium influx in the absence of ATP depletion (79). Berkowitz and Orringer showed that cetiedil also prevents cellular dehydration by inhibiting calcium-dependent potassium efflux in ATP-depleted cells (80).

These *in vitro* studies of cetiedil and the preliminary clinical studies in sickle cell patients along with the favorable safety profile observed in the treatment of chronic cardiovascular diseases (81, 82), gave impetus to the study of this drug in sickle cell crisis. A multicenter, collaborative, double-blind, placebo-controlled study was performed in adult patients in the United States. The duration of crisis was significantly shortened by both the 0.3 and 0.4 mg/kg dosages of cetiedil (7). The 0.4 mg/kg dose also significantly decreased the number of painful sites when compared to the placebo, while being minimally toxic.

In double-blind crossover and double-blind randomized studies performed in children in the Ivory Coast, greater reductions in pain and in the duration of crisis were reported (8). These clinical studies of cetiedil are significant in that they demonstrated in controlled double-blind studies that measurable improvement in painful vaso-occlusive episodes is possible. While this accomplishment, using an approach independent of the chemical modification of hemoglobin S, gives added significance to the findings, optimizing the dosing and uncovering the relative contributions of its mechanisms to the observed improvement would be of great value.

Increasing the Potential for Clinical Utility of Vaso-Erythroactive Drugs

Pharmacokinetic studies suggest that the dosing intervals used in the above studies were not optimal (83, 84). Cetiedil exhibits a biphasic half-life with an early half-life of minutes and a terminal half-life of 3–4 hours. The peak blood levels of 70–200 ng of cetiedil were much lower than those required for an antisickling effect in the *in vitro* studies described above, which were carried out in the 50–400 μM range. Stuart, Stone, Stone, et al. have shown a beneficial effect of cetiedil on the filterability of calcium ionophore-A23187 dehydrated sickle cells at concentrations as low as 1 μmol/1 (85). In the U.S. studies, cetiedil was given at 8-hour intervals, while in the studies conducted in the Ivory Coast it was given at 6-hour intervals. Studies are underway in our facility to determine whether it is possible to maintain safety and increase efficacy by giving cetiedil on a schedule that is more consistent with its pharmacokinetics. Of note is the fact that cetiedil and the vaso-active agent dihydroergotoxine are the only agents that have demonstrated efficacy. Accordingly, as methodology permits, the vascular effects as well as the erythrocyte actions of cetiedil are being explored. These two effects have resulted in the designation of cetiedil as a vaso-erythroactive drug (86).

The drugs that are most similar to cetiedil fall into the chemically heterogeneous class of agents called calcium channel blockers. Like cetiedil, these drugs have been shown to alter cation permeability, dilate blood vessels, and increase red cell deformability, all properties of potential benefit in sickle cell disease (75). Diltiazem, bepridil, verapamil, nifedipine, and nitrendipine have been shown to inhibit sickling or sickling related phenomena in vitro (87–89). There are no published controlled clinical studies in which these vasoerythroactive agents have been evaluated in the treatment of vaso-occlusive episodes. There are reports that nifedipine has beneficial effects on priapism (90) and on sickle retinopathy (91). Thus, these agents, like cetiedil, have shown promise as potentially useful therapies in sickle cell disease and warrant further investigation. A multicenter, double-blind collaborative study of diltiazem in the prevention or attenuation of painful vaso-occlusive events is in progress.

Another kind of agent that has both vascular and erythrocytic effects, Pentoxifylline (trental) is a dimethyl dimethylaxanthine derivative which is used to treat vascular disease such as intermittent claudication and chronic cerebrovascular insufficiency and is reported to have significant hemorheologic properties by virtue of an effect on deformability of sickle erythrocytes (92). A placebo-controlled double-blind study of the drug did not demonstrate any beneficial effects on painful crises or on laboratory parameters previously shown to change during crises (93). It might be possible to exploit the differences among cetiedil, this particular compound, and the heterogeneous class of calcium entry blockers, to dissect out the key elements for an effective therapy.

An entirely different approach can be found in the hemorrheologic drug poloxamer 188 (rheothrx co-polymer, pluronic 68) which exerts its action on erythrocytes and vascular endothelium by lubricating injured cells and thereby decreasing their stickiness (94). It has surfactant activity and blocks adhesion due to pathologic hydrophobic interactions such as are seen in sickle erythrocyte–vascular endothelial interactions (95). Regarding safety, this agent has been utilized in the past as an emulsifying agent and to protect erythrocytes from mechanical or osmotic hemolysis during cardiac bypass surgery (96). Thus, a toxicity literature exists on the compound. The above factors, along with reported properties of improved microvascular flow and enhanced delivery of drugs to damaged tissue, suggest a possible role for this compound in the treatment of vaso-occlusive events.

FUTURE CLINICAL TRIALS

This is a very exciting time for drug development in sickle cell disease in that great strides are being made toward possible curative approaches such as gene therapy (97) or bone marrow transplantation (98) as well as pharmacologic measures to decrease hemoglobin S concentration by increasing fetal hemoglobin (99, 100). Of these approaches, blinded and controlled studies with agents such as hydroxyurea and/or erythropoietin which increase fetal hemoglobin seem nearer. At this time there are more drugs in or near clinical trial for sickle cell disease than at any other period (Table 9.4). Of the agents designed to treat or

Table 9.4
Agents In or Near Clinical Trial

Drug	Mechanism
Hydroxyurea	↑ Fetal Hemoglobin (↓MCH$_s$C)
Erythropoietin	↑ Fetal Hemoglobin (↓MCH$_s$C)
Cetiedil	↓ MCHC, Vasodilator
Diltiazem	↓ MCHC, Vasodilator
BW12C	↑ O$_2$ Affinity
Poloxamer 188	Erythrocyte/Vascular Adherence, Lubricant

prevent painful vaso-occlusive events, cetiedil, poloxamer 188 (RheothRx), hydroxyurea, pentoxifylline (trental), and BW12C have orphan drug status and are in varying stages of development. Diltiazem is currently undergoing clinical trial after favorable safety studies in patients with sickle cell disease. Of note is the fact that these drugs exert their effect by a variety of mechanisms that have pathophysiologic relevance. They either decrease the mean corpuscular hemoglobin (Hb S) concentration (MCHC) by increasing cellular H_2O or fetal hemoglobin, increase oxygen affinity, improve cell deformability, decrease the adhesivity of erythrocytes to endothelial cells, and/or dilate blood vessels and prevent or reverse vasospasm. It is possible that while no single agent or approach will be adequate for total control of the disease, having this array of agents should increase the potential for an effective combination therapy.

Lysine acetylsalicylate, which also has orphan drug status, is being evaluated as a nonnarcotic for treating pain in sickle cell disease after encouraging results in a pilot study. Another parenteral NSAID, ketorolac, has Food and Drug Administration approval for use in post-operative pain and should also be evaluated as an alternative to narcotics in the treatment of moderate and severe acute vaso-occlusive pain in sickle cell disease.

SUMMARY

While many studies have been performed either in the prevention or the treatment of painful crisis, few agents have progressed to controlled clinical trials, and of these, only one has shown measurable improvement during crisis and thus warrants further study. Of note is the fact that this agent, cetiedil, is a multimechanistic drug and has both vascular and erythrocyte effects. It is also interesting that the only other drug that led to modest improvement during a double-blind study is a vasoactive agent. Thus, one could surmise that the vascular component is a significant one and that cetiedil's effects are at least in part related to its vascular actions. A class of compounds called calcium channel blockers have properties that are similar to those of cetiedil regarding erythrocyte and vascular effects. Moreover, there are other agents that employ other mechanisms to act on the vasculature and the erythrocyte. Their evaluation might not only permit the discovery of drugs that are more efficacious but might also contribute to the acquisition of knowledge regarding key elements in a successful therapy.

The many agents that have been evaluated in sickle cell disease pale in comparison to drug development in many disease states. In addition to mechanistic considerations of design, many available agents on pharmaceutical shelves have undergone empirical screening for desired effects in other conditions. In preparation for adding this capability to drug development in sickle cell disease, some steps should be taken to ensure uniformity in evaluations of efficacy. The fact that there are no *in vitro* measures that predict *in vivo* response is problematic. The work that is being done to develop a transgenic mouse as an animal model for sickle cell disease should facilitate the transition from *in vitro* evaluations to *in vivo* studies. In the meantime, simplified and/or automated *in vitro* studies that evaluate oxygen saturation, morphology, and hemorheology should permit the rapid screening of large numbers of compounds. Regarding clinical evaluation, some uniformity in terms of criteria for surrogate end points of efficacy should be established for drugs that fall into different categories and also, in a more general sense, there should be overall criteria for any drug to be labelled efficacious. Thus, the search for objective measures of efficacy should include the assessment of the clinical utility of those alterations that have been reported and attempts to uncover more specific and practical markers and monitors of clinical state.

REFERENCES

1. Dean J, and Schechter AN: Sickle-cell anemia: Molecular and cellular bases of therapeutic approaches. *N Engl J Med* 299 (1978): 752–766, 804–811, 863–870.
2. Ingram V. Sickle cell disease—Molecular and cellular pathogenesis, clinical and epidemiological aspects. In HF Bunn and BG Forget, eds.: *Hemoglobin—Molecular, genetic and clinical aspects*, pp. 453–564. Philadelphia: W. B. Saunders Co., 1986.
3. Aluoch JR: The treatment of sickle cell disease: A historical and chronological literature review of the therapies applied since 1910. *Trop Geogr Med* 36 (1984): S1–S26.
4. Mentzer WC: A review of clinical trials in sickle cell anemia. In: Y Beuzard, S Charache; and F. Galacteros, eds.: *Approches therapeutiques de la drepanocytose (Approaches to the therapy of sickle cell anemia)*. Paris: Les Editions INSERM, 1985.
5. Brewer GJ: Detours on the road to a successful treatment of sickle cell anemia. *Perspects Biol Med* 22 (1979): 250–272.
6. Begue P, Bertrand E, and Bonhamme J: Action de la dihydroergotoxine sur la crises drepanocytaire: Resultats d'une étude multicentrique en double-aveugle nealisée en afrique francsophone, *Noun Presse Med* 7 (1978): 2449–2452.
7. Benjamin LJ, Berkowitz LR, Orringer E, et al.: A collaborative, double-blind

randomized study of cetiedil citrate in sickle cell crisis. *Blood* 67, no. 5 (1986): 1442–1447.

8. Cabannes RA, Sangare C, and Cho YW: Acute painful sickle-cell crisis in children. A double-blind placebo-controlled evaluation of efficacy and safety of cetiedil. *Clin Trial J* 20 (1983): 207–218.

9. Harkness DR: Prospects for therapy at the molecular level: Historical review in their molecular basis of mutant hemoglobin dysfunction, In PB Sigler, ed.: *The molecular basis of mutant hemoglobin dysfunction*, pp. 285–291. Amsterdam: Elsevier/North Holland, 1981.

10. Schechter AN, Nogichi CT, and Rodgers GP: Sickle cell disease. In: G Stamatoyannocoulos, AW Neinhus, P Leder, et al., eds.: *The molecular basis of blood diseases*, pp. 179–218. Philadelphia: W. B. Saunders, 1987.

11. Glader BE, and Nathan DG: Cation permeability alteration during sickling: Relationships to cation composition and cellular hydration of irreversibly sickled cells. *Blood* 51, no. 5 (1978): 823–830.

12. Clark MR, Guatelli JC, Mohandas N, et al.: Influence of red cell water content on the morphology of sickling. *Blood* 55, no. 5 (1980): 823–830.

13. Benjamin LJ: Pain in sickle cell disease. In KM Foley and R Payne; eds.: *Current therapy of pain*, pp. 90–104. Ontario, Canada: B. C. Decker, 1989.

14. Payne R. Pain management in sickle cell disease: Rationale and techniques. In CF Whitten and JF Bertles, eds.: *Sickle cell disease*, p. 565. New York: Ann NY Acad of Sci 1989.

15. Keitel AG, Thompson D, and Itano HA: Hyposthenuria in sickle cell anemia: A reversible renal defect. *J Clin Invest* 35 (1958): 998.

16. Charache S, Lubin B, and Reid CD: *Management and therapy of sickle cell disease*. U.S. Department of Health and Human Services, NIH Publication No. 85–2117, 1985.

17. Davis JR, Vichinsky EP, and Lubin BH: Current treatment of sickle cell disease. In L Gluck and TE Conte, eds.: *Current problems in pediatrics*, p. 64. 1980.

18. Reinhard EH, Moore CV, Dubach R, et al.: Depressant effects of high concentration of inspired oxygen on erythrocytogenes: Observations on patients with sickle cell anemia with description of observed toxic manifestations of oxygen. *J Clin Invest* 23 (1944): 682–698.

19. Embury SH, Garcia JF, Mohandas N, et al.: Effects of oxygen inhalation on endogenous erythropoietin kinetics, erythropoiesis and properties of blood cells in sickle-cell anemia. *N Engl J Med* 311 (1984): 291.

20. Gaston MH, Verter JI, Woods G, et al.: Prophylaxis with oral penicillin in children with sickle cell anemia: A randomized trial. *N Engl J Med* 314 (1986): 1593.

21. Greenbert MS, and Kass EH: Studies on the destruction of red blood cells; observations on the role of pH in the pathogenesis and treatment of painful crises in sickle cell disease. *Arch Intern Med* 101 (1958): 355–363.

22. Greenberg MS, Kass EH, and Castle WB: Studies on the destruction of red blood cells. XII. Factors influencing the role of S hemoglobin in the pathologic physiology of sickle cell anemia and related disorders. *J Clin Invest* 36 (1957): 833–843.

23. Schwartz E, and McElfresh AE: The treatment of painful crises of sickle cell disease: A double-blind study. *J Peds* 64 (1964): 132–133.

24. Barreras L, and Diggs LW: Sodium citrate orally for painful sickle cell crises. *JAMA* 215 (1971): 762–768.

25. Vichinsky EP, Johnson R, and Lubin BH: Multidisciplinary approach of pain management in sickle cell disease. *Am J Ped Hem Onc* 4 (1982): 328–333.

26. Inturrisi CE, and Foley KM: Narcotic analgesics in the management of pain. In M. Kuhar and G. Pasternak, eds.: *Analgesics: Neurochemical, behavioral and clinical perspectives*, pp. 257–288. New York: Raven Press, 1984.

27. Houde RW: Analgesic effectiveness of the narcotic agonist-antagonists. *Br J Clin Phar* 7 (1979): 2975–3085.

28. Shapiro BS: The management of pain in sickle cell disease. *Ped Clin N Amer* 36, no. 4 (1989): 1029–1045.

29. Hardy WR: Sickle cell anemia as a problem in pain management. In LC Marc, ed.: *Pain Control, Practical aspects of patient care*, pp. 1–11. New York: Masson, 1981.

30. Cole TB, Sprinkle RH, Smith SJ, et al.: Intravenous narcotic therapy for children and severe sickle cell pain crises. *Am J Dis Child* 140 (1986): 1255–1259.

31. Leslie ST, Rhodes A, and Black FM: Controlled release morphine sulfate tablets—A study in normal volunteers. *Br J Clin Phar* 9 (1980): 531–534.

32. Schechter NL, Berrien FB, and Kat SM: The use of patient-controlled analgesia in adolescents with sickle cell pain crises: A preliminary report. *J Pain Sympt Mgmt* 3 (1988): 109–113.

33. Miser AW, Narang PK, Dothage JA, et al.: Transdermal fentanyl for pain control in patients with cancer. *Pain* 37, no. 1 (1989): 15–21.

34. Benjamin LJ: Intravenous lysine acetylsalicylate for the treatment of acute pain in sickle cell disorders: Potential alternative to narcotics. *Clin Res* 37, no. 2 (1989): 335A.

35. Yee JP, Koshiver JE, Allbon C, et al.: Comparison of intramuscular ketorolac tromethamine and morphine sulfate for analgesia of pain after major surgery. *Pharmacotherapy* 6, no. 5 (1986): 253–261.

36. Fabry ME, Benjamin L, Lawrence C, Nagel, et al.: An objective sign in painful crisis in sickle cell anemia: The concomitant reduction of high density red cells. *Blood* 64, no. 6 (1984): 559–563.

37. White J, Muller MA, Billimoria F, et al.: Serum alpha hydroxybutyrate levels in sickle cell disease and sickle cell crisis. *Lancet* no. 1 (1978): 532–533.

38. Kenny MW, Meaken M, Worthington DJ, et al.: Erythrocyte deformability in sickle cell crisis. *Am J Clin Pathol* 79 (1983): 667.

39. Benjamin JJ: Biochemical and cellular alterations in sickle cell anemia: Crisis markers and therapeutic monitors. In Y. Beuzard, S. Charache, and F. Galacteros, eds.: *Approaches to the therapy of sickle cell anemia*, INSERM 141, p. 451. Paris: Les Editions INSERM, 1985.

40. Leichtman DA, and Brewer GJ: Elevated plasma levels of fibrinopeptide A during sickle cell anemia pain crisis—evidence for intravascular coagulation. *Am J Hematol* 5 (1978): 185–190.

41. Benjamin LJ, Jones RL, Peterson CM, et al.: Hemostatic alterations in sickle cell anemia: Objective markers of vaso-occlusive crisis. *Blood* 66, no. 5-suppl. 1 (1985): 318A

42. Alkjaersig N, Fletcher A, Hoist H, et al.: Hemostatic alterations accompanying sickle cell pain crises. *J Lab Clin Med* 88 (1976): 440.

43. Devine DV, Kinney TR, Thomas PF, et al.: Fragment, D-dimer levels: An objective

marker of vaso-occlusive crisis and other complications of sickle cell disease. *Blood* 68, no. 1 (1986): 317–319.

44. Mankad VN, Williams JP, Harpen M, et al.: Magnetic resonance imaging, percentage of dense cells and serum prostanoids as tools for objective assessment of pain crises: A preliminary report. In RL Nagel, ed.: *Pathophysiological aspects of sickle cell vaso-occlusion, Progress in Clinical Biological Research* 240 (1987): 337–350.

45. Mankad VN, Williams JP, Harpen M, et al.: Magnetic resonance imaging of bone marrow in sickle cell disease: Clinical, hematologic and pathologic correlations. *Blood* 75, no. 1 (1990): 274–283.

46. Rodgers GP, Schechter AN, Noguchi CT, et al.: Periodic microcirculatory flow in patients with sickle cell disease. *N Engl J Med* 311 (1984): 1534–1538.

47. Sunshine HR, Hofrichter J, and Eaton WA: Requirements for therapeutic inhibition of sickle hemoglobin gelation. *Nature* 275 (1978): 238–240.

48. Stuart J, and Johnson CS: Rheology of sickle cell disorders. *Bailier's Clin Haema* 1, no. 3 (1987): 747–769.

49. Nalbandian RM, Schultz G, Lusher JM, et al.: Oral urea and prophylactic treatment of sickle cell disease. *Am J Med Sci* 261 (1971): 325–334.

50. Nalbandian RM, Schultz G, Lusher JM, et al.: Sickle cell terminated by intravenous urea in sugar solutions—A preliminary report. *Am J Med Sci* 261 (1971): 309–324.

51. Cooperative Urea Trials Group: Clinical trials of therapy for sickle cell vaso-occlusive crises. *JAMA* 228 (1974): 1120–1124.

52. Cooperative Urea Trials Group: Treatment of sickle cell crises with urea in invert sugar, A controlled trial. *JAMA* 228 (1974): 1125–1128.

53. Lipp EC, Rudders RA, and Pisciotta AV: Oral urea therapy in sickle cell anemia: A preliminary report. *Ann Intern Med* 76 (1972): 765–768.

54. Opio E, and Barnes PM: Intravenous urea in treatment of bone pain crisis of sickle cell disease. *Lancet* no. 2 (1972): 160–162.

55. Lubin NH, and Oski F: Oral urea therapy in children with sickle cell anemia. *J Peds* 82 (1973): 311–313.

56. Cerami A, and Manning JM: Potassium cyanate as an inhibitor of the sickling of erythrocytes *in vitro*. *Proc Natl Acad Sci USA* 68 (1971): 1180.

57. Gillette PN, Peterson CM, Lu YS, et al.: Sodium cyanate as a potential treatment for sickle cell disease. *N Engl J Med* 290 (1974): 654–660.

58. Harkness DR, and Roth S: Clinical evaluation of cyanate in sickle cell anemia. *Prog Hematol* 9 (1975): 157–184.

59. Peterson CM, Tsairis P, Ohnishi A, et al.: Sodium cyanate induced polyneuropathy in patients with sickle cell disease. *Ann Intern Med* 81 (1974): 152–158.

60. Diederich DA, Trueworthy RC, Gill P, et al.: Hematologic and clinical responses in patients with sickle cell anemia after chronic extracorporeal carbamylation. *J Clin Invest* 58 (1976): 642.

61. Lee MY, Uvelli DA, Agodoa LCY, et al.: Clinical studies of a continuous estracorporeal cyanate treatment system for patients with sickle cell disease. *J Lab Clin Med* 100 (1982): 344.

62. Klotz IM, Haney DN, and King LC: Rational approaches to chemotherapy: Antisickling agents. *Science* 213 (1981): 724.

63. Shamsuddin M, Mason RG, Ritchey JM, et al.: Sites of acetylation of sickle cell hemoglobin by aspirin. *Proc Nat Acad Sci USA* 71 (1974): 4673.

64. Kokkini G, Bhargava K, Benjamin LJ, et al.: Design of new anti-sickling agents. In J Rose, Y Beuzard, and J Hercules, eds.: *Development of therapeutic agents for sickle cell disease*, INSERM Symposium 9, p. 111. Amsterdam: Elsevier/North Holland Biomedical Press, 1979.

65. Walder JA, Zaugg RH, Walder RY, et al.: Diaspirins that cross-link β chains of hemoglobin: Bis (3,5-dibromosalicyl) fumarate. *Biochemistry* 18 (1979): 4265.

66. Ueno H, Popischil MA, Manning JM, et al.: Site-specific modification of hemoglobin by methyl acetyl phosphate. *Arch Biochem Biophys* 244 (1986): 795.

67. Ueno H, Benjamin LJ, Pospischil MA, et al.: Inhibitions of the gelation of extracellular and intracellular hemoglobins by selective acetylation with methyl acetyl phosphate. *Biochemistry* 26 (1987): 3125–3129.

68. Ueno H, Benjamin L, and Manning JM: Effects of methyl acetyl phosphate on hemoglobin S: A novel acetylating agent directed towards the DPG binding site. In RL Nagel, S Carache, W Eaton, et al.: eds.: *Pathophysiological aspects of sickle cell vaso-occlusion*, pp. 105–110. New York: Alan Liss, 1987.

69. Lewis RA, and Gyang FN: Inhibition of sickling by phenothiazines: Comparison of derivatives. *Arch Int Pharmacodyn Ther* 153 (1965): 158–171.

70. Mohandas N, and Feo C: A quantitative study of the red cell shape changes produced by anionic and cationic derivatives of phenohiazines. *Blood Cells* 1 (1975): 375–384.

71. Jones GL, and Woodbury DM: Spin label study of phenothiazine interactions with erythrocyte ghost membranes. *Pharmacol Exp Ther* 297, no. 1 (1978): 203–211.

72. Mahmood A: A double-blind trial of a phenothiazine compound in the treatment of clinical crisis of sickle cell anemia. *Br J Haematol* 16 (1969): 181–184.

73. Smith E, Rosenblatt P, and Bedo AV: Sickle cell anemia crisis: Report on seven patients treated with priscoline. *J Peds* 43 (1953): 655.

74. Diggs LW, and Williams DL: Treatment of sickle cell crisis with papaverine. Preliminary report. *Southern Med J* 56 (1963): 472–474.

75. Benjamin LJ: Membrane modifiers in sickle cell disease. In CF Whitten and JF Bertles: eds.: *Sickle cell disease*, p. 147. Ann NY Acad Sci, 1989.

76. Cabannes R, Maron P, et al.: Preliminary study of the effects of cetiedil on acute symptoms of sickle cell anemia. *Clin Trials J* 18 (1981): 114–127.

77. Benjamin L, Kokkini G, and Peterson CM: Cetiedil: Its potential usefulness in sickle cell disease. *Blood* 55 (1980): 265–270.

78. Asakura T, Ohnishi ST, Adachi K, et al.: Effects of cetiedil on erythrocyte sickling: New type of anti-sickling agent that may affect erythrocyte membranes. *Proc Natl Acad Sci USA* 77 (1980): 2955–2959.

79. Schmidt WF, Asakura T, and Schwartz E. Effect of cetiedil on cation and water movement in erythrocytes. *J Clin Invest* 69 (1982): 589–594.

80. Berkowitz LR, and Orringer EP: Effects of cetiedil on monovalent cation permeability in the erythrocyte: An explanation for the efficacy of cetiedil on the treatment of sickle cell anemia. *Blood Cells* 8 (1982): 283–288.

81. Barbe R, Amiel M, Ponzeratt B, et al.: Evaluation of cetiedil (Stratene) in peripheral vasodilation. *Clin Trials J* 17 (1980): 20.

82. Divier J.: Cetiedil trial in daily medicine, clinical evaluation of 1143 subjects suffering from artertis of the lower limbs or vasomotor disturbances of the extremities. *Med Pract* 545 (1974): 67.

83. Soeterboak AM, Scaf AHJ, Lammers W, et al.: Human experience of cetiedil, a

new vasodilator with anticholinergic properties. *Eur J Clin Pharmacol* 12 (1977): 205–208.

84. Orringer EP, Powell JR, Cross RE, et al.: A single-dose pharmacokinetic study of the anti-sickling agent cetiedil. *Clin Pharm Ther* 39 (1986): 276–281.
85. Stuart J, Stone PCW, Stone YY, et al.: Oxpentifyline and cetiedil citrate improve deformability of dehydrated sickle cells. *J Clin Pathol* 40 (1987): 1182–1186.
86. Cho YW, and Aviado DM: Clinical pharmacology for pediatricians. II. Anti-sickling agents, with special reference to new vasoerythroactive drugs. *J Clin Pharmacol* 22 (1982): 1–13.
87. Weintraub M, and Ozunu M: Inhibition of *in vitro* sickling by diltiazem. *Clin Pharmacol* 35 (1984): 281.
88. Reilly MP, and Asakura T: Comparison of three membrane-acting anti-sickling agents: Cetiedil, bepridil and tellurite. In Y Beuzard, S. Charache, and F Galacteros, eds.: *Approaches to the therapy of Sickle Cell Anemia*, INSERM 141, pp. 423–428. Paris: Les Editions INSERM, 1985.
89. Onishi ST, Horiuchi KY, Horiuchi K, et al.: Nitrendipine, nifedipine and verapamil inhibit the *in vitro* formation of irreversibly sickled cells. *Pharmacology* 32 (1986): 248–256.
90. Temple JD, Harrington WJ, and Rosenfeld E: Treatment of early priapism with nifedipine, *Blood* 68, no. 1 (1986): 67a.
91. Rogers GP, Roy MS, Noguchi CT, et al.: Is there a role for selective arteriolar vasodilatation in the management of sickle cell disease? *Blood* 71 (1988): 567–602.
92. Seiffge D, Berthold R, and Berthold F: Effect of pentoxifylline on sickle cell thalassemia: Haemorheological and clinical results, *Klin Wochenschr* 61 (1983) 1159–1160.
93. Billett NH, Kaul DK, Connnel MM, et al.: Pentoxifylline (Trental) has no significant effect on laboratory parameters in sickle cell disease, *Nouv Rev Fr Hematol*, 31 (1989): 403–407.
94. Tanford C: *The Hydrophobic Effect: Formation of Micelles and Biological Membranes*, 2 ed. New York: John Wiley, 1980.
95. Smith CM II, Hebbel RP, Tukey DP, et al.: Pluronic F-68 reduces the endothelial adherence and improves the rheology of liganded sickle erythrocytes, *Blood* 69, no. 6 (1987): 1631–1636.
96. Danielson GK, Dubilier LD, and Bryant LR: Use of pluronic F-68 to diminish fat emboli and hemolysis during cardiopulmonary bypass: A controlled clinical study, *J Thoracic Cardiovas Surg* 59 (1970): 178.
97. Bank A, Markowitz D, Lerner N: Gene transfer. A potential approach to gene therapy for sickle cell disease. *Ann NY Acad Sci* 565 (1989): 37–43.
98. Johnson FL, Look AT, Gockerman J, et al.: Bone marrow transplantation in a patient with sickle cell anemia, *N Engl J Med* 311 (1984): 780.
99. Platt OS, Orkin SH, Dover G, et al.: Hydroxyurea enhances fetal hemoglobin production in sickle cell anemia, *J Clin Invest* 74 (1984): 652.
100. Dover GJ, Humphries RK, Ley TJ, et al.: Hydroxyurea induction of hemoglobin F Production in sickle cell disease: Relationship between cytotoxicity and F cell production, *Blood* 67 (1986): 735.

10

Infection in Sickle Cell Disease

Marilyn H. Gaston and Clarice D. Reid

The association of sickle cell anemia and infection has been reported for some time and was included in the fourth case report of sickle cell anemia in this country (1). The earliest recognized clinical infection with a documented organism was salmonella osteomyelitis (2). Shortly thereafter, more cases were described (3, 4), and the decade of the 1950s produced numerous case reports of salmonella osteomyelitis complicating sickle cell anemia. At the decade's end, 33 cases of sickle cell anemia and salmonella infection had been reported and the relationship between these diseases was clearly established (5–12). Hook's review of the literature documented 31 cases with osteomyelitis and 2 patients with salmonella bacteremia without apparent bone localization. *Salmonella paratyphi B* and *Salmonella typhimurium* accounted for 67 percent of the infections, and there were three times as many males as females. The ages ranged from infancy to 27 years, occurring mainly in children and young adults, with a mean age of 7 years. Hook also documented an incidence of sickle cell anemia patients with severe salmonella infections exceeding the expected incidence of osteomyelitis in the black population in the United States by 70 times (13). As more cases were reported (14–17), almost simultaneously an increasing number of reports occurred in the literature regarding cases of severe and fulminant infection in children after splenectomy for hematologic disorders, namely, sickle cell disease, spherocytosis, and thalassemia (18–23). These series documented the increased susceptibility to severe infections (particularly septicemia and meningitis), the overwhelming nature of the infection, and the frequent involvement of the pneumococcal organism.

Within a few years, the clear association between sickle cell anemia and increased susceptibility to infection with other organisms besides salmonella began to emerge. Scott and colleagues repeatedly described the frequency of fever and the problem of infection and recommended a program of prophylactic sulfonamides and intramuscular (IM) gamma globulin for children with sickle cell disease during the winter and spring months to decrease the incidence of respiratory tract infections (24–27). Porter and Thurman reported that infections were the major presenting symptom in sickle cell anemia during the first year of life and was the primary cause of death in 64 children diagnosed with sickle cell anemia before their first birthday (28).

Greer and Schotland studied 400 patients with sickle cell trait or disease and reported 5 cases of meningitis (pneumococcal in 3 and staphylococcal in 2), and 1 case of a brain abscess (E. coli) (29). However, it was the retrospective analysis by Robinson and Watson (30) of 252 patients with sickle cell anemia at the State University of New York Downstate Medical Center over a 10-year period that provided the first information and focused attention on the markedly increased incidence of pneumococcal meningitis in sickle cell anemia. Of those patients, 16 (6.3%) with sickle cell anemia had meningitis, while the rate of bacterial pneumococcal meningitis in New York for the same period was 0.2 percent. Of the patients with sickle cell anemia and proven bacterial meningitis, 13 (87%) were caused by the pneumococcus organism. This association was even more important since 85 percent of the children with bacterial meningitis were under 3 years of age and 61 percent were 2 years of age or less, an age group in which the pneumococcus is not the most common cause of meningitis. Hemophilus influenzae type b is the most common pathogen under age 2. No patient with pneumococcal meningitis was over 6 years of age. This highlighted the common existing factor between the previously reported increased frequency of pneumococcal infections after splenectomy and pneumococcal meningitis in patients with sickle cell anemia.

Simultaneously, African investigators were reporting an observed increased susceptibility to bacterial meningitis and septicemia due to pneumococci and salmonellae (31–33). They recommended routine neonatal testing to enable early application of preventive measures to improve the survival of children in Central Africa (33).

An important retrospective study in 1971 by Barrett-Connor (34) reported on bacterial infection in patients with sickle cell anemia of all ages. It was a comprehensive analysis of 250 infections in 166 patients and a review of the literature. Two-thirds of the patients required at least one hospitalization for bacterial infection over an 11-year period, and bacterial infection was the single most common reason for hospitalization and, in one-fourth of these patients, led to the initial diagnosis of sickle cell anemia. The data demonstrated that the risk for pneumonia and pneumococcal meningitis was increased in this group of patients, with the risk for pneumococcal meningitis being 579 times that of normal children. The risk for salmonellosis was 25 times that for the black population in Dade County, Florida. Of importance was the fact that the greatest risk for life-threatening bacterial infection was for patients under three years of age. Proven pneumococcal infection was not seen in children over three years of age unless they had experienced previous pneumococcal infection. Bacterial infection was the single most common cause of death, especially in the children. In childhood, meningitis and sepsis were the most frequent infections, and the organisms most frequently found were *S. pneumoniae* and *Hemophilus influenzae*. Osteomyelitis was increased in frequency and occurred at all ages. In older age groups, infections with salmonella were more frequent.

By the early 1970s, the increased susceptibility to infection had been well documented. While salmonellosis was the first bacterial infection reported with a recognized increased incidence in sickle cell anemia, it was apparent that the risk from the pneumococcus for meningitis and septicemia was greatly increased, especially in children, and was associated with a high mortality.

PATHOPHYSIOLOGY OF INFECTIONS

The clear association between sickle cell anemia and infection had been documented; however, the etiology remained unclear. To explain the increased incidence of salmonella infection, Hook postulated that several factors might have been responsible for the increased occurrence of salmonella osteomyelitis in patients with sickle cell anemia. The possibility was raised that capillary thrombosis made the gastro-intestinal (GI) tract more vulnerable to invading organisms; that auto-splenectomy may decrease resistance to infection and predispose patients to invasion by salmonella organisms, and that areas of ischemia and necrosis resulting from the sickling process may predispose patients to localization of the organism. In addition, he speculated that ischemia of the bone marrow may lower local resistance and permit the growth of dormant organisms, thus explaining the observation that sickle cell crisis often preceded symptoms of osteomyelitis (13).

Other investigators postulated the possibility of autosplenectomy, and this theory was attractive in view of the evidence for increased pneumococcal infection in postsplenectomized patients. However, this theory was discarded as unlikely because of the enlarged or normal-size spleens in the age groups reported. Nevertheless, at the same time, Howard Pearson and his colleagues observed the paradox of Howell-Jolly bodies in the blood of children with sickle cell anemia who showed splenic hypofunction despite clinical splenomegaly. The loss of uptake of radioactive label was documented with spleen scans even though the spleens were enlarged. The term *functional asplenia* was coined and defined as the lack of uptake of 99m Tc sulfur colloid by clinically enlarged spleens of young children with hemoglobin SS disease. This was suggested as the reason for the heightened susceptibility to bacterial infection (35).

While the spleen was clearly being implicated as the culprit, Winkelstein and Drachman (36) described a deficiency of pneumococcal serum opsonizing activity in this illness and proposed a hypothetical model of the stages in the development of pneumococcal infection in sickle cell disease. Pneumococci from the respiratory tract enter the circulation, and little or no antibody or opsonin is present

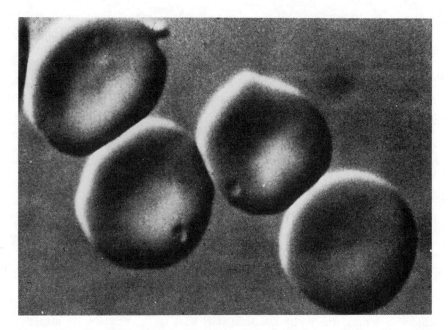

Figure 10.1. Pocked red blood cells. Four red blood cells from a sickle cell disease
patient viewed with Nomarsky optics. Three of the cells exhibit
obvious "pits," while the fourth cell demonstrates a normal surface
morphology.

Source: JT Casper, S Koethe, GE Rodey, A new method for studying splenic retriculoendothelial
dysfunction in sickle cell disease patients and its clinical application, *Blood* 47 (1976): 184.
Reprinted by permission.

in the serum. As a result, the spleen becomes the primary site of clearance for
pneumococci from the circulation. Due to dysfunction of the spleen and the lack
of opsonin, ingestion of the microbes by macrophages of the reticuloendothelial
system is inefficient or ineffective. This also impairs the development of early
antibody or opsonin, which normally facilitates clearance after several hours. In
the absence of adequate clearance, pneumococci lodge in other tissues and mul-
tiply. The lack of serum opsonin prevents adequate phagocytosis and killing of
the pneumococcus, and bacterial multiplication eventually causes overwhelming
infection.

Historically, radiocolloid scans have been considered the "gold standard" for
the diagnosis of functional hyposplenism; this procedure is invasive and expensive. Another test of splenic functioning utilizing quantitation of the percentage
of circulating pocked (vesiculated) red blood cells (Figure 10.1) using interference phase contrast microscopy was described and applied to determine splenic
function (37, 38). This test of pocked RBCs is noninvasive, inexpensive, and

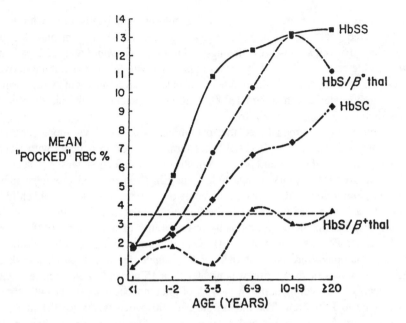

Figure 10.2. Developmental patterns of splenic dysfunction in sickle cell disorders.

Source: HA Pearson, D Gallagher, R Chilcote, et al., Develpmental pattern of splenic dysfunction in sickle cell disorders, *Pediatrics* 76 (1985): 394. Reproduced by permission of *Pediatrics*.

may be performed repetitively. The Cooperative Study of Sickle Cell Disease (CSSCD) demonstrated a strong correlation between nonvisualization of the spleen using technetium 99 spleen scans and pocked (vesiculated) RBCs > 3.5 percent (39). Of major importance is the finding on cross-sectional analysis of pocked RBC data from 2,086 patients of differences in the developmental pattern of splenic dysfunction between the sickle cell disorders. In Hb SS and SB° thalassemia, splenic dysfunction (> 3.5% pocked RBCs) occurred in the first 6–12 months of life. In Hb SB⁺ thalassemia, it occurred less frequently and later. Hb SC disease was intermediate (Figure 10.2) between SS, SB° thalassemia, and SB⁺ thalassemia.

INCIDENCE OF INFECTION

The incidence of infection with organisms other than *Streptococcus pneumoniae* has not been well documented, probably because they do not contribute to the significant morbidity and mortality in sickle cell disease.

Streptococcus pneumoniae

The incidence of meningitis and septicemia caused by *S. pneumoniae* is increased in patients with sickle cell disease, and these infections have been recognized as the major cause of death among children with the disorder, with those under three years of age at highest risk (30, 34, 40). Robinson and Watson described 16 (6.3%) cases of meningitis due to *S. pneumoniae* in 252 patients with sickle cell anemia, with no cases in patients with SC or S thalassemia over a 10-year period, whereas the incidence of this infection in patients with normal hemoglobin was less than 2 in 1,000. Eighty-five percent of the children were less than three years of age (30).

Barrett-Connor demonstrated that pneumonia was 100 times more common and pneumococcal meningitis 579 times more common in patients with sickle cell disease. In this series, proven pneumococcal infection was not seen in children over three years of age unless they had experienced previous pneumococcal infection, and this occurred in only one patient—an 11-year-old child—over the age of five. Of interest is the finding that bacterial infection led to the initial diagnosis of hemoglobinopathy in one-fourth of the patients (34).

Overturf, Powars, and Baroff (41) also documented that children with SS hemoglobinopathy are at great risk for *S. pneumoniae* infections. The risk of acquiring sepsis or meningitis was greater than 15 percent in children less than five years old. In young children the risk of pneumococcal sepsis was 400 times that of normal children. The attack rate per 100 patient years for the first five years of life for meningitis and septicemia was five times greater than in the second 5 years. Prior to 5 years of age, there were only four infections due to bacterial agents other than the pneumococcus among 32 patients. After 5 years of age, beginning with the second decade of life, infections with Gram-negative bacteria became predominant. In contrast to patients with SS hemoglobinopathy, patients with SC hemoglobinopathy had no episodes of meningitis or septicemia before the age of 10 years. After this age, the frequency of serious infections in patients with SC disease was similar to that observed in patients with SS disease. The series reported that children under five years of age had a 40–50 percent chance of dying of pneumococcal sepsis.

Powers et al. (42) also documented, in their comparative analysis of the incidence and subsequent outcome of pneumococcal septicemia in children before and after the establishment of a Comprehensive Sickle Cell Center, the increased incidence of *S. pneumoniae* septicemia and meningitis, and high mortality especially in children less than 6 years of age (Table 10.1). Of importance was the observation that after the sickle cell center was established in 1972, aggressive education and comprehensive care decreased mortality (from over one-third dying before their sixth birthday to no deaths) and progression to meningitis. This occurred despite an increase in the incidence of pneumococcal septicemia from 4.0/100 person years to 8.3/100 person years.

In 1982 the CSSCD reported a large number of children less than five years of age with SS, the majority of whom were followed from birth while participating in a nationwide protocol (43). The incidence of pneumococcal septicemia was 9.3/100 person years, and the mortality of 30 percent was surprising in that comprehensive and aggressive care was provided to these patients beginning at

Table 10.1
Reported Incidence and Mortality of *S. Pneumoniae* Septicemia in Children with Hb SS

Reported by	Age Range	Total Number of Patients (SS)	Incidence of Septicemia		Mortality
			Number of Patients	Per 100 Person Years	
Overturf et al. 1977	12 mos.-5 yrs.	323	20	5.8	35%
Powars et al. 1981	0-5 yrs.	233	34	5.9	35% (prior to 1972)
Gaston et al. 1982	0-5 yrs.	357	35	9.3	30%
Lobel et al. 1982	10 mos.-20 yrs.	143	13	13.3	38%
Gaston et al. 1986	0-3 yrs.	215	15	9.8 (placebo group)	20% (placebo group)
Zarkowsky et al. 1086	0-3 yrs.	459	46	7.98	24%

a very young age, even, in many of the patients, at birth. This continuing high incidence of pneumococcal septicemia and unacceptable mortality laid the groundwork for the Prophylactic Penicillin Trial, which in 1986 reported an incidence of 9.8 per 100 person years and a case fatality rate of 20 percent in the placebo group (44).

Lobel and Bore's series in 1982 (45) also reported the high incidence of pneumococcal septicemia, especially in children under two years of age with SS. The mortality was 38 percent, with all patients demonstrating a fulminant course and adrenal hemorrhage at autopsy (Table 10.1).

The largest series on bacteremia in sickle hemoglobinopathies was reported by Zarkowsky, Gallagher, Gill, et al. for the Cooperative Study of Sickle Cell Disease (CSSCD) in 1986 (46). One hundred seventy-eight episodes of bacteremia that occurred during 13,771 patient-years of follow-up of 3451 patients with sickle hemoglobinopathies were reported. The incidence was highest among children younger than age 2 years with SS and SC. This is the first report documenting the increased incidence in young children with SC disease. For the first 2 years of life, the incidence of bacteremia was similar for SS and SC. Children with SC showed an abrupt decrease after age 2 years, whereas children with SS had a gradual decline in rate from 2 to 3 years, with a more abrupt decrease after 3 years of age.

Another important finding, which was reported for the first time, was children younger than 6 months of age with septicemia. Previous series have not reported severe septicemia prior to the age of 6 months, whereas the CSSCD had three children with infection at 4 and 5 months of age. The mortality from *S. pneumoniae* bacteremia was 24 percent for the 46 cases in children younger than 3 years of age. A review of Table 10.1 reveals that the incidence of pneumococcal septicemia in children with SS, with its associated high mortality, has remained unchanged over the years.

Incidence in Hemoglobin SC

The epidemiology and clinical findings of serious infection in patients with hemoglobin SS have been well documented; the problem in patients with SC has not been as frequently reported. This lack of data is probably related to the need for large numbers to confirm a small magnitude of risk. A study conducted in Jamaica demonstrated a twofold increased rate of infection in children with SC disease as compared with normal children (47), which is still a 200-fold less risk than that noted in age-matched children with SS disease (48). Buchanan, Smith, Holtkamp, et al. (49) noted that children with SC disease may have a greater risk of bacterial infection than normal children but their infection rate was not nearly as high as that observed in patients with SS disease. Of 51 patients with SC disease observed for 370 person-years, there were 7 major bacterial infections. In all the pneumococcal infections there was a well-defined primary focus of infection, in contrast to what is usually seen with pneumococcal infections in SS children. There were no fatalities.

The most frequent complication of probable infectious etiology in SC disease is an illness resembling pneumonia. The overall incidence of pulmonary events in Buchanan's series was 8.1/100 person-years, which is twice as great as the pneumonia attack rate of 4/100 person-years reported in normal infants and children. Lobel and Bore (45) reported three cases of bacterial sepsis among 42 patients with SC disease followed over eight years, with all patients surviving. However, during the same period, there were 25 episodes of septicemia among 143 patients with SS.

In the CSSCD series (46), 1,092 patients with SC had 19 septicemic events, with the greatest incidence in children under three years of age, 3.54/100 patient years. As stated before, the rate of septicemia was the same in children with SS and SC under the age of two years. Two SC patients had sepsis-related deaths: an 11-year-old with pneumococcal sepsis and early meningitis and a 10-year-old who died of *H. influenzae* septicemia within hours of becoming febrile.

CLINICAL MANIFESTATION AND TREATMENT OF INFECTIONS

Infection is the most common cause for hospitalization in children with sickle cell disease and represents the most common cause of death in children with SS hemoglobin, usually from pneumococcal septicemia and/or meningitis in the first five years of life, especially in the first three years.

Patients with sickle cell disease present with a variety of signs and symptoms of infection, all of which are usually more severe than those seen in nonsickle patients. The clinical manifestations vary for patients in different age groups. Fever in the young child is the most frequent indication of infection and requires aggressive follow-up because of the possibility of life-threatening bacterial infection. Fever greater than 39.5° C is not uncommon with severe infection due to encapsulated bacteria. Infectious diseases were documented in 38 percent of febrile events reported in 182 episodes of fever seen in 22 children with sickle cell disease (50). Because of this high association, parents are routinely instructed to seek medical care for any fever, particularly in children under five years of age. If the cause of the fever is undetermined, cultures of blood and urine are recommended (51).

The symptoms may vary from appearing quite mild to an extremely rapid and fulminant course as seen in septicemia. Once this occurs, death is usually the outcome. However, a number of cases of bacterial septicemia have occurred in patients with a diversity of symptoms, including GI tract symptoms, upper respiratory tract symptoms, extremity pain, and lethargy. This type of presentation often has a more gradual onset (52).

The reliability of laboratory findings in infection, particularly the leucocyte count, is debatable. In one series of 22 patients with bacterial septicemia, the white count was frequently normal and only one-third of the patients had an elevated absolute band form count. Patients who subsequently died had significantly lower mean white counts than did surviving patients (45). Other series show a similar lack of utility of the white count in diagnosing serious infections in patients with sickle cell disease. Various hematologic features of infection in sickle cell disease were investigated by Cole, Smith, and Buchanan. They compared the findings in children with proven bacterial infection with a similar cohort experiencing fever without evidence of bacterial infection (53). Although most values of the complete blood count differed from steady state values in the children studied, there were no significant differences between those with or without proven infection. In the absence of specific laboratory or reliable clinical parameters, as a clinical guide to managing children with fever, a high index of suspicion and aggressive treatment is mandatory.

Although it is well known that there is increased susceptibility to pneumococcal septicemia and salmonella osteomyelitis, other bacterial, viral, and granulomatous organisms are found in patients with sickle cell disease. These causative agents will be discussed under the topics of septicemia, specific infections, including pneumonia or acute chest syndrome, osteomyelitis, parvovirus infection, and meningitis.

SEPTICEMIA: CLINICAL MANIFESTATIONS AND TREATMENT

The incidence of septicemia and associated mortality are related to the age of the patient and the type of hemoglobinopathy. In addition, the frequency with which specific pathogens cause sepsis and the association of septicemia with a focus of infection follow age-specific patterns.

Fever in the child with sickle cell anemia and aged younger than 5 years often indicates life-threatening septicemia. Most series describe a sudden onset of fever with few to no associated symptoms (42, 50, 54, 55). The fever is usually greater than 102 degrees (38.9° C) (50), but temperatures below 102 degrees may be seen in early bacterial septicemia. However, soon thereafter—usually after 2–3 hours—the temperature rises rapidly, and this is felt by some to be the hallmark of sepsis (42). On the other hand, some researchers describe a more gradual prodromal illness of 1 to 7 days duration, with the temperature being as low as 37.7° C (99.8° F) (45). In Lobel's series, the temperature was above 40.5° C (104.9° F) in only one-third of the patients and below 40° C in almost half the children.

Elevation of the total white blood cell (WBC) or absolute band form count is variable and is not of great value in diagnosing septicemia. Leukocytosis can frequently be absent and without elevation of the absolute band form count (45). No single aspect of the complete blood count can be used to guide major management decisions in febrile children with sickle cell anemia to differentiate between viral illness and potentially life-threatening infection (53).

Of importance is the fact that there is no clear difference in the above-listed clinical parameters between the children who die and those surviving (45). In the CSSCD (46), of the patients who died, 75 percent had a white cell count less than 15,000/mm3 and there were no statistically significant differences between patients who survived and those who died with regard to sex, temperature on admission, duration of illness, or presence of splenomegaly.

Lobel's series also demonstrated that patients who died were similar to those who recovered with respect to age distribution, type and length of prodromal symptoms, degree of fever, and sites of infection other than the bloodstream. The one exception might have been the finding that the group of fatal cases had a significantly lower mean WBC than the survivors. The mean WBC of 24,250/ml in the survivors was significantly greater than the mean of 11,000/ml in the fatal cases (p < .01). Therefore, since clinical and laboratory parameters can not accurately identify viral versus bacterial infections, nor the fatal cases, all patients must receive prompt and aggressive treatment for presumptive bacterial septicemia and continued efforts to prevent such infections must receive high priority.

Fulminant Septicemia

Evidence that some episodes of pneumococcal septicemia can be fulminant and proceed to death within several hours has been known since the early 1970s (54–59). In addition, the association of pneumococcal sepsis, the syndrome of asplenia, and disseminated intravascular coagulation (DIC) with Waterhouse-Friderichsen syndrome has been documented since 1970 (60). Despite the variability in initial clinical and laboratory data, patients who die have progressive shock and succumb within 24–48 hours of admission. This aspect of pneumococcal septicemia accounts for the associated, and continuing, unacceptably high mortality rate. It occurs as a sudden catastrophic illness with little or no prodrome, sudden onset of fever, no clear-cut clinical sign, and a general benign appearance of the child. Symptoms typically have been present for less than 6–12 hours before presentation, with progression to septic shock and/or death in a matter of hours. The rapid course, often leading to refractory circulatory collapse and death, is consistent with the clinical component of the Waterhouse-Friderichsen syndrome and DIC. Fifty percent of the patients who died in the CSSCD had clinical evidence of DIC, and death occurred within 24 hours of arrival at the hospital. It is important to note that this patient population was considered to be well educated on the need to respond appropriately to low-grade fever and mild symptoms. In addition, these patients were receiving immediate and aggressive care from well-trained professionals with many years of sickle cell experience. Similarly, in the prophylactic penicillin study (PROPS) (44), of the 13 infections in the placebo group, four cases were fulminant in nature, progressing from the onset of fever to septic shock and/or death in less than nine hours. Three of the 4 children died. The fourth child had an associated cerebrovascular accident and remains severely neurologically impaired. The two episodes in the penicillin group were not fulminant and the outcome was good.

The reason for the overwhelming fulminant nature of some cases of pneumococcal septicemia is not clear, and the mechanism that triggers DIC in pneumococcal septicemia has not been elucidated. This is puzzling since all children with sickle cell anemia supposedly have the same reasons for increased susceptibility to the pneumococcal organism. The role of the spleen has been well documented, namely, decreased phagocytic function of the reticuloendothelial cells within the spleen leading to RE "functional asplenia" (35, 61, 62). The failure to clear the bloodstream of pneumococci leads to concentrations that may reach immense proportions in the blood. It is estimated from *in vitro* studies that there must be at least 1 million organisms per milliliter before the pneumococci will be readily apparent within neutrophils on a peripheral blood smear (63). In many fulminant cases of pneumococcemia, the organisms can be seen after applying a gram stain to a buffy coat smear of the blood. Another defect in the immune system is serum opsonic activity related to an abnormality of the properdin pathway (64–68), which is specific for the phagocytosis of pneumococci and related to low levels of both IgG and IgM anticapsular antibodies (65). In the very young patient there is an absence of type-specific antibody which contributes to the increased susceptibility. The question remains, however: Why do only some cases present in such a fulminant, catastrophic manner?

Septicemia in Older Children and Adults

The CSSCD documented reduced rates of bacteremia in all age groups after age five (46). Children with SS who were 6–9 years of age had a rate of 1.05 events/100 patient-years, ages 10–19 had a rate of 0.63/100 person years, and adults over the age of 20 had 0.86/100 patient years. As expected, the rates for patients with SC were reduced even further, being 0.27 for 6–9-year-olds, 0.48 for 10–19, and 0.19 for those over 20 years.

In addition, the pathogens most frequently cultured from the blood differed from younger to older children. Only 19 percent of the bacteremia cases over the age of six years were pneumococcal as compared to 67 percent in children under five years. In older patients, gram-negative organisms are more frequent and more often there is an associated specific focus of infection. E. coli septicemia is associated with urinary tract infections and salmonella bacteremia, with foci in the bone (68).

In the CSSCD, there were only four sepsis-related deaths in the 6–9 year age group and two over the age of 20 in patients with SS. Fatalities from fulminant sepsis are rare in adults with sickle cell anemia. There have been only a few reports in the literature of adolescents (63, 69) and one of an adult (70). Of interest is the fact that two teenagers with Hb SC died from overwhelming sepsis. Deaths from overwhelming septicemia in SC are unusual, and only one other case, a nine-year-old with SC, has been reported (71).

Septicemia with Other Organisms

Hemophilus influenzae

The risk of Hemophilus influenzae septicemia and meningitis is increased in children with sickle cell anemia (SS) compared to normal children. Ward and Smith (72) reported in the mid-1970s that the majority of bacteremias seen by their programs were due to *H. influenzae b,* with all of them occurring in children under four years of age. Sixty percent of their cases were caused by *H. influenzae.*

Powars, Overturf, and Turner (73) reported a fourfold increase in risk for children with SS and aged less than nine years for *H. influenzae* septicemia. Important differences between H. flu septicemia and pneumococcal septicemia are that patients remain susceptible throughout life to the *H. influenzae* organism as opposed to normal children, whose susceptibility is mainly early in life (i.e, less than two years of age). In addition, contrary to the rapid clinical course of pneumococcal infections, *H. influenzae* septicemia has a two to three day prodrome of upper respiratory tract infection, low-grade fever, and otitis media.

As previously mentioned, septicemia from *E. coli* is usually associated with a urinary tract infection and salmonella septicemia with osteomyelitis (46).

Treatment of Septicemia

In young children with fever, diagnostic and therapeutic efforts must be immediate and aggressive. The first step to effective and timely therapeutic measures begins with the education of the child's caretakers to ensure a complete understanding of the implications of fever and to promote confidence in implementing appropriate steps to address the fever and obtain medical advice and attention. In addition, all emergency personnel should be well educated regarding children with fever and sickle cell disease. Blood and throat cultures should be obtained immediately with fever greater than 102° F (38.9° C). A lumbar puncture should be performed with minimal indications to rule out meningitis. The administration of antibiotics should not be postponed awaiting the results of laboratory studies or cultures. An antibiotic effective against *S. pneumoniae* and *H. influenzae* should be immediately administered intravenously and the child should be admitted to the hospital. After the confirmation of *S. pneumoniae* sepsis by a positive blood culture, intraveneous penicillin G at 100,000 units per kg every eight hours should be administered. Therapy should be continued for a minimum of five to seven days.

H. influenzae septicemia should be treated with intravenous ampicillin of 200–250 mg/kg/24 hours. In areas where beta-lactamase–producing *H. influenzae* are frequently isolated, a beta-lactamase–resistant antibiotic, such as cefuroxime (100 mg/kg/24 hours) or cefotaxime, should be used (74). Bacterial meningitis should be treated for 10 days or for at least 7 days after cerebrospinal fluid sterilization has occurred.

If blood, urine, and throat cultures are negative after 3 days and the patient is well, antibiotic therapy can be discontinued and the diagnosis presumed to be a viral illness. If the patient is not well but the cultures are negative, the patient should be reevaluated and treatment continued.

SPECIFIC INFECTIONS: CLINICAL MANIFESTATIONS AND TREATMENT

Pneumonia or Acute Chest Syndrome

Lung involvement is a common acute complication of sickle cell disease, accounting for significant morbidity and mortality (75). The usual presentation is of an acute illness with cough, fever, and physical and radiologic evidence of an acute pulmonic process. Abdominal pain, due to diaphragmatic irritation, is often seen. This clinical entity, generically referred to as acute chest syndrome, includes etiologies of infection and infarction. The acute chest syndrome is generally considered to be primarily of bacterial origin in young patients with this disorder, although in many cases the pathogen is not identified. Other causative organisms are viral or mycoplasma pneumoniae. Several studies in adults attributed clinical findings to infarction secondary to sickling, and this etiology of acute chest syndrome is considered to be more likely in this population (76–78). However, infection should also be considered in adults. The differential diagnosis of pneumonia from infarction or infection remains a clinical problem. Regardless of the etiology, the initial treatment is identical.

Bacterial Pneumonia

Pneumonia of bacterial origin, especially due to *Streptococcus pneumoniae,* is seen more frequently in infants and children than in adults. The most frequently cited evidence for this infectious etiology is the Barrett-Connor series of 166 cases of pneumoniae with only 5 percent reported as infarction (75).

In a large reported series by Poncz, Kane, and Gill (79), of 102 episodes of acute chest syndrome in children, less than 15 percent could be documented to be of bacterial origin. Similar findings of low frequency of bacterial infection were reported in a retrospective review of 100 cases of acute chest syndrome in 57 pediatric patients with clinical and radiographic evidence of pulmonary disease over a five-year period (80). Only 2 of the 93 cases studies had positive blood cultures for *S. pneumoniae.* Both authors point out that current preventive approaches with pneumococcal vaccine and prophylactic penicillin have undoubtedly had some influence on this picture.

Patients should be hospitalized and treated according to the degree of lung involvement and impairment of respiratory function as monitored by arterial blood gases. In progressive disease or respiratory insufficiency, exchange transfusion is indicated. Antibiotic therapy with penicillin, ampicillin, or cephalosporins will be effective for the most common pathogens, with adjustments made to a more specific regimen based on bacterial cultures. Pain must be carefully managed to avoid hypoventilation with narcotic analgesics.

Mycoplasma Pneumonia

The frequency of pneumonia due to *mycoplasma pneumoniae* in sickle cell disease has not been established, and most reports on this infection are from studies of epidemics, but it probably occurs more frequently in the pediatric population (81). Shulman, Bartlett, Clyde, et al. reported five cases of mycoplasma pneumoniae in pediatric patients with sickle cell disease (82). Of particular interest was the unusual clinical severity as compared to mycoplasmal infections in non–sickle cell patients. The pneumonia involved several lobes in four of the five patients, which is atypical for mycoplasma pneumonia. Other findings included marked leucocytosis, pleuritic pain, and respiratory distress and pleural effusion in several patients. In three patients, high fever persisted for seven days. Similar febrile patterns were noted in other patients with a minimal criteria for mycoplasma pneumoniae in the Sprinkle, Cole, Smith, et al. series (80). All five patients had cold hemagglutinin titers suggestive of mycoplasma infection, and high complement-fixation titers of 1:256 or more were found in four patients. Cold agglutinins of anti-I specificity were previously reported in 11 out of 16 episodes of acute anemic crises in children with sickle cell disease, but only two had rising titers to *mycoplasma pneumoniae* (83). Mycoplasma pneumoniae has also been seen as a concurrent infection with parvovirus in a child with Hb SC disease (84). These cases highlight the need to look for nonbacterial pathogens, especially in the absence of clinical response to initial antibiotic therapy with penicillin. The drug of choice for mycoplasma pneumoniae is erythromycin.

Other Pneumonia

Cytomegalovirus (CMV), which is characteristically seen in immunocompromised patients, was reported in a fatal case of pneumoniae in an otherwise healthy young male with sickle cell β thalassemia (85). The presenting clinical symptoms were typical of the acute chest syndrome with fever and persistent cough; however, the radiological findings included cardiomegaly and early pulmonary edema. The course was one of progressive decline ending with disseminated intravascular coagulapathy and death in a period of days. All cultures were negative except for CMV and the patient had no known risk factors. There were no studies of T-lymphocyte function. The authors concluded that "perhaps this patient signals a warning to physicians caring for patients with sickle cell disease to consider CMV as a cause of unexplained overwhelming pneumonia" (85: p. 265).

Fungal infection with *cryptococcus neoformans* has been seen in a 33-year-old black male with sickle cell anemia (86). Cryptococcus was cultured from bronchial aspirates, and no other pathogens were found. Although it was postulated that an underlying immunological predisposition was a T-cell defect, it could not be demonstrated in this patient.

Osteomyelitis

Osteomyelitis is not an uncommon infection in sickle cell disease, occurring most often in the young age group. The clinical manifestations include symptoms of pain, local tenderness, and fever and are indistinguishable from vaso-occlusive crises. The clinical distinction between bone infarction and osteomyelitis is often difficult to make. However, point tenderness with local inflammation and high fever favor the diagnoses of osteomyelitis. In one comparison, clinical and laboratory findings of infection versus infarctions were similar in some areas but showed distinctly different febrile patterns (87). Similar findings reported by Rao, Solomon, Miller, et al. revealed that 75 percent of patients with sickle cell disease and osteomyelitis had temperatures greater than 39° C (88). Leucocytosis occurs in both the infectious and noninfectious processes; however, the absolute band neutrophil count may be of value in the differential diagnosis. The pitfalls in diagnosis based on the clinical findings, even with bone scans, have been well documented by three unusual cases in pediatric patients (89). The one suggestive, consistent finding of infection was an absolute band count greater than five times that in the steady state. Diagnosis is further complicated because conventional X rays obtained in the early stages of disease are of limited value. Later changes reveal osteolysis or periosteal new bone formation. Osteomyelitis can involve any site but most frequently is located in the lower extremity. Multiple site involvement occurs in both salmonella osteomyelitis and in bone infarction. Radionuclide imaging studies maybe a useful tool for diagnosis. There is some evidence that marrow scans may be more useful in the differential diagnosis of infarction versus osteomyelitis than bone scans (90). A normal marrow scan favors osteomyelitis.

Salmonella is the most common pathogen in osteomyelitis in patients with sickle hemoglobinopathies. This observation, which was made in 1951 (91), has been substantiated in a number of other studies (92–94). In a large series of cases involving 63 patients with salmonella osteomyelitis, 57 had sickle hemoglobinopathies (94). In a review of 84 patients with proven positive bacterial culture and SCD, 50 percent had salmonella in contrast to 75 percent staph aureus in nonsickle patients (92). Reports from Africa suggest that poor sanitation plays a role in the pathogenesis of salmonella infection because there is increased exposure to frequent gastrointestinal infections with salmonella. However, asymptomatic intestinal carriage of salmonella could not be documented in 71 patients with sickle cell disease (95). Other researchers have speculated that reported episodes of intravascular sickling and bowel ischemia devitalize tissues in the intestine, facilitating salmonella invasion. The immunological defects and splenic dysfunction in these patients potentially favor propagation of salmonella infection.

There is general agreement that osteomyelitis in sickle cell disease is caused by salmonella; however, a number of other pathogens have been isolated in patients with this complication. These include *Staphylococcus aureus, Streptococcus pneumoniae*, and a number of gram-negative rods. An unusual case describes acute hematogenous osteomyelitis due to anaerobic organisms. The radiographic finding of intramedullary gas was the key factor in suggesting this etiology (96).

A high index of suspicion of osteomyelitis mandates immediate aspiration and culture of the site along with blood and stool cultures. Antibiotics to cover both salmonella and staphylococcus should be administered if given before culture results are available. Subsequent antibiotic therapy depends on determining the specific causative organism.

Parvovirus Infection

An infectious etiology of aplastic crises in patients with chronic hemolytic anemia was suspected for a number of years, primarily because of its single occurrence mainly in young children and the tendency for siblings to be affected. In the mid-1970s a parvovirus-like particle, now designated as B19, was first detected in blood during routine screening for hepatitis B. The antibody to this viral agent was found in a high number of healthy adults, indicating previous subclinical infection (97) but rarely as a result of significant disease.

The first suggestive evidence of the B19 association with aplastic crisis was reported from Kings College Hospital in five children with sickle cell disease. These cases occurred in four families and each had either detectable viral antigen or antibody to parvovirus during some phase of the illness (98). The following year, additional reports of this association from this group confirmed findings of parvovirus-like infection in nine children presenting with aplastic crises over a two-year period. During the same time, a number of sickle cell patients were found to be antibody-positive to B19 without hematological changes, suggesting that infection with this virus does not necessarily result in aplastic crises (99). The latter observation was also made by Gowda, Rao, Cohen, and colleagues in this country (100). Similar outbreaks, clustering in time, were analyzed in Jamaican patients, and 24 of the 28 patients presenting with aplastic crises had evidence of recent parvovirus infection and a higher prevalence of B19 antibodies than in normal sickle cell controls (101). Temporal clustering in these patients and in later reports from Jamaica (102), as well as simultaneous outbreaks of aplastic crisis and erythema infectiosum, confirmed the epidemic pattern of this disease (103).

Initial studies, in 1980–1982, of the relationship of parvoviral infection and aplastic crises in this country were of six adult patients with sickle cell anemia and one with thalassemia intermedia (104). All were antibody-positive and had clinical findings similar to those reported in children with aplastic crises. Documented infection with parvovirus was later demonstrated in all six pediatric patients presenting with aplastic crises at the Children's Hospital in Washington, DC (105). These investigators further postulated that parvoviral infection may be the exclusive cause of aplastic crisis in patients with hemolytic anemia: The mechanism of action of this human virus has been shown in vitro to be an inhibitory effect on hematopoiesis and "may be the direct result of virus cytotoxicity for erythroid progenitors in the bone marrow" (106: p. 428).

The clinical manifestation is usually a prodromal period consisting of a number of nonspecific viral-like symptoms such as malaise, low-grade fever, headache, sore throat, ear ache, and abdominal pain. Within a period of 6–12 days, symptoms of anemia requiring hospitalization and transfusion therapy become evident. Laboratory findings of reticulocytopenia are consistent with bone marrow aplasia. Increased serum iron and fetal hemoglobin levels have been reported, which return to normal levels during the recovery of erythropoiesis, which is usually within 8–10 days (102). The clinical severity of aplasia correlates with the severity of the underlying hemolytic anemia (103). The potential life-threatening nature of this event requires prompt diagnosis and management.

Meningitis

The initial report by Robinson and Watson first alerted the medical community to the increased incidence of pneumococcal meningitis in children with sickle cell anemia (30). Soon thereafter Barrett-Conner reported that the risk for pneumococcal meningitis was 600 times that of normal children (34).

Henneberger et al. (107) reported the descriptive epidemiology of pneumococcal meningitis in New York City. The average annual rate of pneumococcal meningitis for Blacks with sickle cell disease was 60.35 per 100,000 population for those under 25 years of age. This rate was 68 times the rate for Blacks without sickle cell disease (0.89 cases per 100,000 population) and 147 times the rate for whites (0.41 cases per 100,000 population).

The clinical presentation reported by investigators in Nigeria (108) was considered to be similar to that of children with AA hemoglobin, with no difference in the symptoms, laboratory data, morbidity, and mortality. They concluded that even though children with sickle cell disease were clearly more susceptible to pneumococcal meningitis, they were not at an increased risk from its effects.

However, investigators at Kings County Hospital compared cerebro-spinal fluid (CSF) findings in meningitis patients with and without sickle cell anemia and observed 6 of 21 episodes of bacterial meningitis with normocellular CSF in children with sickle cell anemia as compared to 1 of 24 episodes with normocellular CSF in non-sickle cell patients. Their review of the literature suggested that the absence of CSF pleocytosis is a relatively frequent finding in bacterial meningitis in children with sickle cell anemia. Therefore, these authors recommended that patients seen with clinical features of meningitis, such as high fever with vomiting, lethargy, or convulsions, should be treated for meningitis regardless of the CSF leukocyte count until culture results are available (109).

Overturf, Powars, and Baraff (41) reported 27 episodes of bacterial meningitis in 25 of 422 patients with hemoglobinopathies. All cases of purulent meningitis occurred before the age of 15. Of the 27 episodes, 26 occurred in 24 patients of the homozygous SS group, for a rate of 8 percent. One patient with SC hemoglobinopathy had meningitis due to *S. pneumoniae* at age 11. Seventy-four percent of all episodes were due to *S. pneumoniae,* with most occurring in children five years of age or less. The case fatality rate was 10 percent (2 of 20 episodes), for pneumococcal meningitis, and 7.5 percent (2 of 27 episodes) for all meningitis.

PREVENTION OF INFECTION

Early and aggressive treatment has been recommended for treatment of infection in early childhood. However, prevention remains the best approach in our armamentarium against the morbidity and mortality of severe bacterial infection. The first step in achieving this goal is to diagnose babies as early as possible (i.e., in the newborn period) to permit the education of the parents and others in charge of the child's care and to ensure the child's early entry into comprehensive care and the provision of specific measures (i.e., prophylactic penicillin and vaccinations).

Penicillin Prophylaxis

Nasopharyngeal colonization with *S. pneumoniae* is the first step in the development of invasive disease; therefore, any measure to prevent or reduce this initial step will impact on this illness. Overturf, Field, Lam, et al. reported that the nasopharyngeal carriage of pneumococci in normal children varies widely from rates of 6 to 55 percent, and the incidence of nasopharyngeal isolation in children with sickle cell disease was 17.8 percent, with Groups 23 and 6 and type 14 predominating. This is similar to normal children (110). Anglin, Siegel, Pacini, et al. reported a decrease in the carriage of pneumococci from prophylactic penicillin (14.5% vs. 34.4% in age-matched controls) without the emergence of pathogenic bacteria in the nasopharyngeal flora (111).

A multicenter, randomized, double-blind trial found an 84 percent reduction in pneumococcal septicemia in children younger than 3 years of age with sickle cell anemia who received oral penicillin prophylactically (44; see Figure 10.3). Of the 110 patients who received a placebo, 13 developed pneumococcal septicemia compared with only 2 of 105 children who were given penicillin (p = 0.0025). In addition, there were no deaths in the penicillin group. However, in the placebo group 3 children developed fulminant infections that progressed from the onset of fever to death in less than 9 hours despite prompt medical care.

Oral penicillin 125 mg BID up to 3 years of age, and then 250 mg BID thereafter is the preferred form of treatment. With penicillin allergy, erythromycin can be substituted. Ampicillin is not recommended as there are more side effects than

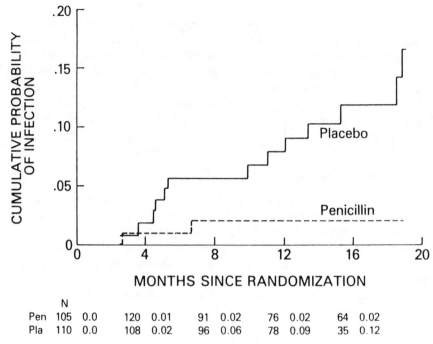

N					
Pen	105 0.0	120 0.01	91 0.02	76 0.02	64 0.02
Pla	110 0.0	108 0.02	96 0.06	78 0.09	35 0.12

Figure 10.3.   Penicillin prophylaxis of pneumococcal infections.

Source: MH Gaston, J Verter, G Woods, et al., Infection in children with sickle cell disease, *N Engl J Med* 314 (1986): 1596. Reprinted by permission of the *New England Journal of Medicine.*

with penicillin, the development of resistant organisms occurs more often, and, most importantly, its effectiveness has not been proven. Bicillin (600,000 to 1.2 million units IM/monthly) has been shown to produce effective levels for only the first 2–3 weeks; in the last week, prior to the next injection, levels fall and the child is at risk for infection (112). Therefore, it is recommended that it be administered every 3 weeks and supplemented in the last week with oral penicillin (113). The other problems associated with IM Bicillin relate to the painful injections, little muscle mass (114), and the lack of sustained compliance with monthly intramuscular injections because of the progressive reluctance of families to continue to allow their children to undergo the painful prophylactic injections. Therefore, IM prophylaxis is less desirable, and the desirability of a painless, continuous, readily available form of penicillin prophylaxis is apparent.

Babies identified at birth as having an FS electrophoretic pattern (SS disease, S-β° thalassemia) should begin to receive prophylactic penicillin at two months of age. Since children with SC disease under the age of two years have the same rate of septicemia as children with SS (43), it is recommended for this group also. The recommended length of time for continuation of the penicillin is currently under investigation. Although data are presently not available that identify the age at which prophylactic penicillin can safely be discontinued, the experience to date indicates that prophylaxis should continue at least to age five or six years.

The Prophylactic Penicillin Study (PROPS) data, albeit a short investigation, demonstrated that orally administered penicillin prophylaxis is safe and, for that period of time, did not encourage the emergence of penicillin-resistant pneumococcal strains or enhanced pharyngeal colonization with *H. influenzae* type b. In addition, no penicillin allergies developed during the course of the study.

Education

Failure of patients to take medication in any long-term prophylaxis program is common and is a real cause for concern (115–117). However, one investigation has demonstrated that penicillin was present in 66 percent of the urine samples, indicating compliance within the previous 12–24 hours (118). This was attributed to an intensive educational program in which repetitive efforts were made to counsel patients and parents about the risks of life-threatening infection. In addition, the authors documented a trend toward improved compliance on subsequent clinic visits as a result of continuing, intensive education. This education should be provided by all members of the health care team (i.e., physicians—especially nurse practitioners, social workers, child health associates, etc.). Education also helps parents to understand the alternatives and enables them to take the responsibility for their health or the health of their children. This encourages a sense of strength and responsibility and decreases their sense of helplessness. In addition, education must be continuous for all persons within the life space of the child, and especially health care workers (e.g., emergency room personnel). Everyone must understand clearly the implications of fever and the steps to be aggressively undertaken.

Still to be determined are the potential long-term risks of penicillin prophylaxis, especially in light of the fact that the prophylaxis is being initiated at such a young age. A potential risk includes the delayed development of humoral immunity to the nonvaccine strains of pneumococcus, which would place children at higher risk of pneumococcal septicemia when they were older and prophylaxis was discontinued. It is theorized that penicillin prophylaxis, by decreasing the carriage rate of the pneumococcus or by decreasing the occurrence of subclinical infection with the organism, may decrease the development of humoral immunity to the pneumococcus. Another concern is the possible emergence of penicillin-resistant pneumococci as a result of long-term prophylaxis.

Immunizations

Pneumococcal Vaccine

A second means of preventing penumococcal disease is by vaccination with the polyvalent pneumococcal vaccine. However, the vaccine is not completely effective in preventing disease because there is poor antibody response to the vaccine in children below two years of age, the time at which the vaccine would be of the greatest use (119, 120). In addition, the vaccine does not contain all the serotypes that cause infections in young children, and some serotypes that are contained are poorly immunogenic. The antigen that most frequently accounts for "vaccine failures" is pneumococcal polysaccharide type 6A which is less immunogenic than others. Other serotypes contained in the vaccine which are less immunogenic are serotypes 19 and 23 (121–124).

Nevertheless, it is recommended that all children with sickle cell disease receive at 2 years of age the pneumococcal polysaccharide vaccine, which has been shown to be effective in eliciting a normal antibody response, increasing pneumococcal opsonizing activity, and reducing the incidence of pneumococcal disease (125–128). It is recommended that either Pneumovax 23 or Pnu-imune-23 be given in a 0.5 ml dose. Both vaccines contain 23 polysaccharide antigens representing 90 percent of the serotypes causing infection in the United States. If given at 24 months it should be repeated again in three years at the age of five (129, 130). Revaccination results in increased levels of antibody and is associated with a low prevalence of severe reactions. Reactions secondary to the immunization are uncommon in children but include local pain at the injection site and sometimes fever. Adults have a higher reaction rate than children, and the reactions may be unusually severe.

In summary, the combination of both prophylactic penicillin and pneumococcal vaccine can significantly decrease the morbidity and mortality from *Streptococcus pneumoniae* in children with sickle cell disease. It is recommended at present that the penicillin be started by three months of age and continued until age five. The pneumococcal vaccine should be administered at two years of age and probably repeated at five years of age. However, this approach is not as effective as we would like. Programs are reporting the occurrence of pneumococcal septicemia despite pneumococcal vaccine and penicillin prophylaxis (131, 132). Reports following splenectomy with follow-up penicillin prophylaxis and pneumococcal vaccination have also demonstrated failures (133, 134). There is no question that these approaches to prevention must be coupled with an intensive and continuous educational program and constant monitoring to promote compliance. There must be constant vigilance to ensure that complacency does not occur in the families and, most importantly, the medical team providing care. There must be constant attention to the need for compliance and continuing concern for any fever, even though the child is receiving penicillin. This is essential for the time being. In the future, perhaps a better conjugated pneumococcal vaccine will eliminate the need for this approach.

Haemophilus b Conjugate Vaccine (ProHIBit)

This vaccine is a combined vaccine of Haemophilus b capsular polysaccharide which is conjugated or bound to diphtheria toxoid (polyribosylribitol phosphate,

PRP/diphtheria toxoid, D-PRP-D) (135). The diphtheria toxoid acts as the conduit protein to enhance antibody response, thus making this newer vaccine more efficacious. PRP-D gives higher mean titers and mean fold tier increase than PRD in all children. Titers in one study showed that 64 percent of children receiving PRP and 94 percent receiving PRP-D were > 1.0 ug/mL. Therefore, PRP-D is more immunogenic (123). It is recommended that a single dose be administered at 18 months of age or at any age up to five years. If the conjugated vaccine is administered, no booster is necessary regardless of the age at immunization. For those children who received the older polysaccharide vaccine prior to their second birthday, revaccination with the Haemophilus b Conjugate vaccine should be given at two years of age.

ACKNOWLEDGMENT

The authors wish to thank Ms. Wanda Ware for her assistance in the preparation of this manuscript.

REFERENCES

1. Mason VR: Sickle cell anemia. *JAMA* 69 (1922): 1318–1322.
2. Carrington GL, and Davison WC: Multiple osteomyelitis due to bacillus paratyphosus B: Demonstration of bacillus in fresh blood preparation. *Bull J Hopkins Hosp* 36 (1925): 428–430.
3. Diggs LW, Pulliam HN, King JC: Bone changes in sickle cell anemia. *Southern Med J* 30 (1937): 249–259.
4. Seidenstein A: Salmonella osteomyelitis. *Bull Hosp Joint Dis* 6 (1945): 126–132.
5. Wigh R, and Thompson HJ Jr.: Cortical fissuring in osteomyelitis complicating sickle cell anemia. *Radiology* 55 (1950): 553–555.
6. Mayer V, and Pohlidal SJ: Salmonella osteomyelitis with concomitant sickle cell anemia. *New York State J Med* 51 (1951): 2785.
7. Ehrenpreis B, and Schwinger HN: Sickle cell anemia. *Am J Roent Genol* 68 (1952): 28–36.
8. Goldenberg IS: Sickle cell anemia. Salmonella enteritides osteomyelitis and remote postoperative wound abscess: Report of case. *Surgery* 38 (1955): 758–763.
9. Ellenbogen NC, Raim J, and Grossman L: Salmonella osteomyelitis: Report of case and review of literature. *Am J Dis Child* 90 (1955): 275–279.
10. Smith WS: Sickle cell anemia and Salmonella osteomyelitis. *Ohio State Med J* 49 (1953): 692–695.
11. Hughes JG, and Carrol DS: Salmonella osteomyelitis complicating sickle cell disease. *Pediatrics* 19 (1957): 184–191.
12. Hook EW, Campbell CG, Weens HS, et al.: Salmonella osteomyelitis in patients with sickle cell anemia. *N Engl J Med* 257 (1957): 403–407.
13. Hook EW: Salmonellosis certain factors influencing interaction of Salmonella and human host. *Bull New York Acad Med* 37 (1961): 499–512.
14. De Torregrosa MV, Depena RB, and Hernandez H: Association of Salmonella caused osteomyelitis and sickle cell disease. *JAMA* 174 (1960): 354.

15. Hendrickse RG, and Collard P: Salmonella osteitis in Nigerian children. *Lancet* no. 2 (1960): 80.

16. Jenkins T: Osteomyelitis in a child with sickle cell anemia. *Cent African J Med* 8 (1962): 212–216.

17. Sarles HE: Osteomyelitis complicating a sickle cell thalassemia syndrome. *Tex Rep Biol Med* 22 (1964): 356–366.

18. King H, and Shumacker HB Jr.: Splenic Studies. I. Susceptibility to infection after splenectomy performed in infancy. *Ann Surg* 136 (1952): 239.

19. Gofstein R, and Gellis S: Splenectomy in infancy and childhood. *Am J Dis Child* 91 (1956): 566.

20. Smith CH, Erlandson M, Schulman I, et al.: Hazard of severe infections in splenectomized infants and children. *Am J Dis Child* 92 (1956): 507.

21. Huntley CC: Infection following splenectomy in infants and children: Review of experience at Duke Hospital in infants and children during a twenty-two year period (1933–1954). *Am J Dis Child* 95 (1958): 477–480.

22. Smith C, Erlandson ME, Stern G, et al.: Postsplenectomy infection in Cooley's Anemia: An appraisal of the problem in this and other blood disorders. *N Engl J Med* 266 (1962): 737–743.

23. Sprague CC, and Paterson JC: Role of the spleen and effect of splenectomy in sickle cell disease. *Blood* 13 (1958): 569.

24. Scott RB, Ferguson AD, and Jenkins M: Studies in sickle cell anemia VIII. Further observations on the clinical manifestations of sickle cell anemia in children. *AJDC* 90 (1955): 682–691.

25. Scott RB, and Ferguson AD: Studies in sickle cell anemia XIV. Management of the child with sickle cell anemia. *Am J Dis Child* 100 (1960): 85–93.

26. Booker CR, Scott RB, and Ferguson AD: Studies in sickle cell anemia XXII. Clinical manifestations of sickle cell anemia during the first two years of life. *Clin Pediatr* 3 (1964): 111–115.

27. Scott RB, and Ferguson AD: Studies in sickle cell anemia XXVII. Complications in infants and children in the United States. *Clin Pediatr* 5 (1966): 403–409.

28. Porter FS, and Thurman WG: Studies of sickle cell disease. Diagnosis in infancy. *Am J Dis Child* 106 (1963): 35–42.

29. Greer M, and Schotland D: Abnormal hemoglobin as cause of neurologic disease. *Neurology* 12, (1962): 114–123.

30. Robinson MG, and Watson RJ: Pneumococcal meningitis in sickle cell anemia. *N Engl J Med* 274 (1966): 1006–1008.

31. Eeckels R, Gatti F, and Renoirte AM: Abnormal distribution of haemoglobin genotypes in Negro children with severe bacterial infections. *Nature* 216 (1967): 382.

32. Eeckels R, Gatti F, Vandepitte J, et al.: Susceptibility to severe infections in children with sickle cell hemoglobinopathies. *Proc 5th International Congress for Infectious Diseases* (Vienna) 3 (1970): 267.

33. Van Baelen H, Vandepitte J, Cornu G, et al.: Routine detection of sickle cell anemia and hemoglobin Bart's in congolese neonates. *Trop Geogr Med* 21 (1969): 412–426.

34. Barrett-Connor E: Bacterial infection and sickle cell anemia. *Medicine* 50 (1971): 97–112.

35. Pearson HA, Spencer RP, and Cornelius EA: Functional asplenia in sickle cell anemia. *N Engl J Med* 281 (1969): 923–926.

36. Winkelstein JA, and Drachman RH: Deficiency of pneumococcal serum opsonizing activity in sickle cell disease. *N Engl J Med* 279, no. 9 (1968): 459–466.

37. Holroyle CP, Oski FA, and Gardner FH: The pocked erytrocyte. Red cell alterations in retriculeondothelial immaturity. *J Med* 28 (1969): 576–579.

38. Casper JT, Koethe S, Rodey GE, et al.: A new method for studying splenic retriculoendothelial dysfunction in sickle cell disease patients and its clinical application: A brief report. *Blood* 47 (1976): 183–188.

39. Pearson HA, Gallagher D, Chilcote R, et al.: Developmental pattern of splenic dysfunction in sickle cell disorders. *Pediatrics* 76 (1985): 392–397.

40. Seeler RA, Metzger W, and Mufson M: Diplococcus pneumoniae infections in children with sickle cell anemia. *Am J Dis Child* 123 (1972): 8–10.

41. Overturf GD, Powars D, and Baraff LF: Bacterial meningitis and septicemia in sickle cell disease. *Am J Dis Child* 131 (1977): 784–787.

42. Powars D, Overturf G, Weis J, et al.: Pneumococcal septicemia in children with sickle cell anemia. *JAMA* 245 (1981): 1839–1842.

43. Gaston M, Falletta J, Verter J, et al.: Infection in children with sickle cell disease. *Ped Res* 16 (1982): 204a.

44. Gaston MH, Verter J, Woods G, et al.: Prophylaxis with oral penicillin in children with sickle cell anemia: A randomized trial. *N Engl J Med* 314 (1986): 1593–1599.

45. Lobel JS, and Bove KE: Clinicopathologic characteristics of septicemia in sickle cell disease. *Am J Dis Child* 136 (1982): 543–547.

46. Zarkowsky H, Gallagher D, Gill F, et al.: Bacteremia in sickle hemoglobinopathies. *J Peds* 109 (1986): 579–585.

47. Topley JM, Cupidor L, Vaidya S, et al.: Pneumococcal and other infections in children with sickle cell hemoglobin C (SC) sickle cell disease. *J Peds* 101 (1982): 176–179.

48. Powars D, Overturf GD, and Wilkins J: Commentary: Infections in sickle cell and SC disease. *J Peds* 103 (1983): 242–244.

49. Buchanan G, Smith S, Holtkamp C, et al.: Bacterial infection and splenic reticuloendothelial function in children with hemoglobin SC disease. *Pediatrics* 72 (1983): 93–98.

50. McIntosh S, Rooks Y, Ritchey AK, et al.: Fever in young children with sickle cell disease. *J Peds* 96 (Feb. 1980): 199–203.

51. Oski F: Pneumococcal infection in sickle cell disease. *Ped Infect Dis* 2, no. 3 (1983): 184–186.

52. Pearson H: Sickle cell anemia and severe infection due to encapsulated bacteria. *J Infect Dis* 136 (1977): 525–529.

53. Cole T, Smith S, and Buchanan G: Hematologic alterations during acute infection in children with sickle cell disease. *Ped Infect Dis* 6 (1987): 454–457.

54. Kabins SA, and Lerner C: Fulminant pneumococcemia and sickle cell anemia. *JAMA* 211 (1970): 467–471.

55. Seeler RA, Metzger W, and Mufsan MA: Diplococcus pneumoniae infections in children with sickle cell anemia. *Am J Dis Child* 123 (1972): 8–10.

56. Haddock JA, David E, and Mashall L: Sickle cell anemia. *JAMA* 212 (1970): 629.

57. Dyment PG, and Donowho EM: Fatal pneumococcemin and sickle cell anemia. *Southern Med J* 64 (1971): 758.

58. Gilman WL, MacDougall LG, and Judisch JM: Sickle cell disease and disseminated intravascular coagulation. *Clin Pediatr* 12 (1973): 600–602.

59. Seeler RA: Deaths in children with sickle cell anemia. *Clin Pediatr* 11 (1972): 643–647.
60. Bisno AL, and Freeman JC: The syndrome of asplenia, pneumococcal sepsis and disseminated intravascular coagulation. *Ann Intern Med* 72 (1970): 389–393.
61. Pearson HA, Cornelius EA, Schwartz AD, et al.: Transfusion reversible functional asplenia in young children with sickle cell anemia. *N Engl J Med* 283 (1970): 334–337.
62. Pearson HA, Gallagher D, Chilcote R, et al.: Development pattern of splenic dysfunction in sickle cell disorders. *Pediatrics* 76 (1985): 392–397.
63. Torres J, and Bisno AL: Hyposplenism and pneumococcemia. *Am J Med* 55 (1973): 851–855.
64. Johnston RB, Newman SL, and Struth AG: Serum opsonins and the alternate pathway in sickle cell disease. *N Engl J Med* 288 (1973): 803–808.
65. Wilson WA, Hughes GR, and Lachman PJ: Deficiency of factor 13 of the complement system in sickle cell anemia. *Br Med J* no. 1 (1973): 367.
66. Bjornson A, Gaston MH, and Zellner CL: Decreased opsonization for *Streptococcus Pneumoniae* in sickle cell disease. *J Peds* 91 (1977): 371–378.
67. Bjornson A, and Lobel S: Direct evidence that decreased serum opsonization of *Streptococcus Pneumoniae* via the alternative complement pathway in sickle cell disease in relation to antibody deficiency. *Clin Invest* 79 (1987): 388–398.
68. Rao RRP, Patel AR, and Sonnenberg M: Five years' experience of bacteremia in sickle cell anemia. *J Infect* 14 (1987): 225–228.
69. McDonald CR, and Eichner ER: Concurrent primary pneumococcal disseminated intravascular coagulation and sickle cell anemia. *Southern Med J* 71 (1978): 858–860.
70. Greene JR, Polk OD, and Castro O: Fulminant pneumococcal sepsis in an adult with sickle cell anemia [letter] *N Engl J Med* 311 (1984): 674.
71. Chileote R, and Dampier C: Overwhelming pneumococcal septicemia in a patient with Hb SC disease and splenic dysfunction. *J Peds* 104 (1984): 734–736.
72. Ward J, and Smith A: *Hemophilus Influenzae* bactermia in children with sickle cell anemia. *J Peds* 88 (1976): 261–263.
73. Powars D, Overturf G, and Turner E: Is there an increased risk of *Hemophilus Influenzae* septicemia in children with sickle cell anemia. *Pediatrics,* 71 (1983): 927–931.
74. Arpi M, Hnberg PZ, and Frimodt-Miler, N: Antibiotic susceptibility of Haemophilus influenzae isolated from cerebrospinal fluid and blood. *Acta Pathol Microbiol Immunol Scand* 94, no. 3 (1986), 167–171.
75. Barrett-Connor E: Pneumonia and pulmonary infarction in sickle cell anemia. *Amer Med Assoc* 229 (1973): 997.
76. Charache S, Scott JC, and Charache P: "Acute Chest Syndrome" in adults with sickle cell anemia: Microbiology, treatment and prevention. *Arch Intern Med* 139 (1979): 67–69.
77. Petch MC, and Sergeant GR: Clinical features of pulmonary lesion in sickle cell disease. *Br Med J* 713, no. 3 (1970): 31.
78. Davies SC, Win AA, Luce PJ, et al.: Acute chest syndrome in sickle cell disease. *Lancet* 8367, no. 1 (Jan. 1984): 36–38.
79. Poncz M, Kane E, and Gill FM: Acute chest syndrome in sickle cell disease: Etiology and clinical correlates. *J Peds* 107 (1985): 861–866.

80. Sprinkle RH, Cole T, Smith S, et al.: Acute chest syndrome in children with sickle cell disease. *Am J Ped Hem Onc* 8, no. 2 (1986): 105–110.

81. Fernald GW, Collier AM, and Clyde W: Respiratory infections due to mycoplasma pneumoniae in infants and children. *Pediatrics* 55 (1975): 327–385.

82. Shulman ST, Bartlett J, Clyde WA, et al.: The unusual severity of mycoplasma pneumonia in children with sickle cell disease. *N Engl J Med* 287 (1972): 164–167.

83. Mann JR, Cotter KP, Walker RA, et al.: Anemia crises in sickle cell disease. *J Clin Pathol* 28 (1987): 341–344.

84. Brownell A, McSwiggan DA, Cubitt WD, et al.: Aplastic and hypoplastic episodes in sickle cell disease and thalassemia intermedia. *J Clin Pathol* 319 (1986): 121–124.

85. Haddad JD, John JF, and Pappas AA: Cytomegalovirus pneumonia in sickle cell disease. *Chest* 86, no. 2 (1984): 265–266.

86. Hardy R, Cummings C, Thomas F, et al.: Cryptococcus pneumonia in a patient with sickle cell anemia. *Chest* 89, no. 6 (1986): 892–894.

87. Syrogiannopoulos GA, McCracken GH, and Nelson JD: Osteoarticular infections in children with sickle cell disease. *Pediatrics* 78, no. 6 (1986): 1090–1096.

88. Rao S, Solomon N, Miller S, et al.: Scintigraphic differentiation of bone infarction from osteomyelitis in children with sickle cell disease. *J Peds* 107 (1985): 685–688.

89. Wethers D, and Grover R: Pitfalls in diagnosis of osteomyelitis in children. *Clin Ped* 22, no. 9 (1983): 614–618.

90. Rao S, Solomon N, Miller S, et al.: Scintigraphis differentiation of bone infarction from osteomyelitis in children with sickle cell disease. *J Peds* 107 (1985): 685–688.

91. Hodges FJ, and Holt JF: Editorial comment. In FJ Hodges, et al., eds.: *The 1951 year book of radiology (June 1950–June 1951)*, p. 84. Chicago: Year Book Publishers, 1951.

92. Givner LB, Luddy RE, and Schwartz AD: Etiology of osteomylitis in patients with major hemoglobinopathies. *J Ped* 99, no. 3 (1981): 411–413.

93. Ortiz-Neu C, Marr JS, Cherubin CE, et al.: Bone and joint infections due to salmonella. *J Infect Dis* 138, no. 6 (1978): 820–828.

94. Adeyokunnu AA, and Hendrickse RG: Salmonella osteomyelitis in childhood. *Am J Dis Child* 55 (1980): 175–184.

95. Rennels MB, Tenney JH, Luddy RE, et al.: Intestinal salmonella carriage in patients with major sickle cell hemoglobinopathies. *Southern Med J* 78, no. 3 (1985): 310–311.

96. Patton HM, Conlan JK, Long RF, et al.: Unusual presentation of anaerobic osteomyelitis. *Am J Med* 75 (Oct. 1983): 724–726.

97. Cossart YE, Field AM, Cant B, et al.: Parvovirus-like particles in human sera. *Lancet* no. 1 (1975): 72–73.

98. Pattison JR, Jones SE, Hodgson J, et al.: Parvovirus infections and hypoplastic crises in sickle cell anemia. *Lancet* 8221, no. 1 (March 21, 1981): 664–665.

99. Anderson MJ, Davis LR, Hodgson J, et al.: Occurrence of infection with a parvovirus-like agent in children with sickle cell anemia during a two-year period. *J Clin Pathol* 35 (1982): 744–749.

100. Gowda N, Rao SP, Cohen B, et al.: Human parvovirus infection in patients with

sickle cell disease and without hypoplastic crisis. *J Peds* 110, no. 1 (Jan. 1987): 81–84.

101. Serjeant GR, Mason K, Topley JM, et al.: Outbreak of aplastic crisis in sickle cell anemia associated with parvovirus-like agent. *Lancet* 8247, no. 2 (Sept. 19, 1981): 595–597.

102. Goldstein R, Anderson MJ, and Serjeant GR: Parvovirus associated aplastic crisis in homozygous sickle cell disease. *Arch Dis Child* 62 (1987): 585–588.

103. Saarinen UM, Chorba TL, Tattersall P, et al.: Human parvovirus B19-induced epidemic acute red cell aplasia in patients with hereditary hemolytic anemia. *Blood* 67, no. 5 (1986): 1411–1417.

104. Koduri R, Rao P, Patel AR, et al.: Infection with parvovirus-like virus and aplastic crisis in chronic hemolytic anemia. *Ann Intern Med* 98 (1983): 930–932.

105. Kelleher JF, Luban JL, Cohen BJ, et al.: Human serum parvovirus as the cause of aplastic crisis in sickle cell disease. *Am J Dis Child* 138 (Apr. 1984).

106. Mortimer PP, Humphries RK, Moore JG, et al.: A human parvovirus-like virus inhibits haematopoietic colony formation in vitro. *Nature* 302, no. 5907 (1983): 426–429.

107. Henneberger PK, Galaid EI, and Marr JS: The descriptive epidemiology of pneumococcal meningitis in New York City. *Am J Epidemiol* 117 (1983): 484–491.

108. Nottidge, VA: Pneumococcal meningitis in sickle cell disease in childhood. *Am J Dis Child* 137 (1983): 29–31.

109. Rao FP, Schmalzer E, Kaufman M, et al.: Meningitis in patients with sickle cell anemia: Normal cellular CSF at initial diagnosis. *Am J Ped Hem Onc* 5 (1983): 101–103.

110. Overturf GD, Field R, Lam C, et al.: Nasopharyngeal carriage of pneumococci in children with sickle cell disease. *Inf and Imm* 28 (1980): 1048–1050.

111. Anglin DR, Siegel JD, Pacini DL, et al.: Effect of penicillin prophylaxis on NP colonization with *S penumaniae* in children with sickle cell disease. *J Peds* 104 (1984): 18–22.

112. Ginsburg CM, McCracken GH, and Ziverghaft C: Serum penicillin concentrations after intramuscular administration of benzathine penicillin G in children. *Pediatrics* 69 (1982): 452–454.

113. Brown A, Miller S, and Agatista P: Care of infants with sickle cell disease. *Pediatrics* 83 (1989): 897–900.

114. John AB, Ramlal A, Jackson H, et al.: Prevention of pneumococcal infection in children with homozygous sickle cell disease. *Br Med J* 288 (1984): 1567–1570.

115. Gordis L, Markowitz M, and Lilienfeld AM: A quantitative determination of compliance in children on oral penicillin prophylaxis. *Pediatrics* 43 (1969): 173–182.

116. Bergman AB, and Werner RJ: Future of children to receive penicillin by mouth. *N Engl J Med* 268 (1963): 1334–1338.

117. Gordis L, Markowitz M, and Lilienfeld A: Why patients don't follow medical *advice:* A study of children on long-term prophylaxis. *J Peds* 75 (1969): 957–968.

118. Buchanan G, Siegel J, and Smith S: Oral penicillin prophylaxis in children with impaired splenic function: a study of compliance. *Pediatrics* 70 (1982): 926–930.

119. Ahonkhai VI, Landesman SH, Fikrig SM, et al.: Failure of pneumococcal vaccine in children with sickle cell disease. *N Engl J Med* 301 (1979): 26–27.

120. Buchanan GR, and Schiffman G: Antibody responses to polyvalent pneumococcal vaccine in infants with sickle cell anemia. *J Peds* 96 (1980): 264–266.

121. Broome CV: Efficacy of pneumococcal polysaccharide vaccine. *Rev Infect Dis* 3-suppl. (1981): S82–S96.

122. Overturf GD, Field R, and Edmonds R: Death from type 6 penumococcal septicemia in a vaccinated child with sickle cell disease. *N Engl J Med* 300 (1979): 143.

123. Broome CV, Facklam RR, and Fraser DW: Pneumococcal disease after pneumococcal vaccination: An alternative method to estimate the efficacy of penumococcal vaccine. *N Engl J Med* 303 (1980): 549–552.

124. Kaplan J, Frost H, Sarnaiks S, et al.: Type-specific antibodies in children with sickle cell anemia given polyvalent pneumococcal vaccine. *J Peds* 100 (1982): 404–406.

125. Platt O, and Nathan D: Disorders of hemoglobin, sickle cell disease. In D Nathan and F Oski, eds.: 3, *Hematology of Infancy and Childhood*, pp. 655–698. Philadelphia: W. B. Saunders, 1987.

126. Ammann AJ, Addrego J, Wara DW, et al.: Polyvalent pneumococcal polysaccharide immunization of patients with sickle cell anemia and patients with splenectomy. *N Engl J Med* 297, no. 17 (1977): 897–900.

127. Overturf GD, Rigau-Perez JG, Selzer J, et al.: Pneumococcal polysaccharide immunization of children with sickle cell disease. I. Clinical reactions to immunization and relationship to pre-immunization antibody. *Am J Ped Hem Onc* 4, no. 1 (1982): 19–23.

128. Chudwin DS, Wara DW, Mathay KK, et al.: Increases in serum opsonic activity and antibody concentration in patients with sickle cell disease after pneumococcal polysaccharide immunization. *J Peds* 102, no. 1 (1983): 51–54.

129. Kaplan J, Sarnaik S, and Schiffman G: Revaccination with polyvalent pneumococcal vaccine in children with sickle cell anemia. *Am J Ped Hem Onc* 8 (1986): 80–82.

130. Weintrub P, Schiffman G, Addiego J, et al.: Long-term follow-up and booster immunization with polyvalent pneumococcal polysaccharide in patients with sickle cell anemia. *J Peds* 105 (1984): 261–263.

131. Buchanan GR, and Smith SJ: Pneumococcal septicimia despite pneumococcal vaccine and prescription of penicillin prophylaxis in children with sickle cell anemia. *Am J Dis Child* 140 (1986): 428–432.

132. Wethers D: Personal communication, July 1988.

133. Evans DK: Fatal post-splenectomy sepsis despite prophylaxis with penicillin and pneumococcal vaccine. *Lancet* no. 1 (1984): 1124.

134. Brivet R, Herer R, Fremaux A, et al.: Fatal post-splenectomy pneumococcal sepsis despite pneumococcal vaccine and penicillin prophylaxis. *Lancet* no. 2 (1984): 356.

135. Frank AL, Labotka RJ, Rao S, et al.: *Haemophilus Influenzae* type B immunization of children with sickle cell disease. *Pediatrics* 82 (1988): 571–575.

11

Neurological Complications of Sickle Cell Disease

Vipul N. Mankad and Paul R. Dyken

Neurological complications are quite common in sickle cell anemia. This would be expected because the brain is highly susceptible to hypoxic damage and also because a decrease in the blood flow in various organs is the major pathophysiologic event in sickle cell disease. This chapter will review the incidence, pathophysiology, clinical manifestations, diagnostic procedures, and conventional treatments of stroke in sickle cell disease. Other neurological abnormalities will also be discussed.

INCIDENCE

There is a wide variation in the reported incidence (6–34%) of neurological abnormalities in sickle cell patients (1–8). There are many reasons for such wide variations in the reports. In addition to different populations under study at various centers, criteria for inclusion in the analysis also vary. For example, patients with seizures but without evidence of vascular accident as the etiology are included in some reports, thus increasing the incidence figures. On the other hand, subtle clinical neurological signs may not have been investigated with sensitive diagnostic and imaging tools in some studies, thus resulting in underreporting of the incidence. Our interpretation of published literature indicates the true incidence of stroke is around 8–10 percent.

PATHOPHYSIOLOGY

Cerebral infarction secondary to decreased blood flow is the most common cause of stroke in sickle cell disease (about 75%), followed by cerebral hemorrhage (about 25%). Although vaso-occlusion in other organs is thought to occur in the precapillary segment of the arterioles, there are many autopsy reports and angiographic studies showing large vessel disease associated with stroke in sickle cell patients (9, 10). On the other hand, there are also reports describing no involvement of the vessel walls of the large arteries themselves but describing retrograde thrombi or dilatation (3). Thus, microvascular as well as large vessel causes of neurological disease are thought to occur in sickle cell patients.

Occlusion of the vaso-vasorum supplying blood to the vessel walls of large arteries has been postulated (10, 11). However, this hypothesis has not been proved and is probably not testable. Since the endothelial cells in the carotid and cerebral vessels are richly supplied with oxygenated blood, hypoxia of the vessel wall is not a plausible hypothesis.

Platelet hyperactivity and/or platelet–endothelial interaction causing atherosclerotic and stenotic changes in the large vessels is another hypothesis. Increased platelet counts, platelet aggregation, and circulating microaggregates have been reported in other patients with stroke, but such studies have not been reported extensively in sickle cell patients (12, 13). In sickle cell patients, increased numbers of platelets and microaggregates of platelets have been found during pain crises compared to controls (14). In addition, Longenecker and Mankad reported increased levels of beta-thromboglobulin, a protein associated with platelet aggregation, in sickle cell patients compared to controls (15). A proaggregatory platelet prostanoid, thromboxane, was also investigated in sickle cell patients. The release of thromboxane per platelet is lower in sickle cell patients than in controls, indicating a refractory state from continuous stimulation of the platelets (15). The precise nature of the role of platelets in the causation of large vessel disease in sickle cell patients is not known.

Fat embolism from areas of bone marrow infarction and antecedent meningitis altering the structure of vessel walls are among other factors postulated to contribute to the etiology of stroke (16, 17). However, cases where these factors can be considered in relationship to stroke are quite rare.

CLINICAL MANIFESTATIONS

The sudden onset of hemiparesis, speech disturbances such as aphasia, visual disturbances, and seizures are common presentations of stroke in sickle cell patients. Only a small proportion of patients exhibit an accompanying or antecedent illness. Pain crisis, pneumonia, mood swings, and frontal headaches have been reported in some patients (1, 7). General anesthesia and pregnancy in sickle cell disease have been associated with stroke as well. There is one report of stroke secondary to angiography (18).

The mean age of occurrence of the first episode of stroke in the population at Los Angeles was 7.7 years (range: 20 months to 16 years) (6). The risk to males and females is approximately equal. Data suggestive of higher incidence in the nonsickle cell siblings of patients with sickle cell disease have been presented but are not conclusive (7). The risk of stroke in various haplotypes of sickle cell disease (Benin, Bantu, Senegal, and Asian, or a combination thereof) needs to be examined. The overwhelming majority of patients with stroke reported in the literature have homozygous sickle cell disease (SS). However, sickle-hemoglobin C disease (SC) is also reported in association with stroke. If the risk factors can be defined, the populations of sickle cell patients at a higher risk of stroke may be investigated with noninvasive or less invasive imaging tools and considered for prophylactic therapy, such as transfusions, or more aggressive therapy, such as bone marrow transplantation.

DIAGNOSTIC PROCEDURES

Although stroke should be considered in any sickle cell disease patient with any combination of neurologic symptoms, including sudden signs or symptoms such as hemiparesis, hemiparesis with seizures, isolated seizures, aphasia, or alteration of consciousness, these presentations may also indicate other potential causes of neurological disease that are also known to be associated with sickle cell disease, such as meningitis. Lumbar puncture represents an important diagnostic procedure to exclude bacterial meningitis. Since neurological and other complications have occurred in sickle cell populations after both arteriography and contrasted computerized tomography (CT) scan, either head magnetic resonance imaging (MRI) scans or noncontrasted CT neuro-imaging is indicated in those suspected of having had stroke (Figures 11.1 and 11.2). Recent studies have shown that arteriography after proper preparation is indicated in a setting of intracranial hemorrhage and in some instances of infarction syndrome, particularly if subdural hematoma, a possible mimicker, has not been excluded as a diagnostic possibility. When an arteriography candidate with sickle cell disease needs such a procedure, it has been shown that adequate preparation with hydration and reduction of hemoglobin S to 30 percent or less of the total hemoglobin is a good preparation prior to arteriography. Thorough evaluation of cardiac status, including the use of echocardiography, should be always considered in the sickle cell patient with presumed stroke to exclude an often coexisting cardiac abnormality. Late neurological reactions to contrast material used in CT scanning (19) have been identified as a possible source of further transient or permanent neurologic dysfunction in sickle cell disease with stroke. Recent work has suggested that transcranial doppler scanning may be an accurate and noninvasive method of evaluating the vascular system in sickle cell disease. Angiographic study by means of MRI have been developed recently and are under investigation (30). Cerebral flow studies using ultrasonography represent a much less invasive method of measuring cerebral blood flow in sickle cell patients with stroke than more complicated and invasive, if not more accurate, methods of study using xenon-133 inhalation (20).

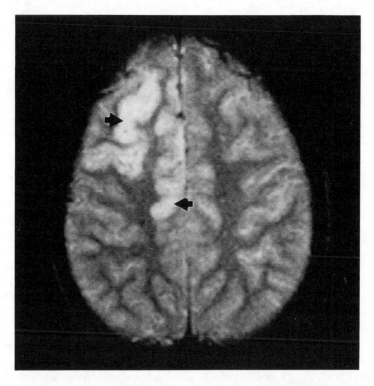

Figure 11.1. T$_2$-weighted MRI of brain in a 10-year-old black female with sickle
cell anemia and left hemiplegia. Increased signals (arrows) in the gyri
of the right cerebral hemisphere (frontoparietal region) represent an
infarct in the distribution of the frontoparietal branch of the middle
cerebral artery.

TREATMENTS

The mainstay of treatment of sickle cell disease patients with ischemic stroke
remains excellent general body care and adequate hydration. The most accepted
form of specific treatment is represented by hypertransfusion. This involves the
partial exchange transfusion of normal matched blood to maintain hematocrit
levels at 30 to 34 percent and the total hemoglobin over 10–11 gm/dl. The
transfusion program is adjusted to maintain hemoglobin S at a level less than
30 percent. Such hypertransfusion intervention may have little effect on the acute
effects of infarction (the prognosis for at least partial recovery is good anyway),
but there is good evidence that it may prevent recurrent infarctions and decrease
the progression of stenotic lesions (21, 22). Usually, the hypertransfusion treatment program must be extended. Long-term blood transfusion requires chelation
therapy to reduce iron overload. Desferioxamine in a dose of 2 gm/m^2 adminis-

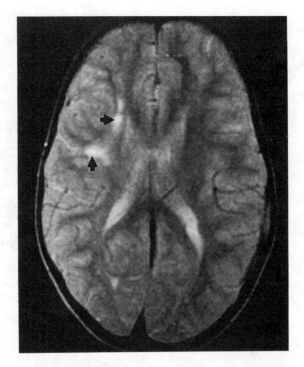

Figure 11.2. T$_2$-weighted MRI of brain in a seven-year-old black female with sickle
cell anemia and left hemiplegia. Increased signal (arrow) in the white
matter of the right cerebral hemisphere is thought to be due to
infarctions involving arterioles.

tered subcutaneously by a continuous pump for 20 hours daily is optimal. However, the compliance with such a program is usually low. When patients stop chelation therapy and the transfusion program after several years of treatment, strokes
generally do not occur. However, the safety of stopping blood transfusions has not
been established. It is the practice at the Comprehensive Sickle Cell Center in Mobile to recommend blood transfusions for prolonged periods of time.

The use of anticoagulants, antiplatelet agents, or corticosteroids have not been
established as helpful for acute as well as maintenance treatment of ischemic
stroke in sickle cell disease.

OTHER NEUROLOGICAL COMPLICATIONS

Although much less commonly seen than stroke in sickle cell disease, spinal
cord infarction and subsequent acute myelopathy have been reported infrequently
(1, 23, 24). Additionally, paraplegia related to cord compression has also been described (25). Another patient had a transverse myelitis from presumed viral cause (7).

Neuropathy as an isolated event has been reported. A unique example is represented by a mental nerve neuropathy ocurring as a result of, or in coexistance with, severe vaso-occlusive pain episodes of the mandible (26). A multiple cranial nerve neuropathy with trigeminal neuralgia and facial palsy was reported in one patient (27). Auditory involvement in the form of hearing loss has been reported in a large series of patients. Todd, Sarjeant, and Sarson (28) observed that 18 of 83 patients with SS disease had hearing losses of at least 25 decibels. It is believed by some researchers that these findings are related to the central auditory system, whereas others believe they are due to both reduced nerve and central auditory function (29). The peripheral neuropathy reported in some cases of SS disease may be related to plumbism. In one series of 15 children with lead poisoning and peripheral neuropathy (which usually manifests as an encephalopathy), 6 had hemoglobin SS or SC disease (1). In these instances, footdrop and peripheral muscle weakness represented the main symptomatology.

Other neurological complications of SS disease include sudden blindness with ophthalmoscopic evidence of retinal occlusive disease and retinal edema. The relationship of retinal vascular disease with stroke is uncertain.

SUMMARY

Cerebral infarction due to vaso-occlusive complications and cerebral hemorrhage cause one of the most devastating complications of sickle cell disease. Investigations include magnetic resonance imaging and/or computerized tomograms and, in selected instances, angiographic studies. Other noninvasive or less invasive procedures are available. In addition to supportive treatment, blood transfusion to prevent the recurrence of stroke is recommended.

REFERENCES

1. Greer M, and Schotland D: Abnormal hemoglobin as a cause of neurological disease. *Neurology* 12 (1962): 114–123.
2. Portnoy BA, and Herion JC. Neurological manifestations in sickle cell disease. *Ann Intern Med* 76 (1972): 643–652.
3. Hughes JG, Diggs LW, and Gillespie CE. Involvement of the central nervous system in sickle cell anemia. *J Peds* 17 (1940): 166–184.
4. Adeloye A, and Odeku LE. The nervous system in sickle cell disease. *Afr J Med Sci* 1 (1970): 33–48.
5. Seeler RA. Deaths in children with sickle cell anemia. *Clin Pediatr* 11 (1972): 634–637.
6. Powers D, Wilson B, Imbus C, et al.: The natural history of stroke in sickle cell disease. *Am J Med* 65 (1978): 461–471.
7. Sarnaik SA, and Lusher JM. Neurological complications of sickle cell anemia. *Am J Ped Hem Onc* 4, no. 4 (1982): 386–394.
8. Adams RJ, Nichols FT, Hartlage P, et al.: Stroke in sickle cell disease. *JMAG* 75 (1986): 271–274.
9. Bridges WH. Cerebral vascular disease accompanying sickle cell anemia. *Am J Pathol* 15 (1939): 353–361.

10. Stockman JA, Nigro MA, Mishkin NM, et al.: Occlusion of large cerebral vessels in sickle cell anemia. *N Engl J Med* 287 (1972): 846–849.

11. Baird RL, Weiss DL, Ferguson AD, et al.: Studies in sickle cell anemia. XXI. Clinicopathological aspects of neurological manifestations. *Pediatrics* 34 (1964): 92–100.

12. Schmidley JW, and Coronna JJ. Transient cerebral ischemia: Pathophysiology. *Prog Cardiovasc Dis* 22 (1980): 325–342.

13. Barnhart MI, Gilroy J, and Meyer JS. Dextran-40 in cerebrovascular thrombosis. *Thromb Diath Haemorrh* 42-suppl. (1970): 321–342.

14. Mehta P, and Mehta J. Circulating platelet aggregates in sickle cell disease patients with and without vaso-occlusion. *Stroke* 10 (1979): 464–466.

15. Longenecker GL, Byers BJ, and Mankad VN. Platelet regulatory prostanoids and platelet release products in sickle cell disease. *Am J Hematol* 40 (1992): 12–19.

16. Wyatt JP, and Orrahood MD. Massive fat embolization following marrow infarction in sickle cell anemia. *Arch Pathol* 53 (1952): 233–238.

17. Seeler RA. Commentary: Sickle cell anemia, stroke and transfusion. *J Peds* 96 (1980): 243–244.

18. Gerald B, Sebes JI, and Langston JW. Cerebral infarction secondary to sickle cell disease: Arteriographic findings. *Am J Radiol* 134 (1980): 1209–1212.

19. Imbus C, Powars D, Pegelow C, et al.: Computerized tomography complications. *Arch Neurol* 35 (1978): 620.

20. Huttenlocker PR, Moohr JW, Jabus L, et al.: Cerebral blood flow in sickle cell cerebrovascular disease. *Pediatrics* 73 (1984): 615–621.

21. Russell MO, Goldberg HI, Hodson A, et al.: Effect of transfusion therapy on arteriographic abnormalities and on recurrence of stroke in sickle cell disease. *Blood* 63 (1984): 162–169.

22. Williams J, Godd JR, Anderson HR, et al.: Efficacy of transfusion for one to two years in patients with sickle cell disease and cerebrovascular accidents. *J Peds* 96 (1980): 205–208.

23. Dowland LP. Neurological manifestations in sickle cell disease. *J Nerv Movt Dis* 115 (1952): 456–457.

24. Russell MO, Goldberg H, Reiss L, et al.: Transfusion therapy for cerebrovascular abnormalities in sickle cell disease. *J Peds* 88 (1976): 381–387.

25. Ammoumi AA, Sher JH, and Schmelka D. Spinal cord compression by extramedullary hemopaetic tissue in sickle cell anemia. *J Neurol Surg* 43 (1975): 483–485.

26. Konotey-Ahula FID. Mental nerve neuropathy: A complication of sickle cell crisis. *Lancet* no. 2 (1972): 388.

27. Asher SW. Multiple cranial neuropathies, trigeminal neuralgia and vascular headaches in sickle cell disease, A possible common mechanism. *Neurology* 30 (1980): 210–211.

28. Todd GB, Serjeant GR, and Sarson MR. Sensori-neural hearing loss in Jamaicans with SS disease. *Acta Oto Laryngologica* (Stockholm) 76 (1973): 268–272.

29. Sharp M, and Orchik D. Auditory function in sickle cell anemia. *Arch Otolaryngol* 104 (1978): 322–324.

30. Witznitzer M, Ruggieri PM, and Masaryk TJ: Diagnosis of cerebrovascular disease in sickle cell anemia by magnetic resonance angiography. *J Peds* 117, no. 4 (1990): 551–555.

12

Hepatobiliary, Renal, and Pulmonary Complications in Sickle Cell Disease

Vipul N. Mankad and Yih-Ming Yang

Multiple organ systems are affected in sickle cell disease either due to vaso-occlusion or hemolytic anemia. Clinical features, pathophysiology, and issues related to diagnosis and management of disorders related to several organs (brain, bones, spleen, and blood) are described in Chapters 2–11.

This chapter describes clinical features of hepatobiliary, renal, and pulmonary disorders commonly seen in sickle cell patients.

HEPATOBILIARY DISORDERS

Hepatobiliary abnormalities are extremely common in sickle cell disease. These include:

1. Hepatomegaly
2. Abnormal liver function tests
3. Hyperbilirubinemia
4. Acute hepatic vaso-occlusive crisis
5. Acute hepatic sequestration crisis
6. Viral hepatitis
7. Gall stones
8. Cirrhosis of the liver
9. Hemosiderosis
10. Acute hepatic failure

Signs and symptoms of several liver disorders may overlap and multiple conditions may coexist. Therefore, it is not always possible to precisely define the nature of liver disease in a specific patient. Hepatobiliary disorders include (1) conditions for which sickle cell patients are at increased risk (i.e., intrahepatic sickling, hepatic sequestration, gall stones, and hepatic failure), (2) viral hepatitis secondary to blood transfusion required for indications related or unrelated to sickle cell disease, and (3) other liver diseases that occur in the general population and coincidently occur in sickle cell patients with the same frequency.

Biopsies of the liver in patients with sickle cell disease reveal sinusoidal dilatation, Kupffer cell hyperplasia, and erythrophagocytosis (1–4). Increased collagen material is found in the basement membrane on electron microscopy. Autopsy studies show focal necrosis, portal fibrosis, and micronodular cirrhosis in a significant number of patients (2). Multiple causes of cirrhosis of the liver may be present, such as hypoxia from sickling, hepatitis, gall stones, congestive cardiac failure, hemosiderosis, and alcohol or drug abuse (5).

Major Clinical Abnormalities

Relatively Asymptomatic Conditions

In steady state patients with sickle cell disease, several abnormalities in the hepatobiliary system are found. Hepatomegaly is present in more than 50 percent of patients with sickle cell disease that are seen in medical centers and is usually found in most cases at autopsy (3, 6). Abnormal liver function tests are found in many sickle cell patients, but the hepatic origin of the abnormality is not always established (5). Elevated total bilirubin, usually in the range of 3–6 mg with increase in both direct and indirect fractions, is found. Marked elevations in bilirubin levels should raise the possibilities of acute intrahepatic sickling, hemolysis, or cholestasis. Serum alkaline phosphatase generally derived from the bones is usually elevated in adults. Prothrombin time of 2 or more seconds greater than the upper limits of normal may be found. Transaminases may be mildly elevated during asymptomatic periods.

Acute Vaso-Occlusive Hepatic Crisis

Seven to 10 percent of hospitalized patients have acute hepatic crisis (7). Nausea, abdominal pain, low grade fever, and increasing jaundice suggest vaso-occlusive hepatic crisis that should be distinguished from viral hepatitis and acute hepatic sequestration crisis. There is often an upper respiratory infection or pain crisis in other locations preceding the hepatic crisis. The liver is enlarged and tender. Transaminases are one to three times normal, bilirubin is 2–13 mg percent, and investigations for hepatitis and cholestasis are negative. Transaminase levels fall more rapidly in this condition than in viral hepatitis. Transient, hypoxic injury due to intrahepatic sickling is thought to cause the syndrome.

Acute Hepatic Sequestration Crisis

Several episodes of acute hepatic enlargement associated with a dramatic fall in hemoglobin and an increase in reticulocytes have been reported in patients with sickle cell anemia (4, 6–8). There is usually no evidence of cardiac failure or gall stones as the contributing causes. Although bilirubin and transaminases are elevated, the abnormalities are not strikingly different from other liver problems in sickle cell disease. Severe anemia may necessitate a transfusion of red blood cells. However, in some instances, the hemoglobin level may spontaneously increase, with a remarkable decrease in the liver size as the patient recovers (8). This usually indicates a return of sequestered red cells to circulation. It may be extremely difficult to separate this condition from acute vaso-occlusive hepatic crisis because the latter may be accompanied by severe anemia as well.

Cholelithiasis and Cholestasis

Bilirubin gall stones are very common in sickle cell anemia and may be detected as early as 2 years of age. In early childhood, ultrasound may detect gall stones in about 10–12 percent of patients. During late adolescence and adult life, the prevalence approaches 40–50 percent. Radionuclide scans using diisopropyl iminodiacetic acid (DISIDA) or other iminodiacetic acid salts show obstruction or patency of the bile duct. Generally, the treatment of asymptomatic gall stones is conservative. However, cholecystectomy is necessary in instances where cholecystitis produces signs and symptoms such as recurrent abdominal pain. Abdominal pain is a vague symptom and not specific for cholecystitis. Since emergency cholecystectomy in a patient with dehydration and electrolyte imbalance is likely to be associated with higher peri-operative risks, elective cholecystectomy is usually advised in patients with gall stones without requiring strong evidence for cholecystitis or cholestasis. Issues concerning anesthesia and surgery are presented in Chapters 14 and 15.

Viral Hepatitis

Due to an increased need for blood transfusions for various complications, sickle cell patients are at a greater risk for transfusion-acquired viral hepatitis. There have been several reports reviewing the clinical presentation and course of viral hepatitis in sickle cell disease (7, 9–11), Symptoms and signs include malaise, nausea, upper abdominal pain, low-grade fever, increased jaundice, and tender hepatomegaly. Average bilirubin in one series was 45 mg percent and transaminases were above 500 U. Serologic evidence for the presence of the antigen or antibody related to type A B, or C hepatitis viruses may be present. Liver biopsy, when available, demonstrates necrosis and cellular disarray with baloon cells and leukocyte infiltration. The patients become asymptomatic within 3–9 weeks (average: 6 weeks). Clinical similarities of viral hepatitis with vaso-occlusive hepatic crisis and cholestasis make the distinction between these entities a diagnostic challenge.

Cirrhosis of the Liver

Cirrhosis of the liver has been reported in 16–29 percent of autopsy specimens (2–4). Four (17%) of 24 patients with autopsy findings of cirrhosis had iron overload (2–4). An additional patient who was diagnosed to have cirrhosis by biopsy had gall stones (12). The patient had received multiple blood transfusions. The bilirubin and transaminase levels were elevated. The patient underwent cholecystectomy after a liver biopsy. Jaundice, hepatic enlargement, and abnormal liver function tests continued and worsened over 4 years. She died of liver failure. A high frequency of cirrhosis of the liver at autopsy suggests progressive liver disease in sickle cell patients.

Acute Hepatic Failure

Fatal cases of acute hepatic failure are characterized by severe jaundice (biluribin levels usually over 100 mg), marked prolongation of prothrombin time, and mild elevation of transaminase levels. An early report by Henderson described five such patients (6). From this report, it is not possible to determine the cause of severe hepatitis. Subsequent reports describe fatal cases in which gall stones and viral hepatitis are reasonably excluded (4, 7). Nonfatal cases of acute hepatic failure have also been reported (13–17).

RENAL ABNORMALITIES IN SICKLE CELL DISEASE

Abnormalities of the kidney were observed and recognized in the first description of sickle cell disease in Herrick's historical case report in 1910 (18). Renal abnormalities in sickle cell disease include:

1. Impaired urinary concentration ability
   a. Hyposthenuria
   b. Enuresis
   c. Nocturia
2. Papillary necrosis
3. Hematuria
4. Proteinuria and nephrotic syndrome
5. Renal failure

The pathology of the kidney in sickle cell disease mainly lies in the medulla, involving both renal tubules and blood vessels. The renal medulla consists of a portion of the loop of Henle and the distal end of the collecting tubules, as well as a portion of the peritubular capillary network. Long, straight capillary loops are called vasa recta. In the normal physiological state, hypoxia and slow blood flow with low pH are present in the medulla since only a very small percentage (1–2%) of total renal blood circulates through the vasa recta, and high osmolality is maintained due to the countercurrent multiplication effect of the loop of Henle for the reabsorption of fluid. This special environment induces sickling of red blood cells, resulting in vaso-occlusion of the vasa recta and leading to tubular infarction and necrosis (19). Microangiographic studies have demonstrated an almost complete loss of vasae rectae in adults with sickle cell disease (19). As a consequence of repeated infarction in the medulla, a urinary concentration defect, hematuria, and papillary necrosis occur. Ischemic damage to the medulla may induce the secretion of vasodilating prostaglandin substances (20) and results in the increase of renal blood flow and glomerular filtration rate (21). It has been suggested that chronic hyperfiltration may damage the glomeruli and lead to mesangial proliferation and glomerulosclerosis which results in proteinuria, nephrotic syndrome, and the deterioration of renal function (22).

Major Clinical Abnormalities

Impaired Urinary Concentration Ability and Tubular Function

All sickle cell patients have decreased urinary concentration function, which manifests as decreased urine specific gravity (hyposthenuria) (19–26), and it may occur as early as 6 months of age. Children usually cannot concentrate their urine at greater than 800 mOsm/kg of H_2O (27). After adolescence the urine-concentrating ability is frequently fixed at 400 mosm/kg of H_2O. The patients usually excrete urine with the same osmolality as that of plasma (isosthenuria). The concentrating defect can be temporarily corrected by transfusion before 5 years of age; the degree of correction decreases after this age and no improvement is seen after 15 to 20 years of age (28).

Hyposthenuria is also observed in persons with sickle cell trait (24) and other sickle cell–related hemoglobinopathies (26). Hyposthenuria is generally milder in sickle cell trait and is developed later in life.

Clinically, enuresis is commonly observed in children and nocturia is frequently experienced in all patients (29). The water loss caused by the concentration defect predisposes patients to dehydration and makes the urine specific gravity or volume unreliable as indicators of dehydration. Vaso-occlusive pain crisis following moderate fluid restriction, such as 1 liter per day for a few days, may occur. Hemostasis, sickling, and vasoocclusion may be precipitated and aggravated by the urine concentration defect.

Serum sodium concentration and free water clearance are usually not affected but hyponatremia due to sodium-loss has been reported (30). Impaired urinary acidification resulting in mild distal renal tubular acidosis (31), impaired potassium excretion (32), and hyporeninemic hypoaldosteronism (33) have been observed.

Hematuria

Hematuria is a well-recognized clinical problem in both sickle cell disease and sickle cell trait. In one study, a majority of hematuria episodes were shown to occur in the left kidney, which is probably due to the fact that intrarenal hemostasis is more likely to occur in the lower left renal vein (34).

Renal pelvis ulceration, vascular dilatation and engorgement, and papillary necrosis are frequent pathological findings. Papillary necrosis is suggested to be the causal anatomic abnormality in many cases of hematuria (35). This is suggested by the evidence that papillary necrosis is observed in about half of sickle cell patients who are subjected to urographic studies (36). However, hematuria can occur without radiographic evidence of papillary necrosis.

Six percent of patients with sickle cell anemia and 3 percent of individuals with sickle cell trait have hematuria (36). Most episodes of hematuria are mild and subside spontaneously. Recurrence is observed in about half the patients and is usually ipsilateral (34). Causes other than sickling disorder need to be excluded in sickle cell patients with hematuria since other etiologies such as infection, malignancy, and coagulation defect may occasionally be encountered (37–41).

Treatment is generally supportive and nonsurgical. Transfusion to replace blood loss may be required in severe bleeding and iron therapy may be needed in frequent, recurrent hematuria. Long-term chronic transfusion has been used to allow the lesion to heal and prevent further bleeding (34). Severe hematuria that is refractory to transfusion may be treated with epsilon aminocaproic acid with caution (42, 43)

Proteinuria and Nephrotic Syndrome

Proteinuria is sometimes observed in sickle cell disease (37, 38, 44–47) and is occasionally seen in sickle cell trait. Proteinuria in patients with sickle cell anemia usually represents glomerular pathology including mesangial proliferation and focal segmental glomerulosclerosis, and is often associated with nephrotic syndrome (22, 48–50). Membranoproliferative glomerulonephritis and, rarely, membranous nephropathy have also been described (48, 76).

Although the pathogenesis of nephrotic syndrome is not clear, it is suggested that chronic glomerular hyperperfusion-induced glomerular injury may play an important role (22, 23). Other causes, such as immunologically mediated, antigen-antibody complex deposits in the glomeruli (45, 48) and reaction to iron deposition (44) resulting in renal glomerular tubular damage have been suggested.

The clinical features of nephrotic syndrome in sickle cell disease is similar to that of other causes except for cholesterol, which is usually not elevated (46). It often progresses to renal failure and bears poor prognosis, with 50 percent mortality (44).

The role of adrenal corticosteroid in the treatment of this complication has not been established (44, 47, 49). It is usually steroid-resistant, although some patients have been reported to have favorable response (44, 47).

Renal Failure

End-stage renal disease has been reported to cause about 10 percent of the deaths in sickle cell anemia (48). Renal failure is an uncommon complication of sickle cell disease which often follows nephrotic syndrome (50). The kidneys are usually atrophic and scarred at this stage.

Patients can be managed with hemodialysis or peritoneal dialysis. Renal transplantation is suggested for end-stage renal failure (51, 52). Survival of the kidney recipients who have the sickle cell disease or trait is comparable with those who have other causes of chronic renal failure (53). Transplantation may increase the hemoglobin levels and may reduce the need for blood transfusions but may also increase pain crises (54).

PULMONARY DISORDERS

General Considerations

Surveys of morbidity and mortality among sickle cell patients throughout the world reveal pulmonary disease to be the leading cause of death and a common reason for hospitalization. Since vaso-occlusive infarct and infectious processes are extremely difficult to distinguish, both are included in the term *acute chest syndrome*. This term describes a sickle cell patient with fever, clinical features suggestive of pulmonary involvement, and a new infiltrate on chest X ray. In Jamaica and Great Britain, acute chest syndrome is second only to pain crisis as a reason for admission to hospitals (55–58). Except for children under age two years, acute chest syndrome was the most common cause of death in patients with sickle cell disease in Jamaica (55). The incidence of acute chest syndrome in Miami, Florida, was estimated to be 21 episodes per 100 patient-years for those followed at that center (59, 60).

In addition to acute chest syndrome, chronic pulmonary insufficiency due to progressive damage to the lungs due to recurrent infection or infarction is also quite common. It may manifest as abnormalities in pulmonary function tests, exercise intolerance, or cor pulmonale.

Major Clinical Abnormalities

Acute Chest Syndrome

Etiology.   There are several causes of acute chest syndrome in children and adults with sickle cell disease. These include:

1. Pulmonary infections
    a. Bacterial pneumonia
        i. *Streptococcus pneumoniae*
        ii. *Hemophilus influenzae*
        iii. *Mycoplasma pneumoniae*
        iv. Other bacteria
    b. Viral lower respiratory syndromes
        i. Respiratory syncytial virus

    ii. Parainfluenza and influenza viruses

    iii. Parvovirus B19

    iv. Other viruses

  c. Adult respiratory distress syndrome and pulmonary edema

2. Pulmonary vaso-occlusive disease

  a. Thrombosis in situ

  b. Pulmonary arterial embolism (thromboembolism, bone marrow necrosis and embolism)

3. Secondary to extra-pulmonary lesions

  a. Pain crisis of ribs or bony cage

  b. Osteomyelitis of the ribs

  c. Hepatobiliary disease

  d. Surgical or traumatic lesions

In early studies of acute chest syndrome, bacterial infections were found to account for the majority of episodes of acute chest syndrome in children, while infarcts accounted for the majority of episodes in adults (59–60). In a more recent, prospective study of 102 episodes of acute chest syndrome over a two-year study period in a children's hospital, 12 percent had bacterial, 8 percent had viral, and 16 percent had mycoplasma pneumonias (61). The remainder of episodes of acute chest syndrome (64.7 percent) were considered undiagnosed (61). In another retrospective study of children, only 2 of 93 blood cultures were positive for *Streptococcus pneumoniae* and none were positive for *H. influenzae* (62). Twenty-six percent of patients investigated in that study for mycoplasma infections had suggestive, but not confirmatory, serologic evidence (62). However, the cold agglutinins demonstrated in many of their cases are neither specific nor sensitive and several patients in that series had a single antibody titer to mycoplasma.

Bone marrow embolism secondary to bone marrow infarction has been reported in early studies (63–65). Pain suggestive of bone marrow infarction frequently precedes acute chest syndrome. However, there are other possibilities to explain the association of pain crisis and acute chest syndrome, such as hypoventilation due to analgesic therapy for pain causing atelectasis. Infarction of the ribs or other bones of the thorasic cage may cause chest pain and fever. Moreover, a precipitating event such as virus infection may initiate vaso-occlusive event in the bones as well as the lungs.

Etiologic investigations are hampered by (1) our inability to establish an infectious agent as the cause of pulmonary process without invasive studies, (2) expense in obtaining laboratory evidence of viral and mycoplasma infection in many cases, and (3) lack of objective tools to diagnose pulmonary infarct. Pulmonary infarcts are diagnosed generally by excluding infectious causes. However, infection may occur in an infarcted tissue. Furthermore, the epidemiology of infections may change as prophylactic antibiotics and specific immunizations are introduced.

Clinical Features and Management. Acute chest syndrome has been reported in association with homozygous sickle cell anemia, hemoglobin SC disease, and sickle-β^0 and sickle-β^+ thalassemia. Symptoms include fever, dyspnea, cough, rhinorrhea, and vomiting. Pain in the extremities, back, or abdomen is commonly associated with acute chest syndrome (62). Physical examination usually reveals tachypnea, retractions, labored breathing, dullness on percussion, decreased breath sounds, and rales (62). Fever persists for 3–4 days in sickle cell anemia patients with acute chest syndrome in contrast to normal children with pneumonia, who usually become afebrile within 24 hours (61–62).

Chest X ray demonstrates infiltrate. The location of pulmonary infiltrates, in decreasing frequency, includes both lower lobes, the right middle lobe, the right upper lobe or lingula, and the perihilar regions, respectively (62). Pleural effusions are present in many instances; their prevalence varies between 15–38 percent in reported studies (61, 62).

Microbiologic studies usually include blood cultures for bacterial pathogens, latex agglutination and/or counter-immunoelectrophoresis for pneumococcal and *H. influenzae* antigen, and serology for mycoplasma complement–fixing antibodies. Cold agglutinins are not specific for mycoplasma infections. Sputum cultures or nasopharyngeal cultures do not correlate with microbial pathogens involved in the lower respiratory tract and, therefore, are of limited usefulness. Bronchoscopic aspiration with a protected brush catheter can be used safely in sickle cell patients to obtain uncontaminated, lower respiratory secretions (66). Studies of acute chest syndrome in adults by this technique revealed bacterial pathogens in about 21 percent of patients. However, the secretions were not routinely cultured for viral and mycoplasma organisms in that study and, therefore, the total incidence of infectious etiology in adult cases of acute chest syndrome remains unknown. In one report, pulmonary findings in two patients were shown to be associated with serologic evidence of B19 parvovirus infection (67).

White blood cell counts are usually elevated, and the degree of leukocytosis is greater in patients with the involvement of multiple lobes (68). Hemoglobin levels drop significantly and the reticulocyte count rises during the episode, suggesting increased hemolysis (61). Thrombocytopenia during the early clinical course is replaced by thrombocytosis when the patient recovers (61).

A definitive diagnosis of pulmonary thromboembolic disease can be made by pulmonary angiography, but this procedure is usually not carried out because of the hazards of injecting hypertonic radiographic solutions. Arterial blood gas studies demonstrate low arterial oxygen tension and are useful for diagnosis and management. Isotopic pulmonary ventilation-perfusion scans provide additional means for the evaluation of patients with suspected thromboembolic disease. A normal pulmonary perfusion scan essentially rules out the diagnosis of thromboembolism. However, a positive scan is only supportive of the diagnosis but does not establish infarction because about 50 percent of asymptomatic patients have been shown to have abnormal perfusion due to previous pulmonary damage (69). Comprehensive pulmonary studies in sickle cell patients during asymptomatic states provide baseline data that would aid in the evaluation of possible thromboembolic chest syndromes without high-risk angiographic studies (69). However, such data are rarely available.

The management of acute chest syndrome usually requires supportive care. This includes the assessment of pulmonary functions, fluid and electrolyte balance, and hematologic status, as well as investigations to identify microbial etiology, if any. Oxygen therapy and respiratory support are indicated in patients with hypoxaemia. Antibiotics are usually given in most febrile patients pending results of blood cultures. A drop in the hemoglobin frequently requires the transfusion of red cells (61). Whether simple transfusions or exchange transfusions decrease the duration or severity of acute chest syndrome has not been established by controlled studies. However, uncontrolled experience suggests beneficial effects of red cell transfusions on the severity of the pulmonary complications. A judicious use of transfusions is indicated in patients who are clinically sick with moderate to severe respiratory distress, have extensive pulmonary involvement (of more than one lobe or accompanied by effusions), or have arterial oxygen of less than 75 mm Hg despite oxygen therapy, or if a patient's condition deteriorates upon other treatments (70).

Chronic Pulmonary Insufficiency

Vital capacity and total lung capacity are reduced in patients with sickle cell disease, especially adolescents and adults (71–77). Occasionally, pulmonary functions suggest obstructive lung disease or impaired gas exchange (74, 75). Resting arterial pO_2 is usually between 70 and 90 mm Hg. Cyanosis is usually not detected because of anemia. Usually arterial pH is normal, but hyperventilation with low pCO_2 may be present. In one study, the calculated alveolar-arterial pO_2 difference was found to be higher in many patients with sickle cell disease due to one of several factors (72): (1) shunting of blood without exposure to the ventilated lung, (2) unequal ventilation–perfusion ratios, and (3) possibly, abnormal diffusion of oxygen across the alveolar membrane. In the same study, cardiac catheterization was performed in 10 patients. Radiologically, cardiomegaly was present in 9 of 10 patients but pulmonary vascular resistance was normal in all cases (72). Cardiac output and blood volumes were elevated, suggesting that cardiomegaly was secondary to high cardiac output and not due to cor pulmonale. However, true cor pulmonale may be found if a larger number of patients is evaluated.

SUMMARY

The hepatobiliary, renal, and pulmonary systems are commonly affected in sickle cell disease due to vaso-occlusion and hemolytic anemia. A progressive involvement of these organs, superimposed by acute complications, may occur frequently.

REFERENCES

1. Rosenblate HJ, Eisenstein R, and Holmes AW: The liver in sickle cell anemia. A clinico-pathologic study. *Arch Pathol* 90 (1970): 235–245.
2. Bauer TW, Moore GW, and Hutchins GM: The liver in sickle cell disease. A clinicopathologic study of 70 patients. *Am J Med* 69 (1980): 833–837.
3. Song YS: Hepatic lesions in sickle cell anemia. *Am J Pathol* 33 (1957): 331–344.
4. Green TW, Conley CL, and Berthrong M: The liver in sickle cell anemia. *Bull J Hopkins Hosp* 92 (1953): 99–122.
5. Schubert TT: Hepatobiliary system in sickle cell disease. *Gastroenterology* 90 (1986): 2013–2021.
6. Henderson AB: Sickle cell anemia: Clinical study of 54 cases. *Am J Med* 9 (1950): 757–765.
7. Sheehy TW: Sickle cell hepatopathy. *Southern Med J* 70 (1977): 533–538.
8. Hatton CSR, Bunch C, and Weatherall DJ: Hepatic sequestration in sickle cell anemia. *Br Med J* 290 (March 9, 1985): 744–745.
9. Barrett-Connor E: Sickle cell disease and viral hepatitis. *Ann Intern Med* 69 (1968): 517–527.
10. Beddell H, Paley SS, and Evans FG: Virus hepatitis complicating sickle cell anemia. *NY State J Med* 51 (1951): 1944–1946.
11. Meyers F, Lam KB, and Ticktin HE: Viral hepatitis complicating sickle cell anemia. *Med Ann DC* 32 (1963): 55–58.
12. Mills LR, Mwakyusa D, and Milner PF: Histopathologic features of liver biopsy specimens in sickle cell disease. *Arch Pathol Lab Med* 112 (March 1988): 290–294.
13. Klion FM, Weiner MJ, and Schaffner F: Cholestasis in sickle cell anemia. *Am J Med* 37 (1964): 829–832.
14. Owen DM, Aldridge JE, and Thompson RB: An unusual hepatic sequela of sickle cell anemia: A report of five cases. *Am J Med Sci* 249 (1965): 175–185.
15. Wade FA: Sickle cell crisis resembling obstructive (cholangiolar type) jaundice. *VA Med Mon* 87 (1960): 474–478.
16. Sheehy TW, Law DE, and Wade BH: Exchange transfusion for sickle cell intrahepatic cholestasis. *Arch Intern Med* 140 (1980): 136–138.
17. Krishnamurthy M, Elguezabal A, Lee CK, et al.: Case report: Bland cholestasis. *Postgrad Med* 64 (1978): 215–217.
18. Herrick JB: Peculiar exongated and sickle-shaped red blood corpuscles in a case of severe anemia. *Arch Intern Med* 6 (1970): 517–576.
19. Statius Van Eps LW, Pinedo-Veels C, DeVries GH, et al.: Nature of concentrating defect in sickle cell nephropathy. Microadeioangiographic studies. *Lancet* no. 1 (1970): 450–451.
20. Pitcock JA, Muirhead EE, Hatch FE, et al.: Early renal changes in sickle cell anemia. *Arch Pathol* 90 (1970): 403–410.
21. DeJong PE, Saleh AW, DeZeeuw, D, et al.: Urinary prostaglandins in sickle cell

nephropathy: A defect in 9-ketoreductase activity? *Clin Nephrol* 22 (1984): 212–213.

22. Tejani A, Phadke K, Adamson O, et al.: Renal lesions in sickle cell nephropathy in children. *Nephron* 39 (1985): 352–355.

23. DeJong P, and Statius Van Eps LW: Sickle cell nephropathy: New insights into its pathophysiology. *Kidney Int* 27 (1985): 711–717.

24. Schlitt L, and Keitel HG: Pathogenesis of hyposthenuria in persons with sickle cell anemia or the sickle cell trait. *Pediatrics* 26 (1960): 249–254.

25. Noll JB, Newman AJ, and Gross OO: Enuresis and nocturia in sickle cell disease. *J. Peds* 70 (1967): 965–967.

26. Perillie PE, and Epstein FH: Sickling phenomenon produced by hypertonic solutions: A possible explanation for the hyposthenuria of sicklemia. *J Clin Invest* 42 (1963): 570.

27. Statius Van Eps LW, and DeJong PE: In RW Schrier and VN Gottschalk, eds.: *Sickle cell disease of the kidney*, 4th ed., pp. 2561–2581. Boston: Little Brown and Company, 1988.

28. Statius Van Eps LW, Schouten H, LaPorte-Wijsman LW, et al.: The influence of red blood cell transfusion on the hypothenuria and renal hemodynamics of sickle cell anemia. *Clin. Chim. Acta* 17 (1967): 449–461.

29. Noll JB, Newman AJ, and Gross S.: Enuresis and nocturia in sickle cell disease. *J. Peds* 70 (1967): 965.

30. Radel EG, Kochen JA, and Finberg L: Hyponatremia in sickle cell disease. A renal salt losing state. *J. Peds* 88 (1976): 800.

31. Oster JR, Lespier LE, and Lee SM: Renal acidification in sickle cell disease. *J Lab Clin Med* 88 (1976): 389.

32. Oster JR, Lanier DC Jr., Vamonde CA: Renal response to potassium loading in sickle cell trait. *Arch Intern Med* 140 (1980): 534.

33. Yoshino M, American R, and Brautbar N: Hyporeninemic hypoaldosteronism in sickle cell disease. *Nephrologie* 31 (1982): 242.

34. Allen TD: Sickle cell disease and hematuria. A report of 29 cases. *J Urol* 91 (1961): 117–122.

35. Diggs LW: Anatomic lesions in sickle cell disease. In H Abramson and JF Bertles, eds.: *Sickle cell disease, diagnosis, management, education and research*, pp. 199–229. St. Louis, MO: C. V. Mosby, 1973.

36. McCall IW, Moule N, DeSai P, et al.: Urographic findings in hemozygous sickle cell disease. *Radiology* 126 (1978): 94–104.

37. Henderson AB: Sickle cell anemia. Clinical study of fifty-four cases. *Am J Med* 9 (1950): 757–765.

38. Lucas WM, and Bullock WH: Hematuria in sickle cell disease. *J Urol* 83 (1960): 733–741.

39. Oksenhendler E, Bourbigot B, Desbazielle F, et al.: Recurrent hematuria in 4 white patients with sickle cell trait. *J Urol* 132 (1984): 1201–1203.

40. Atkinson DW: Sickling and hematuria. *Blood* 34 (1969): 736–737.

41. Brody JI, Levison SP, and Jung CJ: Sickle cell trait and hematuria associated with von Willebrand syndromes. *Ann Intern Med* 86 (1977): 529–533.

42. Bilinsky RT, Kandel GL, and Rabiner SF: Epsilon amino caproic acid therapy of hematuria due to heterozygous sickle cell diseases. *J Urol* 102 (1969): 93.

43. Black WD, Hatch FE, and Acchiardo S: Epsilon amino caproic acid in prolonged

hematuria of patients with sickle cell anemia. *Arch Intern Med* 136 (1976): 678–681.

44. McCoy RC: Ultra structural alterations in the kidney of patients with sickle cell anemia and the nephrotic syndrome. *Lab Invest* 21 (1969): 85–95.

45. Strauss J, Pardo V, and Koss MN: Nephropathy associated with sickle cell anemia: An autogous immune complex nephritis. *Am J Med* 58 (1975): 382–387.

46. Berman LB, and Tublin OO: The nephropathies of sickle cell disease. *Arch Intern Med* 103 (1959): 602–606.

47. Sweeney MJ, Dobbins WT, and Etteldorf JN: Renal disease with elements of the nephrotic syndrome associated with sickle cell anemia. *J Peds* 60 (1962): 42–51.

48. Pardo V, Strauss J, and Kramer H: Nephropathy associated with sickle cell anemia: an autologous immune complex nephritis. *Am J Med* 59 (1975): 650.

49. Berman LB, and Tublin I: The nephropathies of sickle cell disease. *Arch Intern Med* 103 (1959): 602–606.

50. Nicholson GD, Amin UF, and Alleyne GA: Proteinuria and the nephrotic syndrome in homozygous sickle cell anemia. *West Ind Med J* 29 (1980): 239.

51. Chatteryee SN: National study on natural history of renal allografts in sickle cell disease or trait. *Nephron* 25 (1980): 199–200.

52. Gonzalez-Carrillo M, Ridge CJ, Parsons V: Renal transplantation in sickle cell disease. *Clin Nephrol* 18 (1982): 209.

53. Simmons JR, Jr., Gilani D, Johnson CS, et al.: The pattern of mortality in sickle cell disease. *Blood* 50 (1977): 119.

54. Spector D, Zachary JB, Sterioff S, et al.: Painful crisis following renal transplantation in sickle cell anemia. *Am J Med* 64 (1978): 835–839.

55. Thomas AN, Pattison C, and Serjeant GR. Causes of death in sickle cell disease in Jamaica. *Br Med J* 285 (August 28–September 4, 1982): 633–635.

56. Kehinde MO, Marsh JC, and Marsh GW. Sickle cell disease in North London. *Br Med J* 66 (1987): 543–547.

57. Brozovic M, and Anionwu E. Sickle cell disease in Britain. *J Clin Pathol* 37 (1984): 1321–1326.

58. Williams S, Maude BA, and Sergeant GR: Clinical presentation of sickle cell-hemoglobin C disease. *J Peds* 109, no. 4 (1986): 586–589.

59. Barrett-Connor E: Acute pulmonary disease and sickle cell anemia. *Ann Rev Resp Dis* 104 (1971): 159.

60. Barrett-Connor E. Pneumonia and pulmonary infarction in sickle cell anemia. *JAMA* 224 (1973): 997–1000.

61. Poncz M, Kane E, and Gill FM: Acute chest syndrome in sickle cell disease: Etiology and clinical correlates. *J Peds* 107 (1985): 861–866.

62. Sprinkle RH, Cole T, Smith S, et al.: Acute chest syndrome in children with sickle cell disease, A retrospective analysis of 100 hospitalized cases. *Am J Ped Hem Onc* 8 no. 2 (1986): 105–110.

63. Wade LJ, and Stevenson JD: Necrosis of the bone marrow with fat embolism in sickle cell anemia. *Am J Pathol* 17 (1941): 47–54.

64. Hutchinson RM, Merrick MV, and White JM: Fat embolism in sickle cell disease. *J Clin Pathol* 26 (1973): 620–622.

65. Shelley WM, and Curtis EM: Bone marrow and fat embolism in sickle cell anemia and sickle cell-hemoglobin C disease. *Bull J Hopkins Hosp* 103 (1958): 8–18.

66. Kirkpatrick MB, Lorino G, and Bass JB: Results of lower respiratory tract cultures

from sickle hemoglobinopathy patients with acute chest syndrome. *Am Rev Resp Dis* 133, no. 4 (1986): pt. 2.

67. Conrad ME, Studdard H, and Anderson LJ: Case report: Aplastic crisis in sickle cell disorders: bone marrow necrosis and human parvovirus infection. *Am J Med Sci* 295, no. 3 (1988): 212–215.

68. Charache S, Scott JC, and Charache P: Acute chest syndrome in adults with sickle cell anemia. *Arch Intern Med* 139 (Jan. 1979): 67–69.

69. Walker BK, Ballas SK, and Burka ER: The diagnosis of pulmonary thromboembolism in sickle cell disease. *Am J Hematol* 7 (1979): 219–232.

70. Mallouh AA, and Asha M: Beneficial effect of blood transfusion in children with sickle cell chest syndrome. *Am J Dis Child* 142 (Feb. 1988): 178–182.

71. Fowler NO, Smith O, and Greenfield JC: Arterial blood oxygenation in sickle cell anemia. *Am J Med Sci* 234 (1957): 449–458.

72. Sproule BJ, Halden ER, and Miller WF: A study of cardiopulmonary alterations in patients with sickle cell disease and its variants. *J Clin Invest* 37 (1958): 486–495.

73. Rodman T, Close HP, Cathart R, et al.: The oxyhemoglobin dissociation curve in the common hemoglobinopathies. *Am J Med* 27 (1959): 558–566.

74. Bromberg PA, and Jensen WN: Arterial oxygen unsaturation in sickle cell disease. *Am Rev Resp Dis* 96 (1967): 400–407.

75. Femi-Pearse D, Gazioglu KM, and Yu PN. Pulmonary function studies in sickle cell disease. *J Appl Physio* 28 (1970): 574–577.

76. DeJohn PE, and Statius van Eps LW: Sickle cell nephropathy: New insights into its pathophysiology. *Kidney Int* 27 (1985): 711.

77. Kirkpatrick MB, and Bass JB. Pulmonary complications in adults with sickle cell disease. *Pul Perspect* 6, no. 4 (1989): 6–10.

13

Radiological Implications of Sickle Cell Disease

B. Gil Brogdon, Myron L. Lecklitner, Byron C. Machen, and John Powell Williams

Radiologic manifestations of sickle cell disease (SCD) may be found in many organ systems. Most of them are nonspecific. Consequently, the radiologic diagnosis of sickle cell disease is usually of a confirmatory nature if the history is known, and suggestive of the disease if found unexpectedly. The pure radiographic diagnosis of SCD usually is based on a constellation of findings, the classic example perhaps being posterior-anterior (PA) and lateral radiographs of the chest of a young person showing a large heart, increased flow pattern and fibrosis in the lungs, surgical clips below the diaphragm in the region of the gallbladder, and typical "Reynolds' vertebra" in the thoracic spine. An aseptic necrosis of one or both shoulders would be icing on the cake, but such a fortuitous combination of findings is not often one's lot.

Rather, the radiologic findings usually are tantalizing but imprecise, a concatenation of observations that suggest or confirm a diagnosis already known all too well to both the patient and the physician. The radiologic method can be extremely useful, however, in the diagnosis, evaluation, and treatment of the disease and, particularly, its complications.

In this chapter we will deal with the radiologic implications of sickle cell disease in a systematic matrix, exploiting the armamentarium of imaging modalities now available while recognizing that all too often the clinical universe inhabited by the patient and his or her doctor is not so well ordered.

MUSCULOSKELETAL SYSTEM

The affectations of the bones, joints, and soft tissues that are manifest radiographically in SCD principally result from marrow hyperplasia, thrombosis, disturbance of growth, fracture, and infection (1).

These will be described in an orderly fashion, which is somewhat misleading because some of these effects are interdependent, with one resulting from, or associated with, the other. Further, the bony response to the various insults that this disease complex can deliver may be imitative rather than discriminatory.

Marrow Hyperplasia

In the normal fetus, bone marrow begins hematopoiesis in the fourth month, overtakes the liver and spleen by the sixth month, and is totally responsible for red cell production at birth, when all marrow is hematopoietic (2). Conversion to yellow (fatty) marrow begins in the small bones of the hands and feet at birth and follows a gradual, steady course in the normal child, progressing from distal to proximal. The pattern of red–yellow conversion is similar in all long bones (only being more rapid in distal long bones) until age 25, when the adult pattern is achieved: red marrow residing only in the vertebrae, sternum, ribs, pelvis, skull, proximal shafts of the femora and humeri, and, occasionally, the oscalci. This pattern of conversion is delayed and distorted in the patient with sickle cell hemoglobinopathy (3).

Magnetic resonance imaging (MRI) of long bones in normal children demonstrates a homogenous, bright pattern of signals from the marrow tissues, representing fat. In the proximal parts of the long bones, such as the heads and necks of the femurs, the image is homogenous but less bright, consistent with the presence of more hematopoietic tissue and less fat (Figure 13.1). In contrast, MRI of the long bones in patients with SCD shows a patchy, spotty signal pattern in the marrow of the long bones, perhaps owing to the persistence of hematopoietic activity and areas of postischemic fibrosis. This mottled pattern has been found in 100 percent of our subjects with this disease who have been examined by MRI (Figure 13.2).

Hyperplasia of the marrow is thought to be due to hypoxia resulting from hemolysis of the fragile, abnormal sickle cells. The resultant cellular increase causes resorption of minor bony trabeculae in spongy bone and thins the cortex so that the marrow cavity is widened and bridged by a coarsened pattern of major trabeculae (sometimes described as a basket-weave pattern) (4).

This osteoporotic bone is weak and subject to the injuries of osteoporotic bone of whatever cause. In the spine, the weakened vertebral end-plates may be compressed and displaced by interposed disc material to produce the classic fish vertebra deformity: a smooth lenticular concavity sagging evenly from one corner of the vertebra to the other above, a reversed, symmetrical canopy contour in the inferior end-plate (5, Figure 13.3).

In any part of the skeleton, including the long bones, the weakened osteoporotic bone is susceptible to fractures which may occur with only minor trauma. In the calvarium, the diploe may be widened, the outer table thinned disproportionally, and the residual trabeculae perpendicular to the inner table may produce a "hair-on-end" appearance; however, this finding is rare in sickle cell disease (6). The

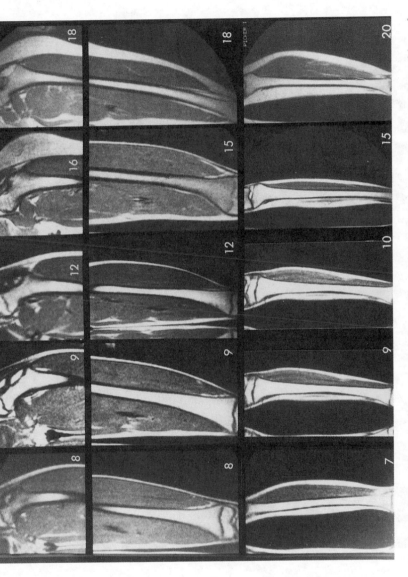

Figure 13.1. Composite of spin echo (SE) magnetic resonance (MR) images of the hips, thighs, and legs of representative, normal control subjects, showing the distribution of homogenous, high-intensity signal fatty marrow. Lower signal areas in the ends of the bone represent residual red marrow. The compact bones of the cortex and physes appears as black, low signal lines. The numbers on each image represent the subject's age in years.

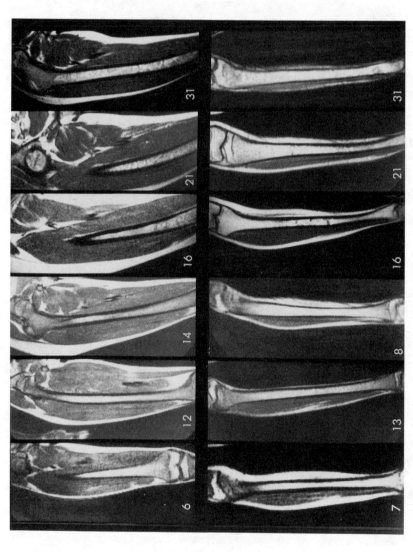

Figure 13.2. Composite of spin echo images of "spotty" marrow pattern sickle cell disease patients, increasing in gradation from left to right. The degree of mottling correlates with age. The overall red–yellow marrow conversion is delayed. The number on each image represents the patient's age in years.

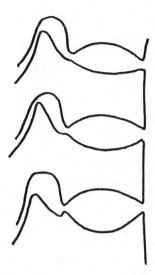

Figure 13.3. Schematic lateral view of vertebral bodies showing typical "fish vertebrae" deformity from marrow hyperplasia and resultant osteoporosis.

trabecular pattern of the mandible and maxilla may become quite foamy as minor trabeculae are resorbed. Residual heavy transverse trabeculae between the tooth roots may produce a "step-ladder" appearance roentgenographically. Malocclusion of the teeth occurs as the softened bone gives way to the repetitive stress of biting and chewing (7, 8).

While the most common skeletal findings in SCD are those related to marrow hypertrophy, they frequently are subtle and nonspecific. More impressive are those bone, joint, and soft tissue changes associated with bone infarction and its sequelae. Unfortunately, here too there are few lesions characteritic of SCD and, viewed in isolation, the roentgen findings usually are indistinguishable from those found in infarctions of other etiologies (9).

Ischemia and Infarction

Hand-Foot Syndrome (Sickle Cell Dactylitis)

Fetal hemoglobin protects the fetus and newborn against sickling of erythrocytes, but during the later months of infancy, infarction of the small bones of the hands and feet is common. The infarction is aggravated by their distance from the lungs and consequent low oxygen concentration of arteriolar blood, exposure to cold, and (in some cultures) constricting bindings and carriers (1, 8). Roentgenograms obtained early during the course of clinical pain, swelling, heat, and tenderness show only soft tissue increase. However, as the clinical symptoms subside in 10–14 days, periosteal elevation and new bone formation, profound osteoporosis, and trabecular coarsening may appear and, in rare instances, the bones may virtually disappear (Figure 13.4).

Restoration to normal may occur in 2 weeks to a month, but residual indications of interference with bone growth—such as shortening and growth arrest lines—can occur as early as 6 months of age.

Acute Ischemia/Infarction

In SCD, erythrocytes that have been deformed as a result of low oxygenation can cause stasis and obstruction in the small vessels. Thus, ischemia and infarction can involve any organ of the body including the long bones, where roentgen manifestations depend on the location of the infarct: (1) the nutrient artery or arteries that enter the diaphysis, divide into proximal and distal branches, and supply the cortex with radial branches; (2) periosteal branches that supply the outer portion of the cortex in the adult and may become an important collateral supply if other sources are compromised, and (3) vessels at the ends of the bones, comprising both metaphyseal and epiphyseal vessels, with the physis acting as a blood barrier in the immature patient. Bohrer (10) argued persuasively that the long bones should be considered in five parts: a large central diaphyseal segment, two small metaphyseal end segments, and two intermediate or diametaphyseal segments.

Since the nutrient artery is the sole supply to the medullary cavity of the long bones, acute medullary infarcts are the most common. If there is no cortical involvement, no acute radiographic changes appear. Medullary infarcts may heal completely or may progress to marrow fibrosis and calcification, with the latter arranged as serpiginous, linear, or crenelated outlines roughly parallel to the endocortex and, presumably, surrounding the injured area (Figure 13.5). The pattern of postmedullary infarct calcification in SCD is not distinctive from that due to other causes (4, 10).

The medullary component of bone can be imaged with Technicium-99m sulphur colloid, which is taken up by the reticulo-endothelial system; the expanded erythron characteristic of SCD is well demonstrated by this method. Conversely, areas of infarction will show sharply demarcated photo-deficient regions of low uptake (11). These abnormalities correlate well with clinical symptoms at times of crisis. Since the areas of photo deficiency are slow to resolve, it may be difficult to distinguish between old and new areas of infarction on initial evaluation. Asymptomatic infarctions are also known to occur, and can be differentiated from the acute change only if serial scans are available. Although the radiation exposure from a single examination may be slight, repeated studies may lead to significant cumulative bone marrow radiation. Less sensitive radionuclide evaluation can be provided by more conventional bone-scanning agents (11).

Cortical infarcts in the long bones imply a compromise of blood supply from

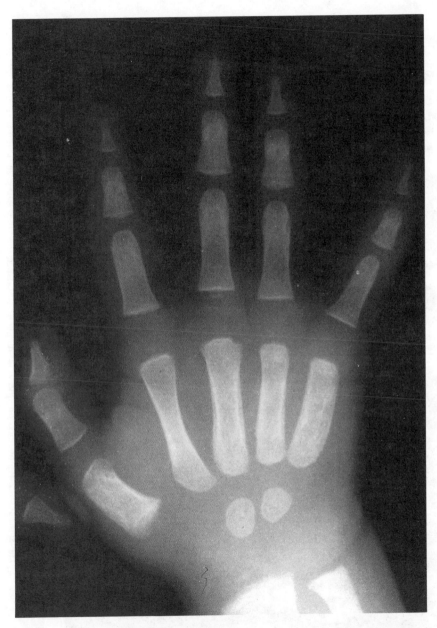

Figure 13.4. Sickle cell dactylitis in hand-foot syndrome. Note the generalized osteoporosis with diminished overall bone density and thinned cortices. The marrow hypertrophy has expanded the marrow cavity, leaving a basket-weave trabecular pattern. There is a fine, unilaminar periosteal elevation with new bone formation along the shafts of most of the metacarpals.

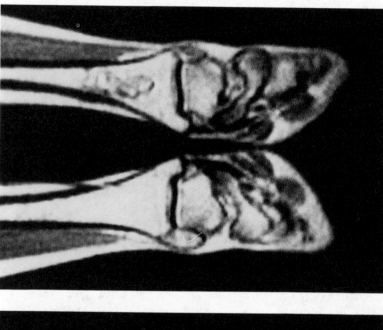

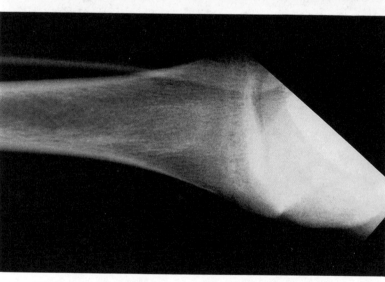

Figure 13.5. Intramedullary calcification. Left: Intramedullary calcification in the distal diametaphysis of the left tibia, presumably representing a healed infarct in a patient with sickle cell disease. Right: The same lesion demostrated on spin echo magnetic resonance imaging. The calcification produces low signal areas, as does the bony cortex.

both nutrient arteries and periosteal vessels, and occur most frequently in the metadiaphyseal regions. Larger infarcts may encompass the central diaphysis as well. Pure metaphyseal infarcts are rare and, as long as it remains open, the physis protects the epiphysis. The bones of the lower extremity, especially the proximal tibia and distal femur, are involved most commonly. Children are affected more than adults, probably because of better periosteal supply in the latter (12).

Roentgenographically, a variety of appearances may result from cortical infarcts of long bones, including subperiosteal new bone formation, localized osteolysis, mottled patterns of osteolysis, osteolysis surrounded by sclerosis, sequestrae or cortical fissuring, and cortical widening with healing (Figure 13.6). Adjacent soft tissue swelling is a usual accompaniment.

Cortical skeletal images can be obtained with Tc-99m Methyl Diphosphonate, and cortical bone scintigraphy is used as the imaging procedure of choice in many clinical settings, being the most sensitive, safe, and noninvasive test for obtaining global, regional, and focal skeletal data of clinical significance (11).

In all affectations of the skeleton (with the exception of trauma), functional changes precede anatomic changes in bone. Because scintigraphy assesses function, there will be increased uptake (a "hot spot") where there is increased osteoblastic activity (e.g., physiologic growth) or pathophysiologic activity (i.e., infarction, infection, or tumor). Since the radioactive tracer is delivered to the bone by its blood supply following intravenous injection, decreased blood flow, such as an infarcted area, may show initially decreased uptake (a "cold spot"; see Figure 13.7). Later, uptake will increase as the body responds to the vascular insult.

Symptomatic acute infarcts of the flat bones and vertebrae are uncommon, but sclerotic changes of healing may be found in the pelvis and vertebrae. A ring-like sclerotic density in the calvarium has been identified as an old infarct in one sickle cell patient (13). However, another study cannot attribute this to any specific disease or etiology, and such ring-like sclerotic density has been reported in a number of patients without sickle cell disease (14).

Magnetic Resonance Imaging (MRI) of bone infarcts in SCD is promising. Spin echo protocols employed during pain crisis have shown increased signal intensity in the area of involvement and, in a few patients, the cortical infarct has been confirmed by biopsy (3, 15; Figure 13.8). The signal change probably is related to edematous tissue reaction about the ischemic area. Using slightly different imaging sequences, Rao, Fishman, Mitchell, et al. (16) demonstrated edema in the spinal marrow of more than half their symptomatic sickle patients. This may allow for a differentiation between new and old infarcts.

Complications of Bone Ischemia

Fractures are a complication not only of cortical thinning due to marrow hyperplasia, but also may result from cortical destruction secondary to osteo-

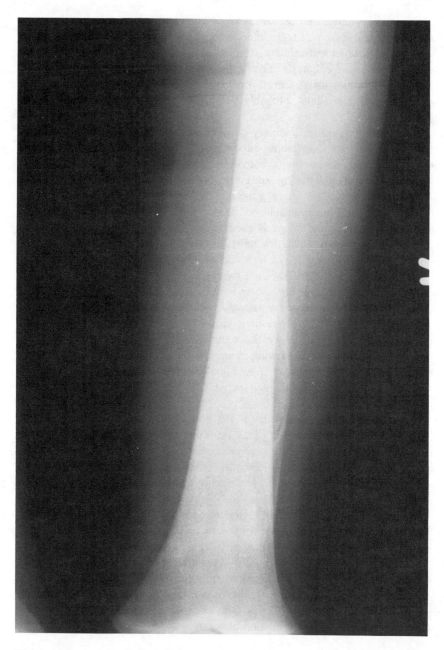

Figure 13.6. Frontal view of the left femur of a young male with sickle cell disease. There is thick periosteal new bone formation along the sclerotic distal diaphysis. These changes resulted from a cortical infarct several weeks previously.

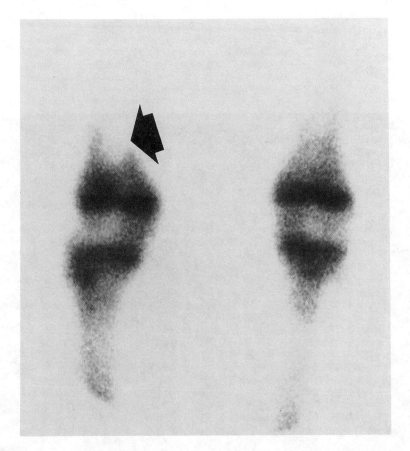

Figure 13.7.   Cortical images of the anterior knees of a six-year-old child with sickle
cell disease. There is a "cold" defect in the distal diametaphysis of the
right femur. Note the "hot" growth areas on both sides of the knee
joint.

Source: ML Lecklitner, Nuclear imaging studies in sickle cell disease, *Ala J Med Sci* 24 (1987):
391, Fig. 2. Reproduced with permission.

necrosis or osteomyelitis. In the latter two instances, the exact etiologic responsibility may be difficult or impossible to assign (17). Full cortical thickness
destruction may be present in up to 50 percent of acute long bone infarcts. If
weight bearing continues, a clinically significant fracture with displacement and
angulation can result (10).

Osteomyelitis occurs with enormously increased frequency in individuals with
sickle cell disease, and certain organisms such as *Salmonella* and *pneumococcus*
are more often seen because of abnormalities in the immune mechanism (10).

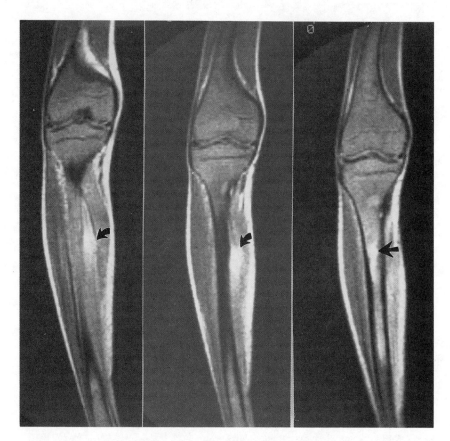

Figure 13.8. Spin echo magnetic resonance images of a nine-year-old male during sickle cell disease pain crisis in the right leg. Left and center: High-intensity signal (curved arrows) in soft tissues. Right: Subcortical marrow posterially (straight arrow) indicates edema of acute cortical infarct (biopsy proven).

Since the same clinical and radiologic constellation may be engendered by osteomyelitis and/or cortical infarction (pain, tenderness, systemic response, swelling, periosteal reaction with new bone in 7–14 days, cortical fissuring, and sequestration), the two conditions may be impossible to differentiate during a single episode in any given patient. In children especially, osteomyelitis is more likely to be nearer the end of the bone than is infarction.

In suspected osteomyelitis, cortical scintigraphy is useful in differentiating the condition from cellulitis, evaluation of bone pain of unknown origin, and selection of aspiration sites with or without biopsy. In the case of osteomyelitis, one must recall that the process begins typically as a myelitis. As a general rule, by the time the patient is symptomatic the bone scan is abnormal. Differentiation of osteomyelitis from osteonecrosis is difficult in non-SCD patients, but the differentiation is particularly difficult in patients with SCD because they are at increased risk for both complications. Although cortical imaging, marrow imaging, and gallium imaging have all been employed in an attempt to differentiate osteomyelitis from osteonecrosis in patients with SCD, the reported results to date indicate that there is a substantial overlap of the scintigraphic findings in both complications of SCD (18).

On the other hand, when the clinical question focuses on osteonecrosis, cortical images may demonstrate "cold lesions" early in the disease process (Figure 13.6). As the disease progresses, "hot lesions" may then appear, which are presumably related to augmented periosteal blood supply (Figure 13.9).

Once a cortical bone scintigram demonstrates a focal area of increased radioactivity, how long does the bone lesion remain "hot"? Matin studied the appearance of skeletal scintigrams in over 200 patients following traumatic fractures (19). He concluded that the minimum time for a fracture to return to normal on a scintigram was 5 months and that approximately 90 percent of fractures had returned to normal within 2 years. Whether the time frame described by Matin applies to skeletal lesions other than fractures is a moot point. In our own experience, "hot" lesions persist for 4–18 months after the patient becomes asymptomatic and can be seen with a skeletal scintigram, and plain films demonstrate healing with normal callus formation.

A cortical scintigram shows an abnormality for a prolonged period. This precludes its use in the follow-up of treated patients with osteomyelitis (11). Rarely, a cortical bone scintigram study may be falsely negative. This usually occurs in the pediatric population. If cortical scintigraphy is so highly sensitive compared to other available imaging modalities, what is the explanation for the possibility of a false-negative study? Most osteomyelitis occurs in the metaphyseal region of the long bones. The metaphysis is contiguous with the epiphysis, and in younger patients the epiphysis is physiologically "hot" because of normal growth. Thus, various small areas of pathophysiologic "hot" spots may go undetected because they abut a physiologic "hot" growth plate. If the clinical suspicion of an acute osteomyelitis remains high, this study should be repeated with gallium-67 citrate, a radiopharmaceutical with high avidity for inflammatory

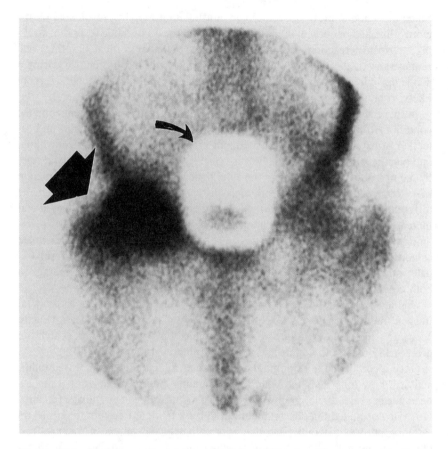

Figure 13.9. Anterior cortical image of pelvis and hips in a 20-year-old patient with sickle cell disease. There is increased osteoblastic activity in the right femoral head (broad arrow) due to osteomyelitis, which is surgically proved. (The curved arrow indicates the artifact of a lead shield positioned over the activity in the urinary bladder.)

Source: ML Lecklitner, Nuclear imaging studies in sickle cell disease, *Ala J Med Sci* 24 (1987): 392, Fig. 3. Reproduced with permission.

tissue. One may ask, "Then why not perform all cases of suspected acute osteomyelitis with gallium-67 citrate?" There are several reasons: Tc-99mMDP is more generally and readily available, costs less than gallium-67 citrate, provides higher spatial resolution, and, most importantly, exposes the patient to a lower radiation dose, approximately one-quarter to one-half the total body radiation dose from gallium-67 citrate (11).

Although it is hoped that MRI protocols can be developed to characterize the differences between bone infarcts and osteomyelitis, current experience would

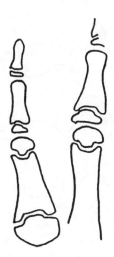

Figure 13.10.   Schematic drawing of typical changes of central growth plate infarcts in the metacarpals and phalanges.

suggest that this will be difficult (20–22). The accumulation of comparative cases in SCD patients will be prolonged and tedious since acute long bone infarcts are 50 times more prevalent than osteomyelitis (23).

Growth disturbance occurs where infarcts affect growing bone adjacent to the physis (5, 10). Central areas of decreased growth occur when the main nutrient artery is compromised. Peripheral growth can continue due to marginal metaphyseal supply. The result is cup-shaped metaphyses and cone-shaped or triangular epiphyses, which are most often seen in the bones of the hand (24; see Figure 13.10).

The same mechanism produces the so-called Reynolds' vertebra in the spine, a vertebral body with a peculiar H-shaped appearance reminiscent of the notched ends of the toy construction logs for children (Figure 13.11). Unfortunately, the Reynolds' vertebra is not specific for SCD (although highly suggestive), being encountered rarely in persons with Gaucher's Disease, paroxymal nocturnal hemoglobinuria, alcoholism, and in young women taking birth control pills (10).

Epiphyseal Aseptic Necrosis

One of the frequently occurring and most disabling skeletal lesions in older children and adults with SCD is aseptic necrosis of the femoral and humeral heads and, rarely, other epiphyses (8, 10, 25, 26). It occurs in 15–30 percent of older patients, being uncommon before age 10. About half have bilateral involvement. Radiographically, aseptic necrosis in SCD is no different than

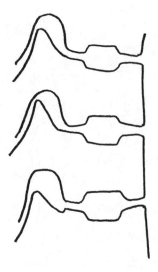

Figure 13.11.   Schematic lateral view of "Reynolds' vertebra" caused by central infarction at the growth plate.

that occurring idiopathically or due to steroid therapy, trauma, alcoholism, Gaucher's Disease, or any of the other causes.

If the hip is involved before the physis closes, the process simulates Legg-Perthes Disease with deformity of the entire epiphysis and broadening and shortening of the femoral neck to produce a mushroom appearance. If the epiphysis is closed, the changes may be more focal.

The earliest roentgenographic finding is the "crescent sign," a tiny, lucent line shaped like a fingernail imprint just beneath the articular cortex. Later, step-like cortical depressions appear, especially at weight-bearing areas of the epiphysis. Irregular areas of radiolucency and sclerosis reflect the jumble of degenerative and reparative processes that follow (Figure 13.12, right).

Symptoms of aseptic necrosis may preceed roentgenographic changes and nuclear scintigraphy may provide early evidence of epiphyseal abnormality (11; see Figures 13.13 and 13.14). Magnetic resonance imaging now is the procedure of choice, (especially for early detection) for avascular necrosis. The hallmark MRI finding is a focal area of homogenous or inhomogenous decreased signal pattern in a subarticular location (27; see Figure 13.12, left).

Cortical thickening and medullary sclerosis often present in the long bones of older SCD patients (10). Repeated episodes of ischemia and infarction are followed by revascularization, resorption, fibrosis, and sclerosis. Because less circulation is required to lay down new bone than to resorb the old, sclerosis is predominant and endocortical thickening, medullary sclerosis, and the "bone within a bone" appearance may ensue.

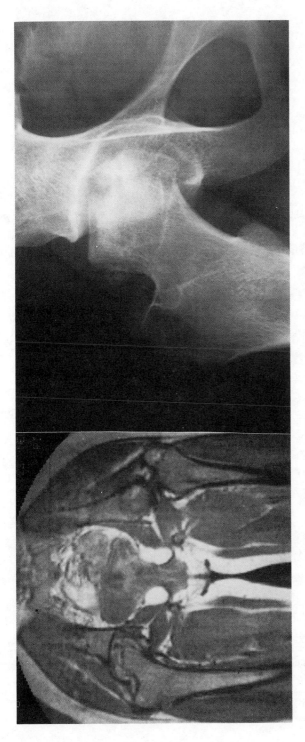

Figure 13.12. Aseptic necrosis. Left: Typical changes of old aseptic necrosis of right hip on spin echo scan. Note the irregular contour of the deformed femoral head, which contains mottled low-intensity areas in the fatty marrow. Right: Confirmatory radiograph with classic findings of advanced aseptic necrosis.

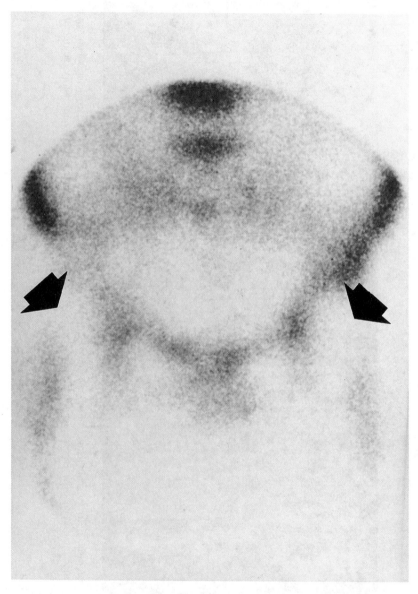

Figure 13.13. Anterior cortical image of pelvis and both hip joints of a 16-year-old patient with sickle cell disease. Nonvisualization of the right femoral head (large arrow) and left femoral head (small arrow) indicates osteonecrosis of both heads, which was confirmed at surgery.

Source: ML Lecklitner, Nuclear imaging studies in sickle cell disease, *Ala J Med Sci* 24 (1987): 393, Fig. 4. Reproduced with permission.

Joint changes of swelling and effusion are common during pain crisis (28, 29). Individuals with SCD may develop gout, septic arthritis from embolism or adjacent osteomyelitis, aseptic osteonecrosis, or hemarthrosis—all of which can produce arthralgia. Radiological findings may be specific or nonspecific according to the particular process present.

THE CHEST

Chest radiography of patients with SCD will demonstrate abnormality in three-quarters of the cases (30). There may be changes in the bones of the thorax and adjacent pectoral girdles. Gallstones, evidence of previous biliary surgery, and abnormalities of the liver and spleen may be seen below the diaphragm. Abnormalities of the heart and lungs are common.

Lung disease associated with SCD includes: (1) pneumonia, (2) pulmonary infarction, (3) pulmonary vascular thrombosis with cor pulmonale in the absence of infarction, (4) embolism of necrotic bone marrow, and (5) alveolar wall necrosis and focal parenchymal scars. Of course, there may be superimposed pulmonary edema and an increased vascular pattern (30, 31). Thus, a variety of radiographic abnormalities may be seen, and frequently, several will be coincident.

These lesions are no different when associated with SCD. The problem is differentiation between "acute chest syndrome" which is associated with occlusive disease and acute pulmonary infarction caused by emboli or pulmonary consolidation from acute infection. It is never easy, and often impossible, to distinguish between infarct and pneumonia, and overlying diffuse patterns of pulmonary edema, interstitial fibrosis, or the increased flow pattern of anemia complicate the picture. Consequently, the radiologist is often most helpful only in excluding the presence of acute focal, segmental, or larger processes in the lung. When those are present, the radiologist will frequently be unable to assign a specific diagnosis or etiology.

The *heart* usually is enlarged. The cardiomegaly may reflect the patient's anemia, increased resistance from occlusive pulmonary disease, papillary muscle infarction, and/or congestive failure. Typically, the symmetrical, multichamber enlargement gives no clue to a specific etiology (30, 32).

THE ABDOMEN

Episodes of abdominal pain are frequent in SCD. Many of these episodes are so-called "sterile crises," but the possibility of gross organ infarction, rupture, infection, or other complications cannot be ignored (33). Plain film studies of the abdomen are usually not helpful. Computed tomography (CT) is an excellent modality for early investigation or screening but is expensive and somewhat time-consuming. Ultrasonography has a role here, especially in evaluating the acute right upper quadrant. Nuclear radiology has a place in evaluating the liver,

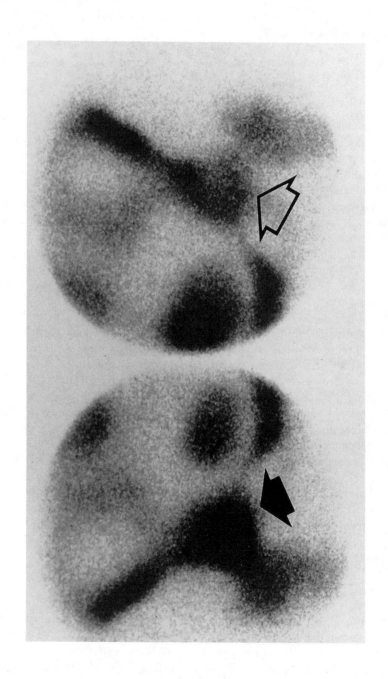

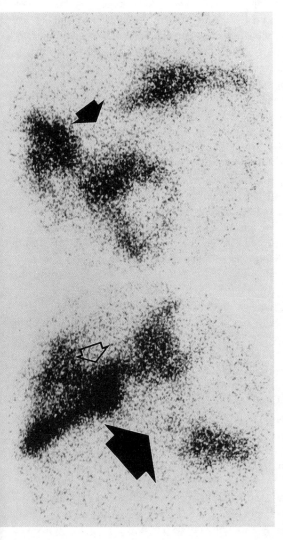

Figure 13.14. Anterior images of hips of patients with sickle cell disease. Left: Anterior cortical images of both hips showing increased abnormal radioactivity in the right femoral head (solid arrow) and normal activity in the left femoral head (open arrow), indicating osteonecrosis of the right femoral head, which was confirmed surgically. Right: Anterior pinhole medullary images of both hips showing nonvisualization of the right femoral head and neck (large arrow) with increased activity in the medial portion of the acetabular lip (open arrow) and nonvisualization of activity in the left femoral head and neck (small solid arrow). This represents surgically confirmed bilateral osteonecrosis of the femoral heads with secondary degenerative changes in the acetabular portion of the right hip joint.

Source: ML Lecklitner, Nuclear imaging studies in sickle cell disease, *Ala J Med Sci* 24 (1987): 393, Fig. 5. Reproduced with permission.

spleen, and biliary system. Our experience with MRI of the abdomen in SCD is so limited as to be inconclusive at this time.

The *spleen* may be seen as enlarged in children during crisis and with acute infection but, over time, focal changes of small infarctions and fibrosis result in a small, shrunken spleen. Granular calcification may appear and the tiny shrunken spleen may be quite dense on either routine films or CT studies; moreover, the density may be further enhanced by siderosis (34). Rupture, hemorrhage, or multiple venous occlusions of the swollen spleen can be demonstrated by CT or angiography (33–35). With obstruction to the flow of sinusoidal blood due to sickling, the diversion of blood through known arteriovenous shunts may produce functional asplenia or lack of splenic uptake in a liver-spleen scan (35).

Biliary Tract disease is frequent in SCD. The abdominal crisis, manifested by pain, jaundice, elevated liver enzymes, and frequently leucocytosis, occurs in 10 percent of all patients. Distinguishing the pain crisis from acute biliary disease is a substantial clinical and radiological problem (36).

Cholelithiasis is associated frequently with SCD. The prevalence of cholelithiasis was 27–29 percent in two studies using ultrasound on sickle cell patients under 18 years of age. Prevalence of gallstones increase with age, being 10 percent at less than ten years and 56 percent from 10–18 years of age (37, 38).

Ultrasound is a very sensitive means of studying the gallbladder and extrahepatic biliary ducts. Gallstones can be identified as echogenic structures with posterior acoustic shadowing within the lumen of the gallbladder. These opacities should move within the gallbladder by gravity. Echogenic, nonshadowing sludge in the gallbladder can also be seen either alone or with gallstones.

The normal sonographic diameter of the common bile duct is 4 mm. Cunningham found that children with sickle cell disease usually do not have biliary enlargement, even in the presence of gallstones or biliary inflammation. When biliary enlargement does occur, it is usually not obstructive (39).

Scintigraphic imaging provides a noninvasive and safe, functional evaluation of the patency and integrity of the biliary system (11). There has been a recent renaissance in hepatobiliary scintigraphic evaluation, attributable to the advent and widespread availability of iminodiacetic acid (IDA) derivatives labelled with technetium-99m.

A host of somewhat simiar IDA compounds—diisopropyl (DISIDA), dimethyl (HIDA), paraisopropyl (PIPIDA), diethyl (DEIDA), and parabutyl (BIDA)—are available, but only Tc-99m–labelled DISIDA is available on an other than investigational basis. Whereas each radiopharmaceutical has its own biokinetics, the main property of IDA radiopharmaceuticals are their action as a bilirubin analogue. Thus, following intravenous injection, Tc-99m IDA compounds can be imaged in assessing the rates and routes of bile flow.

Following intravenous administration of the radiopharmaceutical, there is rapid clearance for the circulation by the liver with rapidly diminishing background (blood pool) activity. Within 15–30 minutes, the gallbladder and common bile duct are visualized. Further imaging demonstrates only a diminution of liver activity and a distal progression of intestinal activity. The finding of nonvisualization of the gallbladder is commonly associated with acute calculous or acalculous cholecystitis or chronic cholecystitis (Figure 13.15) but may also be associated with inadequate fasting, prolonged fasting, and hyperalimentation.

Virtually all patients harboring acute calculous cholecystitis demonstrate nonvisualization of the gallbladder, and chronic calculous cholecystisis is as likely to visualize as not to visualize. Hence, the greatest value of the test is *to rule out* acute calculous cholecystitis. Hepatobiliary scintigraphy is approximately 90 percent sensitive for acute acalculous cholecystitis. There are two guidelines that indicate the diagnosis of chronic cholecystitis in those cases in which the gallbladder visualizes: a small, contracted gallbladder (assuming adequate pretest fasting), and visualization of the gallbladder subsequent to the visualization of intestinal activity (Figure 13.16).

Hepatobiliary scientigraphy likewise evaluates the patency of the common hepatic duct and the common bile duct. If sequential anterior images demonstrate intestinal activity, the common bile duct is patent. Early obstruction demonstrates activity in the intrahepatic or extrahepatic common bile duct without progression into the small intestine (Figure 13.17). The scintigraphic pattern of *late* obstruction of the common bile duct is one of sequential images that appear as a redundant pattern of only hepatic visualization (Figure 13.18).

The most common acute hepatic biliary lesion involving patients with SCD is the syndrome of hepatic crisis that occurs in some 10 percent of patients hospitalized with SCD (40, 41). Within the clinical setting of acute right-upper-quadrant symptoms, signs, and laboratory values, acute cholecystitis, with or without attending choledocholithiasis, may be indistinguishable from sickle cell hepatic crisis, viral hepatitis, or a host of other disorders that may mimic various other hepatic and biliary disorders that are not related to the complications of sickle cell disease. Following is a list of hepatobiliary disorders found seredipitously by scintigraphy:

1. Hepatic Tumors
   a. Primary tumors
      i. Hepatoma
      ii. Hepatoendothelioma
      iii. Cystic duct: adenocarcinoma
      iv. Hepatoblastoma
      v. Hemangioma
   b. Metastatic tumors
   c. Cystic lesions
      i. Simple cyst
      ii. Choledochal cyst

2. Hepatic trauma
   a. Hematoma
   b. Biloma
   c. Fistula
   d. Obstructive hemobilia
3. Infections
   a. Bacterial abscess
   b. Amebic abscess
   c. Pancreatitis
   d. Hepatitis
4. Iatrogenic ligation
   a. Common bile duct
   b. Common hepatic duct
5. Renal lesions
   a. Tumor
   b. Ureteral obstruction
   c. Pyeloureterectasis
6. Gastric lesions
   a. Reflux (11)

Renal abnormalities are common in SCD. McCall, Moule, Desai, et al. (42) found radiographically demonstrable abnormalities in 69 percent of their patients with homozygous SCD. Blunting and clubbing of calices are the most common findings on contrast urography. The clubbing progressively worsens in severity and extent with age but usually is not associated with overlying scarring of the cortex. Cortical scarring has been shown angiographically to be associated with irregularity and absence of cortical arterial vessels. This suggests an ischemic rather than infectious etiology. Papillary necrosis is much less common (23%) and appears as cavitary formation adjacent to one or more papillae. The etiology of papillary necrosis in sickle cell disease is not certain, but it is felt to be due to small vessel obstruction within the papilla where sluggish flow, low oxygen tension, acid pH, and hypertonicity occur. The prevalence of papillary necrosis does not appear to increase with age. The demonstrable urographic abnormalities do not correlate well with symptomatology.

CENTRAL NERVOUS SYSTEM

Central nervous system (CNS) involvement occurs in 13–17 percent of SCD patients (43). Cerebral infarction is a common complication in SC disease and is exceeded only by pain crisis and cardiomegaly as the most common clinical finding (43, 44). The risk of stroke is significantly increased in childhood, with

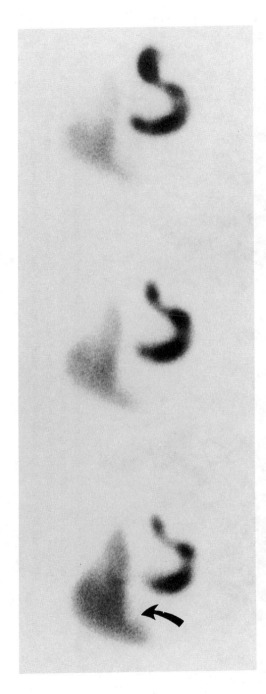

Figure 13.15. Anterior sequential hepatobiliary images at 60 minutes (left), 90 minutes (center), and 120 minutes (right) showing persistent nonvisualization of the gall bladder (curved arrow) throughout the series. Copious intestinal activity is demonstrated. These findings are compatible with acute or chronic cholecystitis. The common bile duct is patent.

Source: ML Lecklitner, Nuclear imaging studies in sickle cell disease, *Ala J Med Sci* 24 (1987): 394, Fig 6. Reproduced with permission.

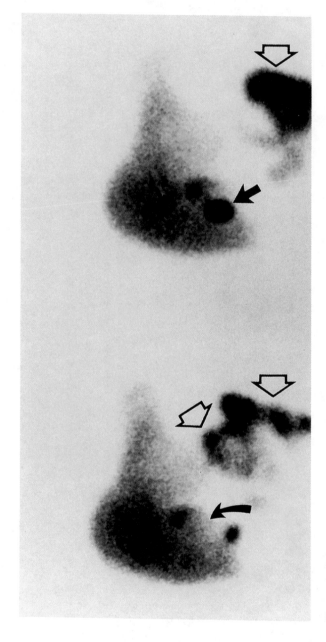

Figure 13.16. Anterior sequential hepatobiliary images at 60 minutes (left) and 90 minutes (right) showing the earlier nonvisualization of the gall bladder (curved arrow), with a subsequent demonstration of the gall bladder (straight arrow) well after the visualization of intestinal activity (open arrows). This indicates chronic cholecystitis and a patent common bile duct, which was confirmed surgically.

Source: ML Lecklitner, Nuclear imaging studies in sickle cell disease, *Ala J Med Sci* (1987): 394, Fig. 7. Reproduced with permission.

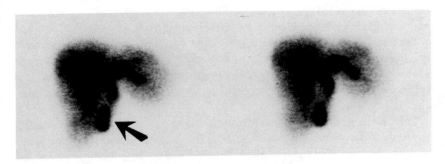

Figure 13.17. Anterior sequential images at two hours and three hours showing visualization of the gall bladder (arrow) and intrahepatic biliary system and persistent nonvisualization of intestinal activity. Thus, acute cholecystitis can be ruled out. Chronic cholecystitis is highly probable, particularly in view of the short duration of total obstruction of the common bile duct. Chronic cholecystitis with impacted calculus at the ampulla of Vater was proved surgically.

Source: ML Lecklitner, Nuclear imaging studies in sickle cell disease, *Ala J Med Sci* 24 (1987): 394, Fig. 8. Reproduced with permission.

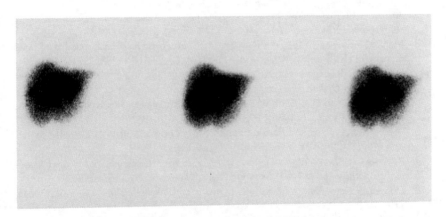

Figure 13.18. Anterior sequential hepatobiliary images at two hour (left), three hours (center), and four hours (right) showing persistent hepatic visualization with no demonstration of gall bladder and no activity in the intrahepatic or extrahepatic biliary components. There is no intestinal activity. This is consistent with long-standing total obstruction of the common bile duct, which was confirmed by intraoperative cholangiography and surgery.

Source: ML Lecklitner, Nuclear imaging studies in sickle cell disease. *Ala J Med Sci* 24 (1987): 394, Fig. 9. Reproduced with permission.

high rates of morbidity, frequent permanent deficit, and a high incidence of repeat infarctions independent of the age of initial onset (45–47).

Intracranial hemorrhage without associated infarction is uncommon but has a grave prognosis. It probably is related to the fragility of the fine collateral vessels (48). Spinal cord infarction has been reported to cause acute myelopathy, and spinal cord compression by extramedullary hematopoietic tissue may cause paraplegia (48, 49).

Cerebral angiography demonstrates stenosis or occlusion of major vessels at the base of the brain, and multiple occlusions often predominate in the distributions of the internal carotid artery. Involvement of the posterior cerebral and posterior fossa distribution is less common. Angiopathic moyamoya or the "puff of smoke" pattern of extensive collateral circulation in the basal region of the brain may be demonstrated (50). Computed tomography is almost ideal for demonstration of cerebral infarction and extra- and intracerebral hemorrhage. MRI shows enormous promise for imaging the brain and spinal cord as it is affected by SCD, and is being used in the investigation of the learning disorders often encountered in children with SCD.

REFERENCES

1. Middlemiss JH, and Raper AB: Skeletal changes in the haemoglobinopathies. *J Bone Jt Surg* 48B (1966): 693–702.
2. Kricun ME: Red-yellow marrow conversion: Its effect on the location of some solitary bone lesions. *Skeletal Radiol* 4 (1985): 10–18.
3. Mankad VN, Yang Y-M, Williams JP, et al.: Magnetic resonance imaging of bone marrow in sickle cell patients. *Am J Ped Hem Oncol* 104 (1988): 344–347.
4. O'Hara AE: Roentgenographic osseous manifestations of the anemias and the leukemias. *Clin Orthop* 52 (1967): 63–82.
5. Reynolds J: A re-evaluation of the "fish vertebra" sign in sickle cell hemoglobinopathy. *Am J Rad* 97 (1966): 693–707.
6. Seber JI, and Diggs LW: Radiographic changes of the skull in sickle cell anemia. *Am J Rad* 132 (1979): 373–377.
7. Reynolds J: *The roentgenological future of sickle cell disease and related hemoglobinopathies,* pp. 87–93. Springfield, IL: Charles C. Thomas, 1965.
8. Diggs LW: Bone and joint lesions in sickle-cell disease. *Clin Orthop* 52 (1967): 119–143.
9. Strecker W, Gilula LA, and Kryiakos M: Case report 479: Ideopathic healing infarct of bone simulating osteosarcoma. *Skeletal Radiol* 17 (1988): 220–225.
10. Bohrer SP: Sickle cell disease. In JM Taveras and JT Ferrucci eds.: *Radiology: Diagnosis—Imaging—Intervention,* Vol. 5, ch. 67, pp. 1–12. Philadelphia: J. B. Lippincott, 1987.
11. Lecklitner ML: Nuclear imaging studies and sickle cell disease. *Ala J Med Sci* 24 (1987): 390–396.
12. Bohrer SP: Acute long bone diaphyseal infarct in sickle cell disease. *Br J Radiol* 43 (1970): 685–697.
13. Middlemiss H: *Tropical radiology,* p. 80. London: William Heinemann, 1961.

14. Keats TE, and Holt JF: The calvarial "doughnut lesion." A previously undescribed entity. *Am J Rad* 55 (1969): 314–318.
15. Mankad VN, Williams JP, Harpen MD, et al.: Magnetic resonance imaging: Percentage of dense cells and serum prostanoids as tools for objective assessment of pain crisis. In N. Nagel, ed., *Patho-physiological aspects of sickle cell vaso-occlusion*. pp. 337–350. New York: Alan R. Liss, 1987.
16. Rao VM, Fishman M, Mitchell DG, et al.: Painful sickle cell crisis: Bone marrow pattern observed with MR imaging. *Radiology* 161 (1986): 211–215.
17. Bohrer SP. Fracture complicating bone infarct and/or osteomyelitis in sickle-cell disease. *Clin Radiol* 22 (1971): 83–88.
18. Alazraki NP, Davis MA, Jones AG, et al.: Skeletal system. In PT Kirchner, ed.: *Nuclear medicine review syllabus*, p. 567. New York: Society of Nuclear Medicine, 1980.
19. Matin P: The appearance of bone scans following fractures, including immediate and long-term studies. *J Nucl Med* 20 (1979): 1227–1231.
20. Modic MT, Pflange W, Feiglin DHI, et al.: Magnetic resonance imaging of muscoloskeletal infections. *Radiol Clin North Am* 24 (1986): 247–258.
21. Fletcher BD, Scoles PV, and Nelson AD: Osteomyelitis in children: Dection by magnetic resonance. *Radiology* 150 (1984): 57–60.
22. Richardson ML: Optimizing pulse sequences for magnetic resonance imaging of the musculoskeletal system. *Radiol Clin North Am* 24 (1986): 137–144.
23. Keeley K, and Buchanan GR. Acute infarction of long bones in children with sickle cell anemia. *J Peds* 101 (1982): 170–175.
24. Barton, CJ, and Cockshott WP. Bone changes in hemoglobin SC disease. *Am J Rad* 88 (1972): 523–532.
25. Lee REJ, Golding JSR, and Serjeant GR: The radiographic features of avascular necrosis of the femoral head in homozygous sickle cell disease. *Clin Radiol* 32 (198): 205–214.
26. Sebes JI, and Kraus AP: Avascular necrosis of the hip in the sickle cell hemoglobinopathies. *J Can Assoc Radiol* 34 (1983): 136–139.
27. Gillespy T III, Genant HK, and Helms CA: Magnetic resonance imaging of osteonecrosis. *Radiol Clin North Am* 24 (1986): 193–208.
28. Espinoza LB, Spilberg I, and Osterland CK: Joint manifestations of sickle cell disease. *Medicine* 53 (1974): 295–305.
29. Schumacher HR, Andrews R, and McLaughlin G: Arthropathy in sickle-cell disease. *Ann Intern Med* 78 (1973): 203–211.
30. Reynolds J. *The roentgenological features of sickle cell disease and related hemoglobinopathies*, pp. 184–218. Springfield, IL: Charles C. Thomas, 1965.
31. Haupt HM, Moore GW, Bauer TW, et al.: The lung in sickle cell disease. *Chest* 81 (1982): 332–337.
32. Rosenthal DS, and Braunwald E. Hematologic-oncologic disorders and heart disease. In E Braunwald, ed.: *Heart disease: A textbook of cardiovascular medicine*, Vol. 1, ch. 48, pp. 1774–1775. Philadelphia: W. B. Saunders, 1980.
33. Magid D, Fishman EK, Charache S, et al.: Abdominal pain in sickle cell disease: The role of CT. *Radiology* 163 (1987): 325–328.
34. Reynolds J. *The roentgenological features of sickle cell disease and related hemoglobinopathies*, pp. 219–245. Springfield, IL: Charles C. Thomas, 1965.

350 B. G. Brogdon, M. L. Lecklitner, B. C. Machen, & J. P. Williams

35. Fishbone G, Nunez D Jr., Leon R, et al.: Massive splenic infarction in sickle cell-hemoglobin C disease: angiographic findings. *Am J Rad* 129 (1977): 927–928.
36. Ariyam S, Shessel FS, and Pickett LK: Cholecystitis and cholelitharis masking as abdominal crises in sickle cell disease. *Pediatrics* 58 (1976): 252–258.
37. Sarnaik S, Slovis TL, Corbett DP, et al.: Incidence of cholelithiasis in sickle cell anemia using the ultrasonic gray-scale technic. *Pediatrics* 96 (1980): 1005–1008.
38. Lachman BS, Lazerson J, Starshak RJ, et al.: The prevalence of cholelithiasis in sickle cell disease as diagnosed by ultrasound and cholecystography. *Pediatrics* 64 (1979): 601–603.
39. Cunningham JJ: Sonographic diameter of the common hepatic duct in sickle cell anemia. *Am J Rad* 141 (1983): 321–324.
40. Diggs LW: Sickle cell crises. *Am J Clin Pathol* 44 (1965): 1–19.
41. Shechy TW: Sickle cell hepatopathy. *South Med J* 70 (1977): 533–538.
42. McCall IW, Moule N, Desai P, et al.: Urographic findings in homozygous sickle cell disease. *Radiology* 126 (1978): 99–104.
43. Huttenlocker PR, Moohr JW, Johns L, et al.: Cerebral blood flow in sickle cell cerebrovascular disease. *Pediatrics* 73 (1984): 615–621.
44. Boros L, Thomas C, and Weiner WJ: Large cerebral vessel disease in sickle cell anemia. *J Neurol Neurosurg Psychi* 39 (1976): 1236–1239.
45. Gerald B, Sebes JI, and Langston JW: Cerebral infarction secondary to sickle cell disease: Arteriographic findings. *Am J Rad* 134 (1980): 1209–1212.
46. Powars D, Wilson B, Imbus C, et al.: The natural history of stroke in sickle cell disease. *Am J Med* 65 (1978): 461–471.
47. Wood DH: Cerebrovascular complications of sickle cell anemia. In AG Waltz, ed.: *Current concepts of cerebrovascular disease-stroke,* Vol. 9, pp. 73–75. Dallas, TX: American Heart Assn., 1978.
48. Sharada SA, and Lusher JM: Neurological complications of sickle cell anemia. *Am J Ped Hem Onc* 4 (1982): 386–394.
49. Ammoumi AA, Sher JH, and Schmelka D: Spinal cord compression by extramedullary hemopoietic tissue in sickle cell anemia. *J Neurol Surg* 43 (1975): 483–485.
50. Seeler RA, Royal JE, Powe L, et al.: Moyamoya in children with sickle cell anemia and cerebrovascular occlusion. *J Peds* 93 (1978): 808–810.

14

Anesthetic Management of Patients with Sickle Cell Disease

Aparna V. Mankad

Sickle cell disease presents a challenge to anesthesiologists and surgeons due to increased risk of morbidity and mortality. Several authors have recognized the risks associated with anesthesia and have reviewed the literature (1–3). The purpose of this chapter is to describe potential peri-operative risks, pre-operative evaluation, the role of pre-operative blood transfusion, anesthetic management, and post-operative complications.

POTENTIAL PERI-OPERATIVE RISKS

Hypoxia during an anesthetic procedure can occur due to various causes: (1) difficulty in establishing an airway during the induction of general anesthesia; (2) an inadequate supply of oxygen due to equipment malfunction or inadvertent error; (3) pulmonary dysfunction, which is of particular concern in sickle cell patients due to the likelihood of previous pulmonary infarcts; (4) decreased oxygen-carrying capacity resulting from anemia, which could be exacerbated during surgery due to hemorrhage; (5) decreased cardiac output; and (6) increased myocardial oxygen demand. Hypoxia is a potential risk factor in any anesthetic procedure, but is of particular concern in patients with sickle cell disease due to increased sickling induced by the deoxygenation of erythrocytes.

Hypothermia due to cold operating room conditions and the use of cold intravenous and surgical irrigation fluids may occur during surgery. Hyperthermia due to environmental conditions and fever is also observed in some patients. Additionally, acidosis due to hypoxia and dehydration due to inadequate fluid replacement may occur during surgery. These factors contribute to increased peri-operative sickling.

Clinical consequences of the above pathologic events may be life-threatening and may place the sickle cell patient at an increased risk of mortality. Death may be due to stroke, cardiac failure, or pulmonary insufficiency (4). Increased morbidity during the post-operative period may include fever, pain crises, cerebrovascular occlusion, acute chest syndrome, wound infection, and anemia (4, 5, 6, 7, 8).

PRE-OPERATIVE EVALUATION

A team approach involving hematologists and other medical specialists, surgeons, and anesthesiologists is highly desirable. The team should develop a plan for the evaluation of the patient, recognize problems early, and attempt a resolution prior to surgery to optimize the patient's condition. The evaluation usually includes (1) general condition, (2) systemic dysfunctions associated with sickle cell disease, (3) location and severity of surgery, and (4) elective or emergency nature of the surgery.

General Condition

If the patient is undergoing a vaso-occlusive crisis, an infectious episode, or another acute complication of sickle cell disease, his or her general condition may not be satisfactory for elective surgery. Therefore, it is desirable to schedule such surgical procedures when the patient is in a stable condition. A complete blood count, reticulocyte count, and hemoglobin electrophoresis are recommended prior to surgery. Solubility tests such as sickledex detect the presence of sickle hemoglobin only and do not differentiate between sickle cell trait (AS) or sickle cell disease (SS, SC, and S-thal). For the purpose of establishing the diagnosis of sickle cell disease and predicting risks, sickledex is not suitable.

Systemic Dysfunctions Associated with Sickle Cell Disease

A thorough history and physical examination will indicate the presence of systemic dysfunctions and assist the physician in individualizing further evaluation. For example, in an adult with a history of recurrent acute chest syndromes, the likelihood of pulmonary insufficiency should be considered. However, in a young child with no history of previous pulmonary complications, extensive laboratory investigations may not be necessary.

Cardiovascular System

Cardiovascular abnormalities manifest clinically by cardiomegaly (9), evidence of hyperdynamic circulation such as full pulse, enlarged laterally displaced apical impulse, anterior parasternal lift, accentuated second heart sound, third heart sound, and murmurs (10). Chronic hemolytic anemia (usual hemoglobin is 7–9 gm %) results in a compensatory rise in cardiac output. A further rise is seen in response to stress and exertion. Patients with sickle cell disease may be able to conduct their usual activities but are reported to have decreased exercise tolerance. During anesthetic procedures, the patient may be subjected to additional stress and, therefore, is at risk of developing cardiac failure (11). Although myocardial ischemia due to vaso-occlusive phenomenon is not common, myocardial fibrosis has been reported as discussed in Chapter 5. Sickle cell patients may develop progressive pulmonary hypertension which results in cor pulmonale (12).

In a young patient (for example, a one-year-old with previous splenic sequestration crisis and a normal cardiovascular examination), a good history and physical examination will suffice. However, in older patients and in those with the clinical features listed above, an extensive evaluation of the cardiovascular system is indicated. This may include (1) chest X ray, (2) EKG, (3) echocardiography, and (4) a cardiac profile, including cardiac output, cardiac index, pulmonary artery pressure measurement, and other parameters obtained through a pulmonary artery catheter.

Pulmonary System

One of the common problems in sickle cell disease is acute chest syndrome. Recurrent pulmonary infarcts, pneumonias, or both reduce pulmonary functions (13). Pulmonary alveolar wall necrosis, exudate or edema fluid in alveoli, and focal areas of fibrotic scarring consistent with persistent pulmonary infiltrates may develop over time (14). The presence of pulmonary infarcts may result in an increased number of bronchopulmonary anastomosis and an increase in right-to-left shunt. These changes result in a progressive reduction in pulmonary vasculature and ventilation perfusion abnormalities, causing reduced oxygen saturation. Resting PaO_2 may be between 70–90 mm Hg (15). In patients in whom pulmonary insufficiency is suspected, the following laboratory investigations are indicated: (1) chest X ray, (2) arterial blood gas analysis, and (3) pulmonary function tests before and after incentive spirometry, deep breathing exercises, and bronchodilatory treatments. Smoking should be discouraged.

Hepatobiliary Functions

Ten percent of patients with sickle cell anemia are hospitalized for the management of hepatic crisis (16). The patient may complain of nausea, vomiting, right-upper-quadrant pain, and increasing jaundice. On examination, a tender, enlarged liver may be found with elevated liver enzymes. The crisis usually resolves in 7–10 days with negative serology (17). Differential diagnosis should include hepatitis, gall stones, cholecystitis and pancreatitis, acute hepatic sequestration of blood, and other causes of acute abdomen. Patients with significant history of hepatobiliary dysfunction should have the following investigations: transaminases, alkaline phosphatase, bilirubin, amylase, PT and PTT to evaluate coagulation, and a hepatitis profile. Fluid and electrolyte status should be evaluated, especially in a patient with vomiting. When possible, the patient should be managed conservatively to stabilize fluids, electrolytes, and hematological status. When liver functions are optimal, elective surgery should be scheduled.

Renal Functions

Glomerular and tubular damage is commonly seen in patients with sickle cell anemia (18, 19). Papillary necrosis is seen in up to 40 percent of patients with or without hematuria. Proteinuria and an inability to concentrate the urine are also commonly seen. This may increase the risk of dehydration in patients with fever, vomiting, diarrhoea, or tachypnea. Under most circumstances, the determination of BUN and creatinine and a urinalysis with a measurement of specific gravity would be sufficient pre-operative evaluations.

Neurological Function

Damage to the central nervous system may cause seizures, stroke due to cerebral infarction or hemorrhage (20), blindness, vertigo, or hearing loss (21). Occasionally, cranial nerve palsy or mental nerve neuropathy may be seen (22). An awareness of potential neurological complications should alert the anesthesiologist in individualizing the anesthetic management.

Location and Severity of Surgery

Peripheral surgery such as skin grafting a small area on one ankle joint or the placement of myringotomy tubes in a young child who has sickle cell disease with minimum organ dysfunction and optimum general health and hematocrit requires little pre-operative preparation (23). Surgery can be done without blood transfusions but does require adequate monitoring. Minor surgery in a patient with multiorgan dysfunction is considered as high risk. Such a patient should have a special pre-operative evaluation and preparation. Major surgical procedures such as cholecystectomy, splenectomy, intracranial or intrathorasic procedures, cesarean sections, and many more will require special evaluation and preparation. Blood transfusion is discussed in a separate section.

Elective versus Emergency Surgery

There is a clear advantage in performing an elective surgery in a prepared patient rather than an emergency procedure in an acutely ill individual. The risks of delaying the surgery should be compared to the risks of anesthesia in an acutely ill patient to determine if emergency surgery is indicated.

ROLE OF PRE-OPERATIVE BLOOD TRANSFUSION

The transfusion of red blood cells increases oxygen carrying capacity. However, the delivery of oxygen to the tissues is not a linear function of the red cell mass (Figure 14.1; see also reference 24). After an optimum hematocrit is

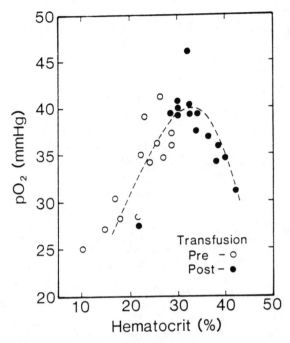

Figure 14.1. Effects of red cell transfusion on venous pO₂ at various hematocrits. The open circles represent pretransfusion hematocrits, while closed circles represent posttransfusion hematocrits. Venous pO₂ increased up to hematocrits of 35 percent and then decreased, probably due to increased viscosity and decreased blood flow.

Source: K Jan, S Usami, and JA Smith, Effects of transfusion on rheological properties of blood in sickle cell anemia, *Transfusion* 22, no. 1: (1982): 19. Reprinted with permission.

reached, the transport of oxygen to the tissues decreases due to increased viscosity and decreased blood flow. The optimum hematocrit is different for red cells carrying hemoglobin A and for those with hemoglobin S (25). Since the whole blood viscosity of blood from the sickle cell anemia patient is high even in oxygenated conditions, the optimum hematocrit in sickle cell anemia is lower than in normal individuals (26). During deoxygenation, the optimum hematocrit of the red cells carrying hemoglobin A does not change. However, upon deoxygenation, the gelation of sickle hemoglobin increases blood viscosity further and, therefore, the optimum hematocrit of deoxygenated sickle blood is even lower (Figure 14.2; 25). Basic and clinical aspects of transfusion in sickle cell disease have been reviewed previously (27).

The effects of red cell transfusions in sickle cell patients are complex, with some favorable and some unfavorable influences. An increased proportion of hemoglobin A would be expected to reduce the likelihood of sickling during hypoxic episodes. Increased oxygen-carrying capacity from transfusion is also

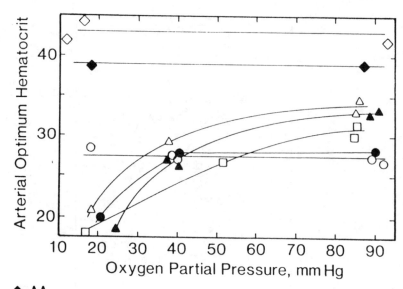

◆ AA
◇ AS
□ SS
● SC
○ CC
△ S-β⁺ Thalassemia
▲ S-β° Thalassemia

Figure 14.2. Oxygen dependence of optimum hematocrits in sickle
hemoglobinopathies. Due to high viscosity even in oxygenated
conditions, the optimum hematocrit of sickle hemoglobinopathies (SS,
SC, and S-thal) is lower. At lower pO_2, viscosity increases further and
optimum hematocrit drops.

Source: F Self, LV McIntire, and BJ Zanger, Rheological evaluation of hemoglobin S and
hemoglobin C hemoglobinopathies, *J Lab Clin Med* 89, no. 3: (1977): 494, Fig. 6. Reprinted
with permission.

an advantage in a patient with anemia, since it will reduce cardiac work load.
However, potential disadvantages of red cell transfusions include the following:
(1) increased viscosity may decrease blood flow especially beyond the optimum
hematocrit; (2) if simple transfusion is used and sickle erythrocytes are not
exchanged, the number of sickle cells in the patient remain the same, and these
cells must negotiate the circulation in a more viscous environment; (3) the patient
is exposed to infections; and (4) the patient may be sensitized to red cell antigens.

Clinical Studies

Many studies have shown a decrease in morbidity and mortality from surgery and anesthesia in sickle cell patients (1, 4, 6, 7, 8). Several investigators have attributed this improvement to modern, state of the art, anesthetic and surgical techniques. In some programs, the improvements have been attributed to pre-operative transfusion therapy with the goal of reducing the percentage of sickle hemoglobin to less than 30 percent (28). However, others have reported good results with simple transfusions directed to correct anemia with no attempt to achieve a specific percentage of sickle hemoglobin. On the contrary, several studies have suggested that transfusion therapy is unnecessary and is associated with acute transfusion reactions, hepatitis, and possible isosensitizations (29–32). Sergeant reported that peri-operative and post-operative complications were minimal in sickle cell patients undergoing surgery even when the hemoglobin level was 7–9 gm percent (33). Homi's findings support these observations and suggest that peri- and post-operative complications were related to pre-operative condition rather than the anesthetic technique or transfusion status of the patient (34).

Since the overall morbidity and mortality of anesthetic and surgical procedures is low, the controversy regarding pre-operative transfusions can only be addressed through a systematic, prospective, randomized, multi-institutional study comparing various protocols, including exchange transfusions, simple transfusions, and no transfusions in the pre-operative preparation. Such a study is currently being conducted by a multicenter preoperative transfusion study group coordinated by the Children's Hospital in Oakland, California. Variations in the anesthetic and surgical practices among the participating institutions may be among the confounding factors in such a study.

Until the results of randomized studies are available, a judicious approach for pre-operative evaluation and preparation is indicated. In sickle cell patients with minimal organ dysfunctions and no major associated disease conditions, anesthesia may be performed without pre-operative transfusions for selected surgical procedures. However, in patients with pulmonary insufficiency, cardiac failure, stroke, renal impairment, hepatic failure, or sepsis, exchange transfusions to reduce the sickle hemoglobin to under 30 percent and the final hematocrit to a maximum of 35 percent is recommended.

ANESTHETIC MANAGEMENT

Premedication

Appropriate analgesics and sedatives can be used when indicated, in order to avoid respiratory depression and hypoxia. The patient should be monitored with pulse oximetry and, if necessary, should receive oxygen during transport to the operating room.

General Intraoperative Management

During the operation, the following conditions should be monitored carefully:

Operating Room Temperature

The ambient temperature should be adjusted to keep the patient euthermic.

Patient's Temperature

In addition to the ambient temperature, the use of warming blankets, radiant lights, warm humidified gases, warm irrigation fluid, and intravenous fluids and blood is recommended.

Hydration

The placement of a large-size intravenous line for hydration on the previous night (1.5 to 2 times the maintenance fluids) is desirable.

Patient Positioning

Patients are positioned carefully with padding at pressure points to avoid circulatory stasis and ischemia.

Monitoring

The basic items to be monitored during the operation include:

Blood pressure,

Pulse rate,

Respiratory rate,

Temperature,

Arterial oxygen saturation,

End-tidal CO_2,

FiO_2.

In patients with multi-organ dysfunctions or during major surgical procedures, all or some of the following monitoring procedures are indicated:

1. An arterial line for blood pressure measurement and arterial blood gas evaluations;
2. A central venous line, with or without Pulmonary artery catheter, for the measurement of central venous pressure, pulmonary artery pressure, pulmonary wedge pressure, mixed venous oxygen saturation, and cardiac profile;
3. Foley's catheter for urine output; and
4. Special procedures such as transesophageal echocardiography, EEG, ultrasonography, fetal heart rate tracing, and tachodynametry in appropriate situations.

Use of the Tourniquet

Although two groups of investigators have reported an uneventful outcome following use of tourniquets (30, 35), intravascular stasis resulting in deoxygenation of red cells, acidosis, and increased sickling are possible. When the tourniquet is absolutely indicated, it is important to exsanguinate the extremity adequately prior to cuff inflation and keep the tourniquet time to a minimum.

Use of Special Techniques

Case reports indicate that if local perfusion is maintained with vasodilatation techniques, hypothermia and hypotension may be achieved safely in patients requiring cardiopulmonary bypass or elective hypotension during anesthesia for intracranial surgery (36, 37).

No data are available comparing general and regional anesthesia in sickle cell patients. The appropriate anesthetic technique should be selected for individual patients (38).

General Endotracheal Anesthesia

Evaluation of the Airway

There must be a careful oropharyngeal examination and study of the neck movement. Any abnormality suggestive of unanticipated difficulty in establishing the airway must be thoroughly investigated. A difficult or a failed intubation in a sickle cell disease patient can have deadly consequences.

Preoxygenation

All patients should receive 100 percent oxygen for 5–7 minutes. This may improve arterial oxygen saturation and may prevent a fall in saturation during endotracheal tube placement.

FiO_2

The recommendations are to keep 30 percent FiO_2 in patients with no cardiopulmonary disease and more than 45 percent FiO_2 for patients with serious cardiopulmonary dysfunctions in order to achieve adequate arterial oxygen saturation (39).

Anesthetic Agents

General anesthesia with potent inhalation agents reduces oxygen consumption and decreases peripheral vascular resistance, allowing good circulation and maintenance of cardiac output. It also reduces V/Q ratio alterations with good oxygenation (40). The percent of irreversibly sickled cells decreases during anesthesia, with the effect lasting for approximately 24 hours (41). Experiments in vitro have shown increased viscosity of deoxygenated sickle red cells treated with clinical concentration of halothane, with no effects on normal, deoxygenated red cells (42). Occasionally, patients have low pseudocholinesterase activity and may require careful use of succinylcholine (43).

Anesthesia Maintenance

The aim of anesthetic maintenance is to prevent hypoxia, hypercarbia, acidosis, hypothermia, venous stasis, and cardiopulmonary depression.

Emergence from Anesthesia

The patient must be fully awake with a return of all protective reflexes and no residual muscle relaxation prior to extubation. The patient should be ventilated with 100 percent oxygen to avoid hypoxia due to nitrous oxide diffusion. The patient should be monitored with pulse oximetry.

The advantages of general anesthesia include: (1) secured airway, which prevents hypoxia, and (2) desired control over respiration and the ability to produce mild respiratory alkalosis.

Regional Anesthesia

Peripheral nerve blocks and major conduction blocks are simple procedures with minimal preparation required. These procedures can provide adequate analgesia or anesthesia for many surgical procedures.

Appropriately used local anesthetics rarely produce respiratory depression. Adequate oxygenation can be maintained with a nasal canula or a face mask. Disadvantages include the following: (1) high spinal or epidural anesthesia with total sympathectomy can lead to severe hypotension, bradycardia, and inadequate ventilation with hypoxia, hypercarbia, and acidosis; (2) compensatory vasoconstriction and decreased oxygen partial pressure in the unblocked area may lead to stasis and vasoocclusive infarction (44); (3) spinal artery thrombosis can occur from sickling, and the complication may be falsely attributed to the regional anesthesia technique; (4) the patient may have weakened vertebrae from osteoporosis which requires a good examination of the back and documentation of findings; (5) prolonged surgery in an apprehensive patient may require the use of large amount of sedatives and narcotics, with a resultant cardiopulmonary depression. If oxygen is not supplemented in such patients, there is a likelihood of the development of hypoxia and hypercarbia.

POST-OPERATIVE CARE AND COMPLICATIONS

During the immediate post-operative period following anesthesia, the patient is at a high risk of developing hypoxia, leading to sickling crisis (45). The patient should be transported to the recovery room with oxygen supplementation and monitoring with pulse oximetry. The patient should be kept warm and well hydrated in the recovery room. Appropriate analgesic therapy should be provided.

Respiration must be adequate and oxygen supplementation and monitoring must be continued for 24–48 hours or until full clinical recovery is achieved. If red cell transfusion is necessary, the product should be warm.

The true rate of post-operative complications is difficult to determine because the literature contains selective reports of major complications. However, the rate of complications in sickle cell patients is probably higher than in individuals with normal hemoglobin electrophoresis. Searle reported a post-operative mortality rate of 7.6 percent in sickle cell patients (2). The complications include (1) fever of unknown origin, (2) acute chest syndrome (respiratory infection, post-operative atelectesis, and pulmonary infarction), (3) congestive cardiac failure, (4) prolonged drug effects in patients with hepatorenal insufficiency, (5) pain crisis, (6) wound infection, (7) transfusion-related problems, and (8) unexpected death. It is not clear whether pre-operative blood transfusions reduce some of the post-operative complications; the question awaits the conclusion of the multi-institutional study.

MANAGEMENT OF PATIENTS WITH SICKLE CELL TRAIT

Although experience with large numbers of sickle cell trait individuals reveals no appreciable increase in morbidity or mortality (2, 46), several fatal cases have also been reported (47, 48). Patients with sickle cell trait have subtle dysfunctions of their organs, especially the kidneys. Under hypoxic conditions, significant sickling may occur due to the presence of 30–40 percent sickle hemoglobin. Therefore, vigilant care should be provided as described above. With the exception of few surgical procedures such as clipping of intracranial aneurism, blood transfusion is not necessary.

SUMMARY

Hypoxia, hypo- or hyperthermia, acidosis, and dehydration may occur during surgery and may contribute to peri-operative sickling. To reduce morbidity and mortality during the peri-operative period, a team approach to evaluate general condition, systemic dysfunctions, the location and severity of surgery, and the elective or emergent nature of the surgical procedure is suggested. Transfusions of red cells in sickle cell patients have some favorable and some unfavorable influences. Until the results of randomized studies are available, a judicious approach for pre-operative transfusions is suggested. General principles of anesthetic management and post-operative care are similar to other situations, with special attention to oxygenation, fluid and electrolyte balance, and monitoring.

REFERENCES

1. Holzmann L, Finn H, Lichtman HC, et al.: Anesthesia in patients with sickle cell disease. *Anesth and Analg* 48 (1969): 566.

2. Searle JF: Anesthesia in sickle cell states. *Anesthesia* 28 (1973): 48–58.
3. Oduro KA, and Searle JF: Anesthesia in sickle cell states: A plea for simplicity. *Br Med J* 4 (1972): 596–598.
4. Murphy SB: Difficulties in sickle cell states: Complications. In F Orkin and L Copperman, eds.: *Anesthesiology;* pp. 476–485.
5. Maduska A, Guinee WS, Heaton JA, et al.: Sickling dynamics of red blood cells and other physiologic studies during anesthesia. *Anesth and Analg* 54 (1975): 361.
6. Goldstein A, and Keats AS. The risk of anesthesia. *Anesthesiology* 33 (1970): 130.
7. Flye MW, and Silver D: Biliary tract disorders and sickle cell disease. *Surgery* 72 (1972): 361–367.
8. Charache S: The treatment of sickle cell anemia. *Arch Intern Med* 133 (1974): 698–705.
9. Linsay J Jr., Meshal JC, and Patterson RH: The cardiovascular manifestations of sickle cell disease. *Arch Int Med* 133 (1974): 643–651.
10. Ng M, Liebman J, Anstorar, et al.: Cardiovascular findings in children with sickle cell anemia. *Dis Chest* 52 (Dec. 1967): 788–799.
11. Gerry JL, Bulkley BH, and Hutchins GM: Clinicopathologic analysis of cardiac dysfunction in 52 patients with sickle cell anemia. *Am J Cardiol* 42 (1978): 211–216.
12. Hales CA, and Mark EF: Clinicopathological conference case 52–1983. *N Engl J Med* 309 (1983): 1627.
13. Bromberg PA: Pulmonary aspects of sickle cell disease. *Arch Int Med* 133 (1974): 652.
14. Haupt HM, Moore GW, Bauer TW, et al.: The lung in sickle cell disease. *Chest* 81 (1982): 332.
15. Bromberg D, and Jenson W: Arterial oxygen saturation in sickle cell disease. *Am Rev Res Dis* 96 (1967): 400.
16. Hartstein G: The patient with sickle cell anemia. *Anesthesiology News* 29 (June 1987; newsletter).
17. Schubert TT: Hepatobiliary system in sickle cell disease. *Gastroenterology* 90 (1986): 2013–2021.
18. Allon M: Renal abnormalities in sickle cell disease. *Arch Int Med* 150 (1990): 501–504.
19. Strauss J, Zilleruelo G., Abitbol C: The kidney and hemoglobin S. *Nephron* 43 (1986): 241–245.
20. Powar SD, Wilson B, Inbus L., et al.: The neural history of stroke in sickle disease. *Am J Med* 65 (1978): 461.
21. Donegan JO, Lobel JS, and Gluckman JL. Otolaryngologic manifestations of sickle cell disease. *Am J of Otolaryn* 3, no. 2 (March 1982): 141–144.
22. Konotey-Okubu FI: Mental nerve neuropathy: A complication of sickle cell crisis. *Lancet* no. 2 (1972): 388–390.
23. Janik J, and Seeler R: Peri-operative management of children with sickle hemoglobinopathy. *J Ped Surg* 15, no. 2 (1980): 117–120.
24. Jan K, Usami S, and Smith JA: Effects of transfusion on rheological properties of blood in sickle cell anemia. *Transfusion* 22, no. 1 (1982): 17–20.
25. Self F, McIntire LV, and Zanger B: Rheological evaluation of hemoglobin S and hemoglobin C hemoglobinopathies. *J Lab Clin Med* 89, no. 3 (1977): 488–497.

26. Chien S, Usami S, and Bertles JF: Abnormal rheology of oxygenated blood in sickle cell anemia. *J Clinical Invest* 49 (1970): 623–634.
27. Schmalzer E, Chien S, and Brown AK: *Am J Ped Hem Onc* 4, no. 4 (1982): 395–407.
28. Lanzkowsky P, Shende A, Karayalcin G., et al.: Partial exchange transfusion in sickle cell anemia. *Am J Dis Child* 132 (1978): 1200–1208.
29. Hilary-Howells T, Huntsman RG, Goys JE, et al.: Anesthesia and sickle cell hemoglobin with a case report. *Br J Anesth* 44 (1972): 975.
30. Gilbertson AA: Anesthesia in West African patients with sickle cell anemia, hemoglobin SC disease and sickle cell trait. *Br J Anesth* 37 (1965): 614.
31. Oduntan SA, and Isaads WA: Anesthesia in patients with abnormal hemoglobin syndromes: A preliminary report. *Br J Anesth* 43 (1971): 1159.
32. Browne RA: Anesthesia in patients with sickle cell anemia. *Br J Anesth* 37 (1965): 181.
33. Serjeant GR: Sickle cell anemia: Clinical features in adulthood and old age: In H Abramson, JF Bertles, and DL Nethens, eds.: St. Louis, MO: C. V. Mosby, 1973.
34. Homi J: Anesthesia in sickle cell disease. *Br J Med* 16 (1979): 1599–1601.
35. Howells TH, Huntsman RG, Boys JE, et al.: Anesthesia and sickle cell hemoglobin. *Br J Anesth* 44 (1972): 975–982.
36. Heiner M, Teasdale SJ, David T, et al.: Aortocoronary bypass in a patient with sickle cell trait. *Can Anaesth Soc J* 26 (1979): 428–434.
37. Ingram CT, Floyd JB, and Santora AH. *Aortic and mitral valve replacement. Anesth and Analg* 61, no. 9 (1982): 802.
38. Aldretee JA: Hematologic disease. In J Katz, J Benumof, and L Kadis, eds.: *Anesthesia and uncommon diseases*, pp. 313–383. Philadelphia: W. B. Saunders.
39. Brody JL, Goldsmith MH, Park SK, et al.: Symptomatic crisis of sickle cell anemia treated by limited exchange transfusion. *Ann Int Med* 72 (1970): 327.
40. Maduska AL, Guinee WS, Heaton JA, et al.: Sickling dynamics of red blood cells and other physiologic studies during anesthesia. *Anesth and Analg* 54 (1975): 361–365.
41. Guinee WS, Heaton JA, Barreras L, et al.: Effects of general anesthesia on sicklemic patients. *Anesthesiology* 29 (1968): 193.
42. Laasberg LH, and Hedley Whyte J: *The red cell*, rev. ed., pp. 168–202. Cambridge, MA: Harvard University Press.
43. Hilkovitz G, and Jacobson A: Hepatic dysfunction and abnormalities of the serum proteins and serum enzymes in sickle cell anemia. *J Lab Clin Med* 57 (1961): 856–867.
44. Bridenbaugh PO, Moore DC, and Bridenbaugh LD: Alterations in capillary and venous blood gases after regional block anesthesia. *Anesth and Analg* 51 (1972): 280–286.
45. Diggs LW: Sickle cell crisis. *Am J Clin Path* 44 (1965): 1.
46. Atlas SA: The sickle cell trait and surgical complications: A matched pair patient analysis. *JAMA* 229 (1974): 1078.
47. Dinh TV, Boor PJ, and Garza JR. Massive pulmonary embolism following delivery of a patient with sickle cell trait. *Am J Obstet Gynecol* 7 (1982): 722–724.
48. Dunn A, Davies A, Eckert G, et al.: Intraoperative death during caesarian section in a patient with sickle-cell trait. *Can J Anaesth* 34, no. 1 (1987): 67–70.

15

Surgical Management of Patients with Sickle Cell Syndromes

John P. Sutton, John J. Farrer, and Charles B. Rodning

The recognition of sickle cell syndromes as distinct clinical entities has occurred only relatively recently, although these hemoglobinopathies have probably existed throughout the evolution of *Homo sapiens,* particularly among the aboriginal populations on the African continent and in the Mediterranean region (1). Since the first case report of a sickle cell syndrome in North America by James B. Herrick (2), a succession of observations have been made in relationship to this syndrome. Although the hemolytic aspects of this disease were recognized in previous case reports (2–5), the concept of a "hemolytic crisis" was not introduced until 1924 by V. P. Sydenstricker (6). In 1927, Hahn and Gillespie (7) demonstrated that erythrocytic sickling was produced by a reduced intravascular oxygen tension and acidosis, and that an abnormal hemoglobin was the incriminating factor. An association of the syndrome with cholelithiasis was noted in several early case reports (3, 8–13), and the osseous manifestations of the disease (medullary expansion, cortical thinning, and sclerosis) were ultimately identified by both post-mortem and roentgenologic analyses (8, 14–17). As clinical experience with this patient population increased, an association with folic acid deficiency secondary to hemolysis was also noted (18–20). The molecular basis of the disease was recognized by Pauling, Itano, Singer, et al. (21), who identified unique, two-dimensional electrophoretic patterns among hemoglobin types, and by Ingram (22) who identified the exact amino acid composition of the hemoglobin chains (valine replacement of glutamic acid at position six of the β-chain distinquished the globin abnormality).

Although the aforementioned features of the disease are secondary to hemolysis, the pathophysiology of visceral infarction has been attributed to hyperviscosity and vaso-occlusive phenomena. Pulmonary (8, 23, 24), renal (25, 26), splenic (27), osseous (8, 28–30), penile (priapism) (31, 32), central nervous system (33, 34), retinal (35), and integumentary (36–40) infarction have been noted by numerous authors as expressions of the natural history of the erythrocytic sickling process. In a hypoxic and acidotic environment, longitudinally oriented aggregates of Hb S form, resulting in distortion of the erythrocytic membrane (41–45), and rendering the cells susceptible to stagnation and phagocytosis (46–49). It is these three pathophysiologic mechanisms—hemolytic anemia, hyperviscosity, and vaso-occlusion—that the anesthesiologist and surgeon must be prepared to address when confronted with a patient with a sickle cell syndrome who requires operative intervention. As discussed in Chapter 14 and reviewed in several articles, a surgeon's sensitivity for possible morbidity or mortality must be heightened for patients with either sickle cell disease, anemia, or trait, particularly when those patients manifest higher levels of Hb S concentration and when stressed by comorbid conditions that predispose to hypoxia and/or hypoperfusion (50–63).

In addition, it is difficult to accurately and precisely define the contribution of organ dysfunction—due to peri-operative erythrocytic sickling episodes or various peri-operative procedures—to the morbidity and mortality observed among groups of patients with a sickle cell syndrome. In part, this is a consequence of variations in patient populations with respect to the severity of disease, comorbidity, and the quality of anesthetic and surgical care. Since the morbidity and mortality rates from routine anesthetic and invasive (operative, endoscopic, and radiologic) procedures are very low in populations with or without sickle cell syndromes, comparisons among the groups to examine the cause-and-effect relationship of any single anesthetic agent or surgical practice would require very large samples of patient populations. It is, therefore, difficult to estimate the risks of anesthetic and surgical procedures in the absence of this type of quantifiable data. This chapter will summarize several studies of surgical management, which were conducted among patient populations with sickle cell syndromes in various types of institutions and will present the authors' recommendations on the basis of the available evidence.

PRE-OPERATIVE ASSESSMENT AND MANAGEMENT

Hematological screening and investigations for a hemoglobinopathy should be performed on all potentially susceptible individuals who are likely to require anesthesia and surgery. Hemoglobin determination, blood film cytological analysis, an Itano test, a sickledex test, hemoglobin electrophoresis, and analysis for *in vitro* erythrocytic sickling can be accomplished within a period ranging minutes to hours (58). The use of laboratory tests for diagnosis and screening is discussed in Chapters 7 and 8.

The outcome for patients with sickle cell syndromes requiring surgery has been improved. Morbidity associated with the natural history of the disease may require intra-abdominal (gastrointestinal, biliary, splenic), genitourinary, orthopedic, ophthalmologic, neurosurgical, thoracic, peripheral vascular, or plastic and reconstructive (skin grafting) surgical procedures. In addition, comorbid conditions unrelated to the primary disease may necessitate emergent, urgent, or elective abdominal, gynecologic, obstetric, otorhinolaryngologic, or dental surgery (64–71). The dilemma that clinicians confront in this regard is the potential for misdiagnosis among patients with a sickle cell syndrome in acute crisis, since any combination of hemolysis, aplasia, infarction, sequestration, and/or infection may mimic other surgical emergencies (58).

Table 15.1 lists the indications for surgery among 65 of 876 (i.e., 7.4%) patients hospitalized with a sickle cell syndrome at the University of South Alabama Medical Center during a 32-month period commencing in January 1986. Experience at any medical institution depends on numerous selection factors, including the availability of services, standard practices of surgical specialists and subspecialists, and referral patterns within a community. However, this retrospective analysis summarizes the common reasons for operative intervention among patients with sickle cell syndromes at a university hospital that provides primary and tertiary care. During this period 39 females (mean age 21 years; age range 2–37 years) and 26 males (mean age 22 years; age range < 1–60 years) required 67 anesthetics and 73 operative procedures to treat a variety of illnesses. Intra-abdominal (cholecystectomy, splenectomy) and obstetric/gyne-cologic (Caesarian section, tubal ligation) were the most frequently performed procedures employing general and regional anesthetic techniques, respectively, among this patient population.

Ideally, operative intervention is deferred until a patient is in a steady state or quiescent phase in terms of the hemoglobinopathy. The assessment of a patient's general condition (history, physical examination, laboratory analysis) is important, with particular attention directed toward cardiorespiratory abnor-malities, recognition of a need for hemodynamic stability, adequate hydration and fluid management, control or eradication of infection, and optimization of nutritional status, hemoglobin level, and Hb S/Hb A ratio. Any or all may require correction and/or support prior to operative intervention (see below).

Among patients with sickle cell disease or anemia, the cardiovascular system is under substantial stress. Severe anemia results in a compensatory rise in cardiac output in both the resting and exertional states, which may progress to cardiac failure or myocardial ischemia. In addition, these patients may have experienced repeated episodes of upper respiratory tract infection and/or pulmonary infarction, which may secondarily cause chronic pulmonary hypertension and right ven-tricular overload or strain.

These patients are also abnormally susceptible to pulmonary infections, and ideally, operative intervention should be deferred if there is evidence of active infection (72–77). Thoracic physiotherapy is an important therapeutic modality in this regard, as is the administration of specific antibiotic medications for established infection. There is no evidence, however, to suggest that the pre-operative administration of broad-spectrum antibiotic medications is of any value

Table 15.1

Anesthetic Techniques and Operative Procedures for 65 Surgical Patients with a Sickle Cell Syndrome Showing Instances of Morbidity

Diagnosis	Anesthetic Technique	Operative Procedure	S-S	S-Thal	$S\text{-}A_2$	S-C	Trait	Total No. Patients
Abdominal								
Cholelithiasis	General	Cholecystectomy	10/(2)	0	1	3/(1)	0	14/(3)
Splenic Sequestration	General	Splenectomy	4	2	0	0	0	6
Appendicitis	General	Appendectomy	0	0	0	0	2	2
Incidental	General	Appendectomy	2	0	0	0	0	2
Cholodocholithiasis	General	Choledochotomy	1	0	0	0	0	1
Colonic Adenocarcinoma	General	Right Hemi-colectomy	1	0	0	0	0	1
Malignancy	General	Exploratory Celiotomy with Biopsy	1	0	0	0	0	1
Inguinal Hernia	General	Herniorrhaphy	1	1	0	0	0	2
Imperforate Anus	General	Posterior Sagittal Anoplasty	0	0	0	0	1	1
Obstetric/Gynecologic								
Pregnancy	Regional	Caesarian Section	4/(4)	2/(2)	0	1	1	8/(6)
Undesired Fertility	Regional	Tubal Ligation	5/(2)	1/(1)	0	0	0	6/(3)
Uterine Leiomyoma	Regional	Abdominal Hysterectomy	0	0	0	0	1	1
Uterine Leiomyoma	Regional	Vaginal Hysterectomy	0	0	0	0	1	1

Table 15.1 (continued)

Diagnosis	Anesthetic Technique	Operative Procedure	S-S	S-Thal	S-A$_2$	S-C	Trait	Total No. Patients
Menometrorrhagia	Regional	Uterine Dilatation/Curretage	0	0	0	0	1	1
Retained Products of Conception	Regional	Uterine Dilatation/Curretage	0	0	0	0	1	1
Ruptured Ectopic Pregnancy	General	Salpingo-oophorectomy	0	0	0	1	0	1
Traumatic Vaginal/Cervical Lacerations	Regional	Repair	0	1	0	0	0	1
Genitourinary								
Priapism	Regional	Shunt	0	0	2/(1)	0	0	2/(1)
Priapism	Regional	Corporectomy	0	0	1/(1)	0	0	1/(1)
Undescended Testicle	General	Orchiopexy	0	0	1	0	0	1
Orthopedic								
Avascular Necrosis Femoral Head	General	Fusion	0	0	0	2	0	2
Septic Arthritis	General	Debridement/Drainage	1/(1)	0	0	0	1	2/(1)
Compound Fracture Tibia/Fibula	General	Debridement/Irrigation	1/(1)	0	0	0	0	1/(1)

	Anesthesia	Procedure						
Ophthalmologic								
Traumatic Hyphema	Intravenous	Trabeculostomy	0	0	0	0	3	3
Neurosurgical								
Intracranial Hemorrhage	General	Decompression	1/(1)	0	0	0	0	1/(1)
Thoracic								
Pericarditis	General	Pericardial Window	1/(1)	0	0	0	0	1/(1)
Pulmonary Carcinoma	General	Lobectomy	0	1	0	0	0	1
Ororhinolaryngologic								
Ventilary Dependency	Local	Tracheostomy	0	0	1	0	0	1
Tonsillitis	General	Tonsillectomy	1	0	0	0	0	1
Plastic/Reconstructive								
Integumentary Ulcer	General	Graft	2	0	0	0	0	2
Eponychia/Paronychia	Local	Drainage	0	0	0	1	1	1
Peripheral Vascular								
Chronic Renal Insufficiency	Regional	Vascular Access	2/(2)	0	0	0	1	3/(2)
TOTAL			37	8	5	8	15	73

Note: Numbers in parentheses indicate instances of morbidity in the total number.

in the context of prophylaxis against wound sepsis for this patient population vis-à-vis any other patient population (58).

A note of caution must be stressed in relationship to the use of arteriographic contrast preparations such as ionic meglumine iothalamate. Several authors have observed increased erythrocytic sickling with use of these hypertonic solutions *in vitro* (78–81), and *in vivo,* its use has been associated with an increased incidence and prevalence of acute neurological damage and death (79). Consequently, several authors have recommended either partial exchange transfusion with the reduction of Hb S levels below 20 percent prior to the use of ionic meglumine iothalamate (53, 82) or have advocated the use of nonionic media, such as iopamidol, if arteriographic analysis is required (80).

INTRA-OPERATIVE ANESTHETIC MANAGEMENT

The decision regarding the type and technique of anesthesia—local, regional, and/or general—is predicated more on the magnitude of the operative procedure than on the presence of a hemoglobinopathy. The need for an adequate quantity and duration of analgesia, amnesia, relaxation, and exposure influences that decision. Independent of the anesthetic technique employed, the capability of carefully monitoring the patient utilizing clinical, non-invasive, or invasive diagnostic instruments (cardiac monitor, peripheral nerve stimulator, thermal probe, urimeter, intra-arterial monitor, central venous monitor, and pulmonary capillary wedge pressure monitor) is essential. Effective communication with laboratory personnel for various analyses and products—such as clinical chemistry, cytology, and blood bank—is relevant. An extensive literature concerning anesthesiologic practices is available (47, 53–56, 83–92) and is reviewed in Chapter 14.

INTRA-OPERATIVE SURGICAL MANAGEMENT

Attention to other intra-operative phenomena may also be important. Proper positioning of the patient, adequate crystalloid fluid maintenance and resuscitative therapy, and the avoidance of arterial hypoxia, hemoconcentration, vasoconstriction, and intravascular stasis are rational goals, although again, they are not unique to this patient population. Quantitative scientific data in this regard is limited. Nevertheless, the physiologic rationale of this approach is to maximize tissue oxygen supply and minimize tissue oxygen demand.

The value of intravenous alkalinization is controversial. Although there are theoretical reasons for administering alkaline solutions (e.g., leftward shift of the oxyhemoglobin dissociation curve), no benefit from its routine use or to control or prevent vaso-occlusive crises has been demonstrated clinically to date (50–53). The use of an occlusive tourniquet for extremity surgery is even more problematic because of the induction of a static intravascular reservoir of erythrocytes that inevitably sickle. Although research in this regard is also limited, basic assumptions would suggest that if the use of a tourniquet cannot be avoided, morbidity may be reduced by: (1) preprocedure partial exchange transfusion, (2) use of an Esmarch bandage to completely exsanguinate the limb, and (3) minimization of the area and duration of stasis (93, 94).

Cholelithiasis, acute splenic sequestration, priapism, renal papillary necrosis, hematuria, and osteomyelitis are pathologic entities more frequently encountered among patients with sickle cell syndromes which may require operative intervention. Accordingly, they are considered in some detail because of the risk of these entities in this patient population.

Cholelithiasis

It is difficult to be dogmatic when making recommendations regarding the appropriate therapy for patients with sickle cell syndromes who also manifest cholelithiasis. The medical literature that addresses these issues predominantly represents retrospective analyses of limited numbers of patients. Nevertheless, that literature and the authors' experience would suggest that increased hemolysis of sickled erythrocytes predisposes patients with sickle cell syndromes to bilirubinate cholelithiasis (95–109). The reported incidence/prevalence varies from 6 to 70 percent, predicated on the age of the patient population and the diagnostic modalities utilized for detection. Biliary colic, cholecystitis, pancreatitis, and serum bilirubin, and hepatic enzyme abnormalities are observed in a significant number of these patients. By contrast to cholelithiasis occurring in a general patient population, extra-hepatobiliary pathology occurs at an earlier age and may be more symptomatic among patients with sickle cell syndromes.

Patients with an acute extra-hepatobiliary syndrome are initially managed with nasogastric decompression, intravenous crystalloid fluid replacement therapy, and analgesic and antibiotic medications. Early elective operative intervention minimizes the risk of recrudescence of symptoms and signs of extra-hepatobiliary pathology, and has been reportedly accomplished with negligible morbidity and mortality (95, 96, 100, 102–104, 107–109). Some authors have also suggested that the subsequent management of abdominal pain crises is simplified in the postcholecystectomy phase (100, 104). In addition, emergent or urgent operative intervention has been associated with higher morbidity (100). Therefore, the concensus of opinion favors early elective cholecystectomy. It should also be emphasized that bilirubinate cholelithiasis is not responsive to bile salt administration, and that the role of investigational extracorporeal shock wave lithotripsy as a palliative therapeutic modality is uncertain at present.

Splenic Sequestration

During the first five years of life, acute splenic sequestration of erythrocytes is a more common cause of mortality among patients with sickle cell disease or anemia, second in frequency only to septicemia (110). Forty-nine percent of patients with one episode of acute splenic sequestration develop a recurrence within 10 years (111, 112). While transfusional therapy provides immediate palliation and may prevent recurrence, it also may predispose a patient to the morbidity of transfusional therapy *per se* (see below) (111, 113). Substantive evidence also suggests that an enlarged spleen becomes dysfunctional at an early age (114). Therefore, although the data currently available is largely anecdotal and retrospective, involving a limited number of patients, splenectomy after the first episode of acute splenic sequestration is a rational recommendation (111, 112).

Priapism

Priapism—a sustained and painful erection—has been reported to occur in approximately 42 percent of all males with sickle cell disease or anemia (115–119). It accounts for 3.7 percent of all hospital admissions for males with sickle cell disease or anemia (120–123). Among priapetics, sickle cell disease or anemia is present in 24.8 percent (124–134), constituting the most frequently identified etiology of priapism. Among African-American adult patients with priapism, 34 percent have sickle cell disease or anemia (124, 126, 127, 130–135); while 67–100 percent of African-American pediatric patients with priapism are so diagnosed (132, 133, 136).

Priapism in this patient population is characterized by frequent recurrences and presents in two distinct patterns: "stuttering" priapism and "major episode" priapism (119, 137). "Stuttering" priapism consists of transient (< 6 hrs) clusters of erections (2–3/week for weeks; then remission; and then recurrence) and will progress to "major episode" priapism in 28 percent of instances (119). By contrast, "major episode" priapism (erection persistent > 24 hrs) frequently, but not invariably, brings the patient to medical attention. Thirty percent of patients with sickle cell disease or anemia with priapism requiring hospitalization report prior episodes (120, 121, 123, 138–140), while 42 percent of all priapetics report prior episodes (124, 126, 127, 130, 131, 133, 134, 141, 142). Prior spontaneous resolution may lead the patient to delay seeking therapy.

The onset of priapism associated with sickle cell disease or anemia is generally a nocturnal event associated with sleep far more frequently than with sexual activity (119, 143). Rarely is it concurrent with other manifestations of sickle cell disease or anemia (137, 144). It may occur in either homozygous or heterozygous individuals, with the latter accounting for 26 percent of instances (126, 132, 133, 135, 137, 139, 145). In a given patient, hematological parameters at the time of priapism are usually consistent with intercrisis values (143, 144). An elevated Hb F level seems to have an ameliorating effect on the incidence of priapism; a less significant effect is noted with microcytosis and decreased platelet and reticulocyte counts (119, 146). Fever is present in 60 percent of these patients (135), while leukocytosis (with immature forms) and urinary retention are less common (120, 135).

There is a paucity of well-controlled and randomized clinical trials regarding the management of priapism associated with sickle cell disease or anemia. A study by Serjeant, deCeulare, and Maude (147) is one notable exception in that it demonstrated that stilbesterol could eliminate "stuttering" priapism but had no effect on the subsequent development of "major attack" priapism. Those authors also observed a 20 percent incidence of gynecomastia in the treated patient population. Based on a current incomplete understanding of the pathophysiology of priapism, initial medical management of the primary disease is the most rational and successful approach (136, 137, 142–144, 148). During normal nocturnal erections, blood enters the cavernosal sinusoids, which dilate and afford passive compression of the exiting venules (149–151). Although the process is normally dynamic, at full erection there is transient stasis. During conditions of mild acidosis and hypercarbia (as during sleep), perhaps augmented by mild hemoconcentration due to a commonly encountered urinary concentrating defect (152), sickling may occur within the sinusoids. Vaso-occlusion may further enhance stasis perpetuating a vicious cycle. Direct intracavernosal measurements during priapism have revealed acidosis, hypercarbia, and hypoxia (145). Aspirated cavernosal blood during priapism contains irreversibly sickled erythrocytes, which are not present in simultaneously aspirated blood from other peripheral sources (149).

The goal of initial medical management for priapism is to rapidly reverse metabolic and hematologic factors that predispose to erythrocytic sickling and to create an environment favorable to resuspension of sickled erythrocytes. Current therapeutic recommendations have been extrapolated from observations regarding acute splenic crises (153). Specific initial measures include (137, 138, 142–144).

1. vigorous hydration at two to three times maintenance levels

2. oxygen supplementation

3. alkalinization

4. analgesia

5. rapid transfusion to restore Hb to 10–12 gms percent range and/or exchange transfusion to reduce the percent of Hb S < 30 percent

Frequently, the above regimen will result in diminished pain and partial detumescence. Persistent pain represents persistent ischemia, and if unrelieved, the patient is at risk for cavernosal cytolysis, fibrosis, and impotence. Early surgical intervention is advised when symptoms—particularly pain—persist or worsen. The majority of contemporary authors adhere to the above medical regimen followed by surgical intervention at 24–48 hours if medical management is unsuccessful (128, 132, 137, 144). The surgical procedure that most authors advocate is a cavernosal-glanular shunt, because of its reputed technical ease and lower morbidity, and if that procedure is unsuccessful, the performance of a cavernosal-spongiosum shunt (128, 133, 137, 138).

Surgical procedures must be performed under strict aseptic technique, including the administration of perioperative antibiotic medications (128). Circumferential and/or pressure dressings must be used judiciously (125, 133). If urethral compression and urinary retention are present, a percutaneous suprapubic catheter is utilized. Morbidity associated with all invasive procedures (including simple aspiration and irrigation) include penile skin slough, abscess, and necrosis, and urethrocavernosal fistulae (125, 137).

The ultimate parameter of successful management of priapism is retained potency. While Winter (136), with the largest clinical experience reported in the medical literature, stated that 50 percent of patients will be impotent regardless of therapy, other researchers are less pessimistic (136, 143). Bertram, Webster, and Carson (128) agreed with Winter that the empirical choice of a particular therapeutic modality had little influence on potency rates; however, they observed that early recognition and early institution of therapy were the most important prognostic factors. In addition, a prior history of priapism seems to portend a poor result (127). Indeed, even among priapetics who never manifest a "major episode," erectile dysfunction, including complete impotence, is present in 56 percent of instances (119).

Other innovative techniques for the treatment of priapism related to sickle cell syndromes have recently been described. One is erythrocytopheresis; unfortunately, results are not dissimilar to the protocols of hydration/transfusion, and the reported morbidity is greater (154). Intracorporeal norepinephrine injection—taking advantage of recently elucidated knowledge of erectile neuropharmacology—has been employed, but experience is too limited to date for substantive conclusions (145). Other approaches have either produced indifferent results or lack a rational basis; these include the application of leeches; hot or cold penile packs; hot or cold enemas; hypotensive anesthesia; the administration of amyl nitrate, ketamine, corticosteroid, or anticoagulant medications; indwelling drains; vigorous rectal massage; or internal pudendal arterial embolization or ligation (125, 133, 143, 144).

The management of impotence in this patient population is primarily surgical. The characteristic intense fibrosis renders prosthetic surgery challenging, but current recommendations include the optimization of hematological parameters, the administration of prophylactic antibiotic medication, and the use of a semirigid (rather than inflatable) prosthesis (155).

Renal Papillary Necrosis and Hematuria

Other genitourological manifestations of sickle cell syndromes rarely require surgical intervention. These include delayed sexual maturation, eneuresis, malefactor infertility, bacterial cystitis, renal vein thrombosis, papillary necrosis, and hematuria (156–161). *Papillary necrosis* in sickle cell disease is conventionally managed as in association with other conditions, including temporary ureteral stenting in the event of significant obstruction. *Hematuria* in association with sickle cell syndrome is a unique condition. Often massive, it is usually unilateral, usually from the left side, and is noted more frequently among heterozygotes (158, 160, 161). Management is initially nonoperative and includes parenteral administration of epsilon-aminocaproic acid, intra-renal pelvic silver nitrate irrigation, or a regimen of sodium bicarbonate, furosemide, acetazolamide, potassium chloride, and crystalloid fluid administration (162, 163). Surgical therapy, which should be instituted only in the event of life-threatening hemorrhage, includes arterial embolization, endoscopic cauterization, or segmental nephrectomy (158, 161).

Osteomyelitis

Osteomyelitis secondary to *Salmonella species* or *Staphylococcus aureus* is not infrequent among patients with sickle cell disease or anemia (164–166). The differential diagnosis of a painful, swollen, and tender extremity must include an acute vaso-occlusive crisis vis-à-vis osteomyelitis. This is often a diagnostic dilemma for a clinician. Although an acute crisis is more common and often manifests itself at multiple sites, osteomyelitis must be considered among patients with sickle cell disease or anemia because of the morbidity and mortality of untreated infection. Imaging by conventional roentgenographic evaluation or by the utilization of radionuclide agents has not been shown to be beneficial in this differential diagnosis. Newer imaging modalities such as computerized axial tomographic analysis and magnetic resonance imaging have not been sufficiently evaluated to date. In a patient with impressive signs of inflammation localized to one area, the possibility of infection should be assessed by percutaneous needle aspiration under sterile conditions. If pus is aspirated, emergent operative debridement and drainage and administration of appropriate antibiotic medications for a protracted period are mandated.

POST-OPERATIVE MANAGEMENT

In the early post-operative period, oxygen supplementation is important since hypoventilation and hypoxia (the lowest arterial oxygen tensions) are likely to occur during that phase of recovery (90). Before extubation, adequate neuromuscular function must be proven by clinical tests (sustained head raising, ability to perform a vital capacity maneuver, etc.) and/or assessment of response to peripheral nerve stimulation. Adequate hydration, hemodynamic stability, and normothermia should be achieved and maintained to reduce the risk of erythrocytic sickling. Early reambulation and active exercise may reduce the attendant risk of phlebothrombosis.

As reported in the literature, the incidence of post-operative morbidity has ranged from 7–32 percent (55, 83), undoubtedly influenced by both pre-operative comorbidity and the peri-operative experience. Table 15.2 summarizes the incidence/prevalence of post-operative morbidity among the patient population at

Table 15.2
Morbidity and Mortality among the University of South Alabama Medical Center Patient Population (17 Patients)

Diagnosis	Morbidity	Mortality
Respiratory		
Acute Chest Syndrome	1	
Asthma	1	
Atelectasis	2	
Bronchiolitis	1	
Bronchopneumonia	2	
Pulmonary Edema	3	
Urological		
Acute Cystitis	4	
Miscellaneous		
Pain Crisis	1	
Drug Dependency	1	
Delayed Wound Healing	1	
Cardiac Dysrhythmia	2	
Seizure	1	
Pelvic Septic Thrombophlebitis	1	
Hemolytic Transfusion Reaction	1	
Death		1
TOTAL	23	1

this institution. Twenty-three instances of morbidity were observed among 17 patients. Of particular note were: (1) the morbidity observed was reversible with appropriate therapy in all but one patient (see below), and (2) no instance of wound sepsis was noted, although delayed wound healing of an integumentary ulcer postgrafting was observed in one patient.

The incidence of post-operative mortality as reported in the literature has ranged from 0–7.6 percent (83, 169). Several authors have suggested that peri-operative mortality is more influenced by a patient's comorbidity than by a properly conducted peri-operative course (167–171). The experience at this institution is comparable in that the one patient who succumbed (1/65; 1.5 percent) manifested posttraumatic intracranial hemorrhage which was not reversed by aggressive partial exchange transfusional therapy and emergency decompressive craniotomy.

UTILIZATION OF BLOOD COMPONENTS

The two major rationales for the transfusion of blood components among patients with sickle cell syndromes are the maintenance of oxygen-carrying capacity and the dilution of circulating Hb S containing erythrocytes, with the latter accomplished by a primary dilutional effect and a secondary bone marrow–suppressive effect. Symptomatic anemia may occur secondary to pathological conditions associated with sickle cell disease or anemia, such as crisis (acute splenic sequestration, hemolysis, aplasia, vaso-occlusion), sepsis, and/or chronic renal insufficiency, and is usually readily responsive to timely erythrocyte transfusion (71, 172–176). In addition, hemorrhagic hypovolemia and anemia secondary to other pathologic entities not unique to this patient population (trauma, peptic ulcer disease, pseudodiverticulosis coli, etc.) are properly treated similarly.

Several investigators have advocated some type of transfusion for patients with sickle cell syndromes as part of their pre-anesthetic and pre-operative preparation. Acute transfusion, repeated transfusion, and partial exchange transfusion either immediately (88) or 10–15 days prior to surgery (83, 176) have been advocated to decrease the Hb S concentration to the 30–50 percent range. Blood for transfusion should be relatively fresh (acid-citrate-dextrose–preserved blood less than 48 hours old, or citrate-phosphate-dextrose–preserved blood less than 7 days old) and warmed prior to and during administration (172). There is some evidence that pre-operative blood transfusion to a hematocrit of 25–30 percent (173) or hemoglobin concentration of 15 grams/dl (174) may be equally as effective as partial exchange transfusion in preventing peri-operative erythrocytic sickling crises, although the patient must be monitored closely for circulatory overload if the latter technique is employed.

The efficacy of these techniques in reducing peri-operative morbidity and mortality is, however, unproven. The number of controlled clinical trials is very limited in this regard, but one study by Fullerton, Philippart, Sarnaik, et al. (176) revealed no benefit of the aforementioned transfusional techniques in relationship to peri-operative morbidity. The risk–benefit analysis must also address the incidence of morbidity associated with transfusion itself—transfusion reaction, iron overload, antigenic sensitization, bone marrow suppression, and viral disease transmission (hepatitis, acquired immune deficiency syndrome, etc.). Likewise, the cost–benefit analysis remains undefined when one considers the logistical support that transfusional therapy requires. Dobson (58) has suggested the following principles of hematological therapy:

1. Ascertain the patient's normal hemoglobin level and operate only if it is steady;

2. Consider other treatable causes of anemia;

3. Consider transfusion if:

   a. The Hgb level is less than 7 grams/dl;

   b. Major surgery is planned and transfusion is not contraindicated;

   c. Major blood loss is expected; or

   d. Cardiac failure secondary to anemia is present; and

4. Consider partial exchange transfusion if there is a substantial risk of intraoperative hypoxia.

A prospective, randomized, and controlled clinical trial of transfusional therapy was initiated by Dr. Vichinsky and his colleagues at multiple institutions in 1989 to assess its role among this patient population who require operative intervention. At present, and until this type of data becomes available, the only tenable conclusion is a reiteration of the basic tenets: maximize oxygen-carrying capacity and minimize hypoxemia.

SUMMARY

There is a paucity of quantifiable research in relationship to recommendations for the anesthetic and surgical care of patients with sickle cell syndromes. The available data, including our retrospective analysis, suggests that the anesthesiologist and surgeon must be prepared to deal with three basic pathophysiologic mechanisms associated with this entity—anemia, hyperviscosity, and vaso-occlusion. Adequate oxygen supplementation, intravenous crystalloid and erythrocytic replacement therapy, and avoidance of metabolic acidosis, hypotension, hypothermia, and intravascular stasis are rational goals. Simple and partial exchange transfusional therapies are unproven aspects of this multimodality treatment regimen.

REFERENCES

1. Konotey-Ahulu FID: The sickle cell disease. Clinical manifestations including the "sickle crisis." *Arch Intern Med* 133 (1974): 611–619.
2. Herrick JB: Peculiar elongated and sickle-shaped red blood corpuscles in a case of severe anemia. *Arch Intern Med* 6 (1910): 517–521.
3. Washburn RE: Peculiar elongated and sickle-shaped red blood corpuscles in a case of severe anemia. *Va Med Semi-Monthly* 15 (1911): 490–493.
4. Cook JE, and Meyer J: Severe anemia with remarkable elongated sickle-shaped red blood cells and chronic leg ulcer. *Arch Intern Med* 16 (1915): 644–651.
5. Mason VR: Sickle cell anemia. *JAMA* 79 (1922): 1318–1320.
6. Sydenstricker VP: Further observations on sickle cell anemia. *JAMA* 83 (1924): 12–13.
7. Hahn EV, Gillespie EB: Sickle cell anemia. Report of a case greatly improved by splenectomy. Experimental study of sickle cell formation. *Arch Intern Med* 39 (1927): 233–254.
8. Graham GS: Case of sickle cell anemia with necropsy. *Arch Intern Med* 34 (1924): 778–800.
9. Hamilton JF: A case of sickle cell anemia. *US Vet Bur Med Bull* 2 (1926): 497–500.
10. Hein GE, McCalla RL, and Thorne GW: Sickle cell anemia. With report of a case with autopsy. *Am J Med Sci* 173 (1927): 763–772.

11. Matthews WR: Pathology of sickle cell anemia. *New Orleans Med Surg J* 88 (1936): 671–678.

12. Mallory TB: Sickle cell anemia. Case records of the MGH. *N Engl J Med* 225 (1941): 626–630.

13. Schaefer BF: Sickle cell anemia and cholelithiasis. *Med Ann DC* 11 (1942): 392–396.

14. Diggs LW, Pulliam HN, and King JC: The bone changes in sickle cell anemia. *Southern Med J* 30 (1937): 249–258.

15. Vogt EC, and Diamond LK: Congenital anemias, roentgenologically considered. *Am J Roentgenol* 23 (1930): 625–630.

16. Le Wald LT: Roentgen evidence of osseous manifestations in sickle cell (drepan-ocytic) anemia and in Mediterranean (erythroblastic) anemia. *Radiology* 18 (1932): 792–798.

17. Grinn AG: Roentgenologic bone changes in sickle cell and erythroblastic anemia. *Am J Roentgenol* 34 (1935): 297–309.

18. Zuelzer WN, and Putzley J: Megaloblastic anemia in infancy. In SZ Levine; ed.: *Advances in pediatrics,* Vol. 6; pp. 243–306. New York: Year Book Publishers, 1953.

19. Jonsson U, Roath OS, and Kirkpatrick CIF: Nutritional megaloblastic anemia of infancy. *Blood* 15 (1959): 535–547.

20. Maclver JE, and Went LN: Sickle cell anemia complicated by megaloblastic anemia of infancy. *Br Med J* 1 (1960): 775–779.

21. Pauling L, Itano HA, Singer SJ, et al.: Sickle cell anemia, A molecular disease. *Science* 110 (1949): 543–548.

22. Ingram VM: Abnormal human haemoglobins. 1. The comparison of normal human and sickle-cell haemoglobins by "finger printing." *Biochim Biophys Acta* 28 (1958): 539–545.

23. Wollstein M, and Kreidel KV: Sickle cell anemia. *Am J Dis Child* 36 (1928): 998–1011.

24. Steinberg B: Sickle cell anemia. *Arch Pathol Lab Med* 9 (1930): 876–897.

25. Yates WM, and Mollari M: The pathology of sickle cell anemia. Report of a case with death during an "abdominal crisis." *JAMA* 96 (1931): 1671–1675.

26. Baird JA: Sickle cell anemia: Report of a case with multiple infections and necropsy. *Med Bull Vet Admin* 11 (1934): 169–171.

27. Diggs LW: Siderofibrosis of the spleen in sickle cell anemia. *JAMA* 104 (1935): 538–541.

28. Danford EA, Marr R, and Elsey EC: Sickle cell anemia with unusual bone changes. *Am J Roentgenol* 45 (1941): 223–226.

29. Kraft E, and Bertel G: Sickle cell anemia. Case report with unusual roentgen findings. *Am J Roentgenol* 57 (1947): 224–231.

30. Legant O, and Ball RP: Sickle cell anemia in adults: Roentgenographic findings. *Radiology* 51 (1948): 665–675.

31. Diggs LW, and Ching RE: Pathology of sickle cell anemia. *Southern Med J* 27 (1934): 839–845.

32. Obendorf CP: Priapism of psychogenic origin. *Arch Neurol Psychiatr* 31 (1934): 1292–1296.

33. Sydenstricker VP, Mulherin WA, and Houseal RW: Sickle cell anemia. Report of two cases in children, with necropsy in one case. *Am J Dis Child* 26 (1923): 132–154.

34. Anderson WW, and Ware RL: Sickle cell anemia. *Am J Dis Child* 44 (1932): 1055–1070.

35. Welch RB, and Goldberg MF: Sickle cell hemoglobin and its relation to fundus abnormality. *Arch Opthal* 75 (1966): 353–362.

36. King AD: Sickle cell anemia. *Arch Dermatol Syphilol* 33 (1936): 756.

37. Netherton EW: Sickle cell anemia with ulcer of the leg. *Arch Dermatol Syphilol* 34 (1936): 158–159.

38. Schwartz WF: Sickle cell anemia associated with ulcers on the leg. *Arch Dermatol Syphilol* 37 (1938): 866–867.

39. Cummer LL, and LaRocco CG: Ulcers of the legs in sickle cell anemia. *Arch Dermatol Syphilol* 42 (1940): 1015–1039.

40. Serjeant GR: *Sickle cell disease.* Oxford: Oxford University Press, 1985.

41. Bertles JF: Haemoglobin interaction and the molecular basis of sickling. *Arch Intern Med* 133 (1974): 538–543.

42. Finch JT, Perutz MF, Bertles JF, Dobler J: Structure of sickled erythrocytes and of sickle-cell haemoglobin fibers. *Proc Natl Acad Sci* (USA) 70 (1973): 718–722.

43. Finch JT: Sickle cell haemoglobin fibres. *Nature* 272 (1978): 496–497.

44. White JG: Ultrastructural features of erythrocyte and haemoglobin sickling. *Arch Intern Med* 133 (1974): 545–561.

45. Milner PF: Oxygen transport in sickle cell anemia. *Arch Intern Med* 133 (1974): 565–574.

46. Eaton WA, Hofrichter J, and Ross PD: Delay time of gelation: A possible determinant of clinical severity in sickle cell disease. *Blood* 47 (1978): 621–627.

47. Serjeant GR, Serjeant BE, and Milner PF: The irreversibly sickled cell; determinant of haemolysis in sickle cell anemia. *Br J Haematol* 17 (1969): 527–533.

48. Malfa R, and Steinhardt J: A temperature-dependent latent-period in the aggregation of sickle-cell deoxyhaemoglobin. *Biochem Biophys Res Comm* 59 (1974): 887–893.

49. Moguchi CT, and Schechter AW: The intracellular polymerization of sickle haemoglobin and its relevance to sickle cell disease. *Blood* 58 (1981): 1057–1068.

50. Lehmon H: Anaesthesia in sickle cell traits. *Br Med J* 1 (1973): 290.

51. Searle JF: Anaesthesia and sickle-cell haemoglobin. *Br J Anaesth* 44 (1972): 1335–1336.

52. Searle JF: Anaesthesia in sickle cell states. A review. *Anaesthesia* 28 (1973): 48–58.

53. Howells TH, Huntsman RG, Boys JE, et al.: Anaesthesia in sickle cell haemoglobin. *Br J Anaesth* 4 (1972): 975–987.

54. Holzmann L, Finn H, Lightman HC, et al.: Anesthesia in patients with sickle cell disease. A review of 112 cases. *Anesth Analges* 48 (1969): 566–572.

55. Oduntan SA, and Isaacs WA: Anaesthesia in patients with abnormal haemoglobin syndromes: A preliminary report. *Br J Anaesth* 43 (1971): 1159–1165.

56. Oduro KA, and Searle JF: Anaesthesia in sickle cell states: A plea for simplicity. *Br Med J* 4 (1972): 596–598.

57. Molulsky AG: Frequency of sickling disorders in U.S. blacks. *N Engl J Med* 288 (1973): 31.

58. Dobson MB: Anesthesia for patients with hemoglobinopathies. *Int Anesth Clin* 23 (1985): 197–211.

59. Jones SR, Binder RA, and Donowho EM: Sudden death in sickle cell trait. *N Engl J Med* 283 (1970): 323–325.

60. Diggs LW: The sickle cell trait in relation to the training and assignment of duties in the Armed Forces. *Aviat Space Environ Med* 59 (1984): 358–364.

61. Oduro KA: Anaesthesia in Ghana. *Anaesthesia* 24 (1969): 307–316.

62. Atlas AS: The sickle cell trait and surgical complications. *JAMA* 229 (1974): 1078–1080.

63. Sears DA: The morbidity of sickle cell trait: Review of the literature. *Am J Med* 64 (1978): 1021–1031.

64. Somanothear S: Anaesthesia and hypothermia in sickle cell disease. *Anaesthesia* 31 (1976): 113.

65. DeLeval MR, Taswell HF, Bowie EJW, et al.: Open heart surgery in patients with inherited hemoglobinopathies, red cell dyscrasias, and coagulopathies. *Arch Surg* 109 (1974): 618–622.

66. Riethmuller R, Grumdy EM, and Radley-Smith R: Open heart surgery in a patient with homozygous sickle cell disease. *Anaesthesia* 37 (1982): 324–327.

67. Fox MA, and Abbott TR: Hypothermia cardiopulmonary bypass in a patient with sickle cell trait. *Anaesthesia* 39 (1984): 1121–1123.

68. Donegan JO, Lobel JS, and Gluckman JL: Otolaryngologic manifestations of sickle cell disease. *Am J Otol* 3 (1982): 141–144.

69. Ijaduola GTA, and Akinyanja OO: Chronic tonsillitis, tonsillectomy and sickle cell crises. *J Laryn Oto* 101 (1987): 467–470.

70. Wessberg GA, Epker BN, Bordelon JH, et al.: Correction of sickle cell gnathopathy by total maxillary osteotomy. *J Max Fac Surg* 8 (1980): 187–194.

71. Cheatham ML, and Brackett CE: Problems in management of subarachnoid hemorrhage in sickle cell anemia. *J Neurosurg* 23 (1965): 488–493.

72. Kabins SA, and Lerner C: Fulminant pneumococcemia and sickle cell anemia. *JAMA* 211 (1970): 467–469.

73. Barrett-Connor E: Bacterial infection and sickle cell anemia: An analysis of 250 infections in 166 patients and a review of the literature. *Medicine* 50 (1971): 97–112.

74. Seeler RA: *Diplococcus pneumoniae* infections in children with sickle cell anemia. *Am J Dis Child* 123 (1972): 8–13.

75. Evans HE: *Shigella* bacteremia in a patient with sickle cell anemia. *Am J Dis Child* 123 (1972): 238–245.

76. Shulman ST: The unusual severity of mycoplasma pneumonia in children with sickle cell disease. *N Engl J Med* 287 (1972): 164–167.

77. Barrett-Connor E: Pneumonia and pulmonary infarction in sickle cell anemia. *JAMA* 224 (1973): 997–1003.

78. Richards D, and Nulsen FE: Angiographic media and the sickling phenomenon. *Surg Forum* 22 (1971): 403–404.

79. Rao VM, Rao AK, Steiner RM, et al.: The effect of ionic and nonionic contrast media on the sickling phenomenon. *Radiology* 144 (1982): 291–293.

80. Rao KRP, and Lee MS: Risks associated with angiography in patients with sickle cell disease. *Radiology* 147 (1983): 600.

81. Cattell WR: Excretory pathways for contrast media. *Invest Radiol* 5 (1970): 473–486.

82. Leppik IE, Thompson CJ, Etheir R, et al.: Diatrizoate in computed cranial tomography: A quantitative study. *Invest Radiol* 12 (1977): 21–26.

83. Homi J, Reynolds J, Skinner A, et al.: General anaesthesia in sickle cell disease. *Br Med J* no. 1 (1979): 1599–1601.

84. Lang RD, Minnich V, and Moore CV: Effect of oxygen tension and of pH on the sickling and mechanical fragility of erythrocytes from patients with sickle cell anemia and sickle cell trait. *J Lab Clin Med* 37 (1951): 789.

85. Hirch R, Hirch A, and Lubbers DW: Transcutaneous measurement of blood PO_2 (TPO_2). Method and application in perinatal medicine. *J Perinatal Med* 1 (1973): 183.

86. Swanstrom S, Ellisaga IU, Cardona L, et al.: Transcutaneous PO_2 measurements in seriously ill newborn infants. *Arch Dis Child* 50 (1975): 913–919.

87. Rieber EE, Veliz G, and Pollack S: Red cells in sickle cell crisis: Observations on the pathophysiology of crisis. *Blood* 49 (1977): 967–974.

88. Burrington JD, and Smith MD: Elective and emergency surgery in children with sickle cell disease. *Surg Clin N A* 56 (1976): 55–71.

89. Nunn JF, and Payne JP: Hypoxaemia after general anaesthesia. *Lancet* 2 (1962): 631–632.

90. Maduska AL, Guinee WS, Heaton JA, et al.: Sickling dynamics of red blood cells and other physiologic studies during anesthesia. *Anesth Analges* 54 (1975): 361–365.

91. Ohuishi T, Asakura T, Pisani RL, et al.: Effect of anesthetic on the stability of oxyhemoglobin. *Biochem Biophys Res Comm* 56 (1974): 535–542.

92. Gilbertson AA: Anaesthesia in West African patients with sickle cell anemia, haemoglobin SC disease, and sickle cell trait. *Br J Anaesth* 37 (1965): 614–622.

93. Stein RE, and Urbaniak J: Use of the tourniquet during surgery in patients with sickle cell hemoglobinopathies. *Clin Orthop* 151 (1980): 231–233.

94. Bentley PG, and Howard ER: Surgery in children with homozygous sickle cell anaemia. *Ann Roy Coll Surg Eng* 61 (1979): 55–58.

95. Barrett-Connor E: Cholelithiasis in sickle cell anemia: Surgical considerations. *Am J Med* 45 (1968): 889–895.

96. Cameron JL, Maddrey WC, and Zuidema GD: Biliary tract disease in sickle cell anemia: Surgical considerations. *Ann Surg* 174 (1971): 702–710.

97. Phillips JC, and Gerald BE: The incidence of cholelithiasis in sickle cell disease. *Am J Roentgenol Rad Ther Nucl Med* 113 (1971): 27–28.

98. Hargrove MD, Jr.: Marked increases in serum bilirubin in sickle cell anemia. *Am J Dig Dis* 15 (1970): 437–444.

99. Flye MW, and Silver D: Biliary tract disorders and sickle cell disease. *Surgery* 72 (1972): 361–367.

100. Stephens CG, and Scott RB: Cholelithiasis in sickle cell anemia. Surgical or medical management. *Arch Intern Med* 40 (1980): 648–651.

101. Kudsk KA, Transbaugh RF, and Sheldon GF: Acute surgical illness in patients with sickle cell anemia. *Am J Surg* 142 (1981): 113–117.

102. Rennels MB, Dunne MG, Grossman NJ, et al.: Cholelithiasis in patients with major sickle hemoglobinopathies. *Am J Dis Child* 138 (1984): 66–67.

103. Pokorny WJ, Saleem M, O'Gorman RB, et al.: Cholelithiasis and cholecystitis in childhood. *Am J Surg* 148 (1984): 742–744.

104. Rambo WM, and Reines HD: Elective cholecystectomy for the patient with sickle cell disease and asymptomatic cholelithiasis. *Amer Surg* 52 (1986): 205–207.

105. Soloway RD, Trotman BW, Maddrey WC, et al.: Pigment gallstone composition in patients with hemolysis or infection/stasis. *Dig Dis Sci* 31 (1986): 454–460.

106. Schubert TT: Hepatobiliary system in sickle cell disease. *Gastroenterology* 90 (1986): 2013–2021.

107. Rutledge R, Croom RD III, Davis JW Jr., et al.: Cholelithiasis in sickle cell anemia: Surgical considerations. *Southern Med J* 79 (1986): 28–30.

108. Ware R, Filston HC, Schultz WH, et al.: Elective cholecystectomy in children with sickle hemoglobinopathies. Successful outcome using a preoperative transfusion regimen. *Ann Surg* 208 (1988): 17–22.

109. Malone BS, and Werlin SL: Cholecystectomy and cholelithiasis in sickle cell anemia. *Am J Dis Child* 142 (1988): 799–800.

110. Seeler RA, and Shwiaki MZ: Acute splenic sequestration crisis (ASSC) in young children with sickle cell anemia. *Clin Ped* 11 (1972): 701–704.

111. Topley JM, Rogers DW, Stevens MCG, et al.: Acute splenic sequestration and hypersplenism in the first five years in homozygous sickle cell disease. *Arch Dis Child* 56 (1981): 765–769.

112. Emond AM, Collins R, Darvill D, et al.: Acute splenic sequestration in homozygous sickle cell disease. Natural history and management. *J Ped* 107 (1985): 201–206.

113. Rao S, and Gooden S: Splenic sequestration in sickle cell disease: Role of transfusion therapy. *Am J Ped Hem Oncol* 7 (1985): 298–301.

114. Solanki DL, Kletter GG, and Castro O: Acute splenic sequestration crises in adults with sickle cell disease. *Am J Med* 80 (1986): 985–990.

115. Gillenwater JY: Priapism as the first and terminal manifestation of sickle cell disease. *Southern Med J* 61 (1968): 133–138.

116. Karayalin G: Priapism in sickle cell disease: Report of five cases. *Am J Med Sci* 264 (1972): 289–296.

117. Rothfelf SH, and Major D: Priapism in children: A complication of sickle cell disease. *J Urol* 105 (1971): 307–313.

118. Snyder GB, and Wilson CA: Surgical management of priapism and its sequelae in sickle cell disease. *Southern Med J* 59 (1966): 1393–1399.

119. Emond AM, Holman R, Hayes RJ, et al.: Priapism and impotence in homozygous sickle cell disease. *Arch Intern Med* 140 (1980): 1434–1437.

120. Hasen HB, and Raines SL: Priapism associated with sickle cell disease. *J Urol* 88 (1962): 71–76.

121. Campbell JH, and Cummins SD: Priapism in sickle cell anemia. *J Urol* 66 (1951): 697–703.

122. Rothfield SH, and Mazor D: Priapism in children: A complication of sickle cell disease. *J Urol* 105 (1971): 307–308.

123. Getzoff PL: Priapism and sickle cell anemia. *J Urol* 48 (1942): 407–411.

124. Farrer JF, and Goodwin WE: Treatment of priapism: Comparison of methods in fifteen cases. *J Urol* 86 (1961): 768–775.

125. Snyder GB, and Wilson CA: Surgical management of priapism and its sequelae in sickle cell disease. *Southern Med J* 59 (1966): 1393–1396.

126. Howe GE, Prentiss RJ, Cole JW, et al.: Priapism: A surgical emergency. *J Urol* 101 (1969): 576–579.

127. Iarocque MA, and Cosgrove MD: Priapism: A review of 46 cases. *J Urol* 112 (1974): 770–773.

128. Bertram RA, Webster GD, and Carson CC: Priapism: Etiology, treatment, and results in a series of 35 presentations. *Urology* 26 (1985): 229–232.

129. Bennett AH, and Pilon RN: Non-incisional therapy for priapism. *J Urol* 125 (1981): 208–209.

130. Ercole CJJ, Pontes JE, and Pierce JM: Changing surgical concepts in the treatment of priapism. *J Urol* 125 (1981): 210–211.

131. Pryor JP, and Hehir M: The management of priapism. *Br J Urol* 54 (1982): 751–754.

132. Wasmer JM, Carrion HM, Mekras G, et al.: Evaluation and treatment of priapism. *J Urol* 125 (1981): 204–207.

133. Macaluso JN, and Sullivan JW: Priapism: Review of 34 cases. *Urology* 26 (1985): 233–236.

134. Fuseleir HA, Ochsner MG, and Ross RJ: Priapism: Review of simple surgical procedures. *J Urol* 123 (1980): 778.

135. Nelson JH, and Winter CC: Priapism: Evolution of management in 48 patients in a 22-year series. *J Urol* 117 (1977): 455–458.

136. Winter CC: Priapism. In MI Resnick and E Kursh; eds.: *Current therapy in genitourinary surgery,* pp. 376–379. Toronto: B. C. Decker Publishers, 1987.

137. Tarry WF, Duckett JW, and Snyder HM: Urological complications of sickle cell disease in a pediatric population. *J Urol* 138 (1987): 592–594.

138. Noe HN, Wilimas J, and Jerkins GR: Surgical management of priapism in children with sickle cell anemia. *J Urol* 126 (1981): 770–771.

139. Karayalcin G, Imran M, and Rosner F: Priapism in sickle cell disease: Report of five cases. *Am J Med Sci* 264 (1972): 289–293.

140. Sousa CM, Catoe BL, and Scott RB: Studies in sickle cell anemia. *J Peds* 60 (1962): 52–54.

141. Hinman F Jr.: Priapism: Reasons for failure of therapy. *J Urol* 83 (1960): 420–428.

142. Grace DA, and Winter CC: Priapism: An appraisal of management of twenty-three patients. *J Urol* 99 (1968): 301–310.

143. Seeler RA: Intensive transfusion therapy for priapism in boys with sickle cell anemia. *J Urol* 110 (1973): 360–361.

144. Baron M, and Leiter E: The management of priapism in sickle cell anemia. *J Urol* 119 (1978): 610–611.

145. Lue TF, Hellstrom WJG, McAnnich JW, et al.: Priapism: A refined approach to diagnosis and treatment. *J Urol* 136 (1986): 104–108.

146. Al-Awamy B, Taha SA, and Naeem MA: Priapism in association with sickle cell anemia in Saudi Arabia. *Acta Hemat* 73 (1985): 181–182.

147. Serjeant GR, deCeulare K, and Maude GHL: Stilbesterol and stuttering priapism in homozygous sickle cell disease. *Lancet* no. 2 (Dec. 7, 1985): 1274–1276.

148. Sagalowsky AI: Priapism. *Urol Clin N. A* 9 (1982): 255–257.

149. Lue TF, and Tanahgo EA: Physiology of erection and pharmacological management of impotence. *J Urol* 137 (1987): 829–836.

150. Newman HF, and Northup JD: Mechanism of human penile erections: An overview. *Urology* 17 (1981): 399–408.

151. de Tejada IS, Goldstein I, and Drane RJ: Local control of penile erection. *Urol Clin N. A* 156 (1988): 9–15.

152. Diggs LW: Sickle cell crises. *Am J Clin Path* 44 (1965): 1–19.
153. Seeler RA, and Shwiaki MZ: Acute splenic sequestration crisis (ASSC) in young children with sickle cell anemia. *Clin Ped* 11 (1972): 704–707.
154. Walker EM, Mitchum EN, Rous SN, et al.: Automated erythrocytophoresis for relief of priapism in sickle cell hemoglobinopathies. *J Urol* 130 (1983): 912–916.
155. Bertram RA, Carson CC, and Webster GD: Implantation of penile prostheses in patients impotent after priapism. *Urology* 26 (1985): 325–327.
156. Osegbe DN, Akinyanju O, and Amaku EO: Fertility in males with sickle cell disease. *Lancet* no 2 (1981): 275–276.
157. Wethers DL: Problems and complications in the adolescent with sickle cell disease. *Am J Ped Hem Onc* 4 (1982): 47–53.
158. Klein LA, and Bennett AH: Other renal diseases of urologic significance. In H Harrison, RF Gittes, A Perlmutter, et al., eds.: *Campbell's Urology*, 4th ed., vol.III, pp. 1983–1990. Philadelphia: W. B. Saunders, 1978.
159. Das S: Renal vein thrombosis. In JJ Kaufman; ed.: *Current urologic therapy*, p. 6. Philadelphia: W. B. Saunders, 1986.
160. Dowd JB, and Gregoriades C: Surgical management of renal papillary necrosis. In JJ Kaufman; ed.: *Current urologic therapy*, pp. 54–56. Philadelphia: W. B. Saunders, 1986.
161. McKinnes BK: The management of hematuria associated with sickle hemoglobinopathies. *J Urol* 124 (1980): 171–174.
162. Meyersfield SA, Morganstern SL, Seery W, et al.: Medical management of refractory hematuria in sickle cell trait. *Urology* 8 (1976): 112–113.
163. Bahnson RR: Silver nitrate irrigation for hematuria from sickle cell hemoglobinopathy. *J Urol* 137 (1987): 1194–1195.
164. Diggs LW: Bone and joint lesions in sickle cell disease. *Clin Orthop.* 52 (1967): 119–131.
165. Engle CA: Osteomyelitis in the patient with sickle cell disease. *J Bone Joint Surg* 53 (1971): 1–12.
166. Hook WE: *Salmonella* osteomyelitis in patients with sickle cell anemia. *N Engl J Med* 257 (1957): 403–409.
167. Janik J, and Seeler RA: Perioperative management of children with sickle cell states. *J Pediatr Surg* 15 (1980): 117–120.
168. Gilbertson AH: The management of anaesthesia in sickle cell states. *Proc Roy Soc Med* 60 (1967): 621–627.
169. Dean J, and Schechter AN: Sickle cell anemia: Molecular and cellular bases of therapeutic approaches (first of three parts). *N Engl J Med* 299 (1978): 752–763.
170. Dean J, and Schechter AN: Sickle cell anemia: Molecular and cellular bases of therapeutic approaches (second of three parts). *N Engl J Med* 299 (1978): 804–811.
171. Dean J, and Schechter AN: Sickle cell anemia: Molecular and cellular bases of therapeutic approaches (third of three parts). *N Engl J Med* 299 (1978): 863–870.
172. Charache S: The treatment of sickle cell anemia. *Arch Intern Med* 133 (1974): 698–705.
173. McPhillips FL, and Bickers JN: Operations on patients with sickle cell anaemia at Charity Hospital in New Orleans. *SGO* 135 (1972): 870–872.
174. Szentpetery S, Robertson L, and Lower RR: Complete repair of tetralogy associated

with sickle cell anaemia and G–6-PD deficiency. *J Thorac Cardiovasc Surg* 72 (1976): 276–279.

175. Green M, Gall RJC, Huntsman RG, et al.: Sickle cell crisis treated by exchange transfusion. *JAMA* 231 (1975): 948–953.

176. Fullerton MW, Philippart AI, Sarnaik S, et al.: Perioperative exchange transfusion in sickle cell anemia. *J Pediatr Surg* 16 (1981): 297–300.

Part III

PSYCHOSOCIAL ASPECTS OF SICKLE CELL DISEASE

16

Diagnosis and Management of Psychosocial Problems in the Sickle Cell Disease Patient and Family

Kermit B. Nash

Sickle cell disease is a chronic, inherited disorder of hemoglobin in the red blood cells. The term *sickle cell disease* refers to a group of genetic disorders characterized by a predominance of hemoglobin S (Hb S) and symptoms related to anemia and/or vaso-occlusion. In the United States, the most common conditions are homozygous sickle cell anemia (SS), sickle-thalassemia, and sickle hemoglobin C disease. Though there are many variations of the disease, sickle cell anemia is the most symptomatic. Intermittent severe episodes of excruciating pain involving the extremities (back, abdomen, and chest) are the primary symptoms of the disease (1).

Sickle cell disease is most often found in persons of African and Mediterranean ancestry. In the United States, the disease is found most frequently in black Americans. Approximately 50,000 individuals in the United States have sickle cell disease (2). It is estimated that sickle cell disease occurs in 1 out of every 400–500 black American births.

The medical severity of sickle cell disease varies among affected individuals. However, different periods of the life span are associated with vulnerability to different aspects of the disease process. Pneumococcal infections in infants, stroke in children, growth retardation of adolescents, and osteoarthritis in adults are likely complications of the disease.

There is no cure for sickle cell disease. Persons with the disease must live daily with the threat of disability, discrimination, and death (3). The current approach to treatment in sickle cell disease is entirely palliative. Management remains primarily supportive and symptomatic. Nevertheless, considerable progress has been made in recent years in understanding the molecular and cellular events for sickling of the red blood cells in persons with sickle cell disease. In 1983 a study conducted by the Sickle Cell Branch of the Division of Blood

Disease and Resources, National Heart, Lung and Blood Institute, effectively demonstrated the value of oral penicillin in preventing pneumococcal septicemia in children with sickle cell anemia (4). As a result of this study, most states implemented newborn screening programs. Family counseling, education, and follow-up services should be provided as well. Improvements in medical care, nutrition, education, and screening have reduced mortality and morbidity associated with sickle cell disease. The potential life expectancy of individuals with sickle cell disease has expanded significantly (3).

Persons with sickle cell disease may experience problems associated with those affected by other chronic diseases: loss of school or work time, unpredictable bouts of pain, fear of impending death, changes in self-image, and social isolation. Thus, the psychosocial aspect of illness in sickle cell disease is a major factor in the individual's overall well-being. Increasingly, attention is now being paid to the impact of the disease on the quality of lives that have been prolonged by advanced technology (5).

The psychosocial dimensions are characterized and defined by the interaction of the medical diagnosis and treatment. The internal reactions of individuals and families, as well as how they perceive themselves and how others perceive them, are considered. The most frequent model utilized for the treatment of chronic diseases such as sickle cell disease is the biomedical molecular biology and its basic scientific discipline. The biomedical model assumes that disease is accounted for by deviations from the norm that can be explained by biomedical and neurophysiological processes (6). Implicit in the model is the expectation that disease be dealt with as an entity that is independent of social behavior and processes. The biomedical model also implies that mental and somatic phenomena are distinct (7).

The distinction between disease and illness, by some analysis, is that disease is a biomedical condition or entity and that illness is a subjective reaction to a physical state (8). Kleinman (9) suggested that, in chronic disorder, the focus of clinical management is more frequently caring for the behavioral and social difficulties associated with those disorders than curing the biological abnormalities underlying them. Thus, it is the subjective reaction and not the physical state that is the measure of the person's illness (10). Lack of compliance with the medical regimen, patient dissatisfaction with the quality of care, and the large and still growing numbers of medical-legal suits offer ready evidence that these clinical tasks are not well performed (9).

Illness problems are psychosocial in nature. For heuristic purposes, these problems can be grouped into several major categories. These include problems related to:

1. Different psychosocial and cultural influences on the symptoms' pattern and course of sickness;
2. Patient and family beliefs and values about the cause, nature, and significance of the sickness;

3. Family malfunctioning that either has preceded or has resulted from a given sickness episode;

4. Conflicts and labelling of specific sickness episodes and in the sanctioning of a particular type of sick role (chronic, etc.);

5. Financial pressures associated with a sickness and its treatment;

6. Choices and interactions with different health care institutions as part of the health care–seeking process;

7. Miscommunication between patient and caregivers; and,

8. Divergent patient and practitioner evaluations of therapeutic outcome and quality care (9).

The biomedical model is useful as a research tool. However, it leaves no room for the consideration of social, psychological and behavioral dimensions of illness. The biopsychological model, by contrast, provides a blueprint for research, a framework for teaching, and a design for action in the real world of health care (7). This model focuses on the clusters of symptoms experienced by people in discomfort and takes into account the social, psychological, and biological factors that influence the onset of disease and variations in the course of the disease. The added dimension of the biopsychosocial model expands the biomedical model by including the patient and his or her attributes as a human being (11). Thus, it is more likely that the problems for which people seek care and what they define as illness will be incorporated in the assessment and treatment of the patient. Perhaps the interaction of the biological, psychological, and social entities of disease and illness can best be illustrated through the illness dynamic (12; see Figure 16.1).

In considering the psychosocial dimension as it expands from the individual to the family, and to the community at large, the epidemiological circular model of illness and disease widens the traditional medical model by positing an interaction of agent, host, and environmental factors as equally necessary for the occurrence of the disease (13). Thus, understanding the causes of disease and illness points to broad and interacting sets of factors that contribute to the individual and family situation (14; see Figure 16.2). These factors arise from within and outside the family and, more often than not, converge to create a situation of extreme need and inability to adapt to chronic illnesses (15).

PSYCHOSOCIAL IMPLICATIONS

The psychosocial implications are characterized and defined by the interactions of the medical diagnosis and treatment. Prenatal and newborn screening have increased the likelihood of earlier knowledge of these interactions. When a diagnosis of a chronic genetic disorder is made, the reactions of parents must be handled, as well as what this might potentially do to the relationships between the child and his or her parents. Also the roles of the parents and the resources

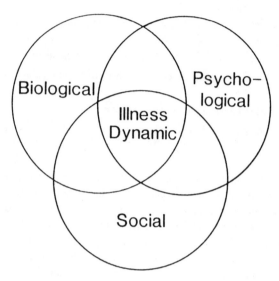

Figure 16.1.   Illness dynamic.

Source: Based on concepts in SA Green, *Mind and Body: The Psychology of Physical Illness* (Washington D.C.: American Psychiatric Press, 1985).

necessary to cope with the disease must be examined. Issues of denial, fear and anxiety, anger and hostility, withdrawal, and depression are some of the feelings internalized by parents that can interfere with parenting and/or following the recommended medical regimens. No matter at what point the diagnosis occurs, there is a profound influence on the psychosocial domain of sickle cell patients and their families (16, 17). Problems are frequently intensified by the lack of adequate information and counseling, lack of a support system, by the varying quality of medical facilities, and by the fragmentation of services.

Like other hereditary diseases, sickle cell may interfere with normal growth and development. Parents are frequently overprotective as they try to prevent recurrences of painful episodes in their offspring (18). These attempts are further compounded by the guilt that surrounds the hereditary nature of the illness. Affected offsprings are often given an inaccurate prognosis of a shortened life span, which, in turn, affects the motivation to achieve and encourages family members to foster dependency.

As the child with sickle cell moves from infancy to the toddler stage and then to preschool, the parents' reactions to sickle cell are frequently translated by the child into behaviors and attitudes of helplessness, dependency, and lower self-esteem and/or self-worth. Parents often must not only cope with the child's disease but also sacrifice the emotional and material needs of other siblings. This

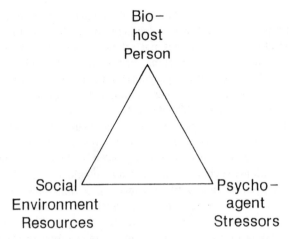

Bio-
host
Person

Social   Psycho-
Environment   agent
Resources   Stressors

Figure 16.2.   A unifying model for medical and psychiatric social work.

Source: Based on concepts in JE Turnbull and KB Nash, A unifying model for medical and psychiatric social work, paper presented at the National Association of Social Workers Annual Meeting, New Orleans, 1985.

sometimes can result in a drain on the family resources which may impact parents to the point that they perceive themselves as functioning ineffectively. For the child, the psychological impact of unpredictable and painful episodes, impending death, and social isolation may be devastating (19).

Experiences during infancy and early childhood can either promote or prevent the attainment of optimal development potential. As the child moves out of the home into the wider community, the reinforcement of negative attitudes and behavior may occur. Physical attributes may lead to teasing while school attendance may be marked with absenteeism, leading to poor school performance and educational deficits. This sometimes leads to social isolation and loneliness, which not only affects how the child feels about him- or herself but also affects interactions with peers and other adults. Through these formative years, the child with sickle cell disease may frequently experience limitations imposed by others but interpreted by the child as reflections of his or her own inadequacy. These communications and/or interpretations may be exhibited in the form of infantile depression, academic failure, social isolation, and so forth (19).

The puberty and adolescence stage of human development is an emotional and turbulent period for any child. It is a stage of transition that encompasses the biological, psychological, and social aspects of the individual. The adolescent period is characterized by rapid changes in physical development. Physical growth in adolescents with sickle cell disease commonly lags behind that of peers. For the adolescent with sickle cell disease whose physical differences are apparent, the challenges of adolescence are often intensified. Having smaller physical attributes may further reinforce the adolescent's feeling of being different than peers (20). Further, as the adolescent approaches high school, he or she may not feel adequate to compete, not only because of what may be a marginal academic record but how they feel about themselves and the prognosis of their life. The minority status of the disease can be expected to further compound the already tremendous challenges faced by the chronically ill adolescent (21).

Psychosocial issues for the late adolescent and young adult sickle cell disease patients become focalized on issues of careers, vocation, dating, and marriage. The ramifications for these issues are compounded by the way in which they are viewed by institutions, such as school, potential employers, and human service agencies. Stereotypes and myths still exist that impose limitations such as the ability to do physical work, prolonged absences, which interact negatively on how the individual may view him- or herself and, correspondingly, on his or her aspirations and hopes. Questions of dating and marriage are frequently marred by the carrier state and worries about genetic transmission as well as the ability to earn a living (22). If an individual decides to marry and start a family, complications of the disease may alter traditional family roles. Issues of dependence and confinement may mean altering usual activities which may, in turn, impact family dynamics negatively. The interplay of these internal feelings and external realities constitutes the complex nature of the psychosocial dimensions.

The population of sickle cell disease patients over age 35 has received relatively little attention in the past. Until recently, individuals with sickle cell disease were not expected to live beyond age 20. During this period of life, changes in social support systems due to deaths, illness, and old age in general are more likely to occur. The successful adjustment of the individual over 35 years of age with sickle cell disease will depend primarily on the individual's coping abilities, vocational opportunities, medical services, and social services (including recreation and leisure). A pilot study conducted by the Duke University Comprehensive Sickle Cell Center revealed that this population is increasing rapidly in numbers (unpublished data). Many individuals with sickle cell disease in this age group lack effective life skills and manifest acquired or learned maladaptive responses to their disease. The difficulties involved in establishing and maintaining relationships, in conjunction with possessing inadequate life skills and coping with the adversities of having a chronic illness, places this population in double jeopardy (23).

As more and more individuals with sickle cell disease are living longer, families are now confronted with providing financial and home health care for adult children. These external realities cause additional stress throughout the life span for which there may be valid concerns among individuals with sickle cell disease and their families. These concerns are related to such basic needs as housing and transportation which influence decisions about medical care, continuation of disability payments, and involvement with a comprehensive rehabilitation program. Thus, restrictions on work, insurance and social security income (SSI)/medicaid interfere with optimal functioning and may have a profound effect on family relationships.

In summary, chronic illness is a life-long stressor that influences an individual and his or her family's psychosocial functioning. Different periods of the life cycle are vulnerable to specific psychosocial problems. For example, the young adult who has survived chronic childhood illness may experience difficulties with social relationships and vocational development. Likewise, the adolescent may experience difficulties with school- and peer-related problems. Families of sickle cell disease must continuously contend with modification of their activities, increased financial burden, and overall intrafamily tension and conflict. Institutional stresses such as fragmented services, racism, and inadequately trained and insensitive health care providers further compound the situation for the sickle cell disease patient and his or her family.

PSYCHOSOCIAL CARE

Psychosocial care involves the provision of a range of services which encompasses education, counseling, support, and the provision of linkages to community resources. The goal of these services is to help patients and their families maintain, reestablish, or improve the aspects of their personal and life situations by developing a greater sense of self-confidence, self-dependence and awareness. Included in such goals are education and counseling about the disease, personal problems, marital problems, parent-child relations, intra- and interfamilial relationships, school problems, employment problems, help with financial assistance, medical expenses, drugs, appliances, convalescent or nursing home care, transportation, overnight stay in the hospital, and utilizing appropriate resources (e.g., social agencies) to assist with these problems.

The ultimate aim of psychosocial care is to help the patient and his or her family with the illness-related problems of the disease. This occurs through assistance with accepting and following medical recommendations, helping patients and families understand the illness and how all family members can be involved in helping the patient to accept changes in social functioning as a result of illness and/or disability and to make appropriate adjustments in roles, employment, and so on.

Psychosocial care is based primarily on the patient's medical diagnosis and the diagnostic impression of the patient and his or her family's social and psychological functioning. Christ (24) suggested that the framework for psychosocial assessment be organized throughout areas of potential sources of stress to enhance understanding of the patient's and his or her family's maladaptive response to diagnosis and treatment. Sources of stress outlined by Christ are:

1. The ecological framework of the treatment system,
2. An expression of underlying psychopathology,
3. A reactivation of underlying conflicts,

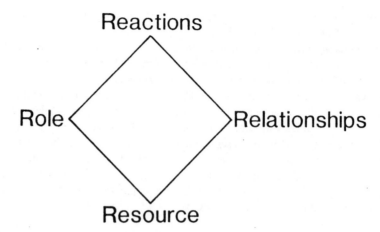

Figure 16.3.   Social diagnosis in health care.

4. A reaction to specific stress; and

5. A dis-synchrony of coping among patients, family, and health care staff.

Key questions that must be considered include the physical condition and level of functioning, attitudes and adjustment, family and social relations, and the socioeconomic situation as it impacts on the individual and the family. A useful paradigm for psychosocial assessment suggested by Doremus is the "four R's": reaction, role, relations, and resources (25; see Figure 16.3). This paradigm allows for the exploration of both internal and external factors that affect the individual, his or her family, and significant others. Because no one form of intervention is appropriate to all patients and families, an accurate assessment is necessary to help patients and families reduce stress, cope with illness and disability, and effectively utilize resources to maximize their adjustment.

PSYCHOSOCIAL INTERVENTIONS

The family remains the chief nurturing and sustaining unit of society. Within the context of the family, a child is socialized and develops sociocultural, gender, and economic roles necessary to function in society. Thus, a logical point of intervention for patients with sickle cell disease is the family system. There are certain basic assumptions that health care professionals need to be cognizant of in order to maximize the opportunity for change within the family system. These assumptions are:

1. There are predictable points of family stress;

2. Families vary in their level of tolerance for the patient's physical condition;

3. Families under stress tend to hold to previously proved patterns of behavior, whether they are effective or not;

4. Families usually go through a grief-loss process following the diagnosis of a disabling condition;

5. Families play a significant role in the encouragement of the family member with a chronic illness to participate in particular therapies;

6. Families react to particular illness behavior;

7. Families may have difficulty adjusting to a chronic physical illness because they either have incorrect or inadequate disease-related information;

8. Where there is a chronic illness, families must adjust to changes and expectations for each other; and

9. A family's perception of the illness event has the most influence upon its ability to cope (26).

The selection of appropriate interventions flows from clearly formulated problems, collaborative practices, social contracts and established goals. These interventions occur through the rendering of services, which can be both direct (micro) and indirect (macro).

Parents who have learned of their child's diagnosis of sickle cell disease through amniocentesis or newborn screening need education, counseling, and support. Not knowing what the disease is, who it affects, or how it can be medically cared for creates a vacuum that can cause stress. Once the parents have some cognitive understanding of the disease, it is important to offer counseling in order to help them with their internal feelings. "What is it that I have given my child?" is a question that, unless resolved, may generate feelings of guilt and anger.

Support, along with other interventions, is particularly needed after the birth of the child. This support can take the form of family or a support group in order for parents to realize that they are not alone in their situation. Such interventions enable parents to sort through their roles, reactions, relationships and resources. Interventions to mobilize other resources if needed might include assistance with transportation, supplemental nutritional programs, financial assistance, and referrals for other services (e.g., legal, mental health, etc.). Case management service may be required in order to coordinate resources needed by the patient and family.

As the infant grows, it may be necessary to use many of the interventions that have already been mentioned to meet the emotional, social, and economic needs of the family. It may be necessary to hold counseling sessions with the small family or have family members involved with a support group. As the child grows and reaches school age, interventions may be necessary with the school as well as individual teachers. These interventions require educational sessions on what sickle cell disease is as well as helping teachers understand the emotional components and reasons why the child might be behaving in a certain way, particularly dysfunctional attitudes in behavior such as resignation, passivity, and withdrawal. Services may include inservice training not only for teachers but for school personnel in general and developing the linkage in order to attend to the child's emotional and physical needs.

Psychosocial interventions can focus on the strengths of the child in helping parents reinforce these strengths in order to minimize the assault on self-esteem and the child's lowered aspirations. It is important to help the child deal with his or her perceived differences on the part of others in the playground situation, where he or she may be viewed as different, thus equipping him or her with the skills necessary to deal with teasing and avoid becoming stigmatized. Perhaps one of the greatest psychosocial interventions during this phase is to dispel the myths and enable parents, as well as the institution of the school, to begin to allow the child to draw his or her own limits rather than having limitations superimposed. Educational services and counseling sessions provided to significant others and to those in the wider community may be of further help in the reinforcement of a positive self-image.

As the youngster approaches adolescence, anticipatory education and counseling can be given to the individual, the family, and school personnel. Recognizing that at different developmental stages there are different issues, particularly as youngsters enter adolescence, there will be the delayed onset of the menses and puberty, as well as concerns regarding sexuality. Again, education, support, and counseling can help the individual and family handle the reactions to this physiological phenomenon as well as helping the individual handle his or her role and relationships with significant others and peers. Constructive interventions to begin helping the individual focus on realistic vocational aspirations can include appropriate referrals to vocational rehabilitation and, if need be, scholarship sources.

As the individual moves through the life cycle, there are continued readjustments as a result of the complicating factors of the disease process. For some, it may mean "early retirement" on disability, while for others, hospitalization may increase or decrease. Correspondingly, the concomitance of emotional individual and family reactions with frequently changing roles and relationships and, not infrequently, a drain on resources, both emotional and economic, may require the utilization of outside support services. Today, 20 is less common than 40 as the anticipated age of demise (3). Consequently, as people live longer, different psychosocial problems arise as they approach different life stages and all require psychosocial care. For example, the elderly population of sickle cell patients have operated for years with the support of their families and limited resources. However, family support once available to patients may become limited because of the death of family members, age-related disabilities, and/or old age in general. Individual, group and family counseling should be offered as well as services to meet special needs (e.g., midlife crisis, retirement planning, etc.).

Throughout the life cycle, the patient and family interact not only with the health care delivery system, but also with the delivery systems, of social, psychological, and economic services. These transactions are often necessary in order to obtain services, programs, and information and to effectively cope with disability. However, it has been noted that frequently there are barriers to necessary resources (27). These barriers include the location of services, hours of service, behaviors of providers, and a lack of collaborative agreement among providers on the type of service that will help alleviate patient/family problems (28). Although the health care professional believes that psychosocial support services are beneficial, the support service professional is often frustrated by barriers to service delivery (27). Issues such as poor communication among agencies and patients, fragmentation of services, bureaucratic inefficiency, and a lack of adequate financial support of service agencies to meet the needs of patients continue to be central themes for support service professionals.

TASK AND FUNCTION OF PSYCHOSOCIAL CARE PROVIDERS

Those providing psychosocial interventions must have a knowledge of human behavior, crisis intervention theory, the impact of chronic illness on the individual and family, the medical care delivery system, community resources, interdisciplinary team practices, and an appreciation for cultural nuances. Further, the provider must be able to conduct individual, group, and family counseling.

The providers of these services will at any point in time have multiple tasks and roles in order to help the patient and family cope and adapt to illness-related problems (15). The provider of psychosocial care must have the ability to deal with ambivalence, resistance, and dependency of the patient and family. The specific task of the provider of psychosocial care includes:

1. Providing emotional support;
2. Providing instructions in coping skills, individually and in groups;
3. Providing opportunities for choice, decision making, and action;
4. Encouraging organizations to be responsive to the emotional needs of the patient and family;
5. Organizing and working with the natural support system;
6. Providing information, time, and space for effective coping; and
7. Developing new programs and services to meet patient and family needs.

While working directly with the client and family, the provider of psychosocial care may as well be a mobilizer, teacher, coach, enabler, and facilitator. While focusing on the environment, the psychosocial care provider may be a mobilizer, collaborator/mediator, organizer, facilitator, innovator, and finally, but not least, an advocate.

As has been repeatedly suggested throughout this chapter, the impact of sickle cell disease on the patient and family is a complex problem that involves an interaction of many forces and influences. Historically, there has been a paucity of research on the psychosocial aspect of sickle cell disease. Briscoe (29) reviewed the research on the psychosocial ramifications of sickle cell disease for the past twenty-five years and summarized her findings in order to alert social and behavioral scientists to the need for their greater involvement with this chronic illness. She noted that past research identified significant factors related to adjustment; however, research activities had major methodological problems. These problems included: (1) the need for appropriate control groups, (2) the need for larger samples, and (3) the need for attention to changes in the individual's psychosocial situation over time. However, since 1986 researchers have increasingly turned their attention to the psychological, social, and environmental factors associated with sickle cell disease.

Nevertheless, the pattern of services provided for sickle cell disease to a large extent affect the patient and family's overall functioning. Investigators studying the affects of the provision of services on the biopsychosocial functioning of the sickle cell patient and family are faced with even more difficulties than those who study the impact of the disease on biopsychosocial functioning in general. A review of the literature reveals limited research focusing specifically on the impact of the provision of psychosocial care. Thus, there is little information available as a point of departure for research.

In summary, we are beginning to develop a knowledge base of specific psychosocial problems associated with sickle cell disease. Continuous research to delineate psychosocial problems unique to sickle cell disease patients and their families is encouraged. However, the provision of psychosocial care and the systematic evaluation of such care are needs that cannot continue to be ignored.

REFERENCES

1. Kinney TR, and Ware R: Advances in the management of sickle cell disease. *Ped Consult* 7, no. 3 (1988): 1–6.
2. Vichinsky E, Hurst D, and Lubin B: Update on sickle cell disease. *Hos Med* 15 (1988): 131–149.
3. Charache S, Lubin B, and Reid CD: *Management and therapy of sickle cell disease.* NIH publication no. 84–2117. Bethesda, MD: Department of Health and Human Services, 1985.
4. Gaston MH, Verter JI, Woods G, et al.: Prophylaxis with oral penicillin children with sickle cell anemia. *N Engl J Med* 134 (June 1986): 1593.
5. Nash KB: Overview of humanistic progress in sickle cell anemia during the past 10 years. *Am J Ped Hem Onc* 5 (1983): 352–359.
6. Mechanic D: Social psychological factors affecting the presentation of bodily complaints. *N Engl J Med* 286 (1972): 1132.
7. Engel GL: The need for a new medical model: A challenge for biomedicine. *Science* 196, no. 4286 (1977): 129–135.

8. Fabrega H: Disease and social behavior: An interdisciplinary perspective. Cambridge, MA: MIT Press, 1974.

9. Kleinman A: Culture, illness and cure: Clinical lessons from anthropoligic and cross-cultural research. *Ann Intern Med* 58 (1977).

10. McKinley JB, and Dutton DB: Social psychological factors affecting health service utilization. In SJ Mushklin, ed.: *Consumer incentives for health care,* pp. 251–301. New York: Prodist, 1974.

11. Engel GL: The clinical application of the bio-psychosocial model. *Am J Psych* 137 (1980): 535–544.

12. Green SA: *Mind and body, The psychology of physical illness.* Washington, DC: American Psychiatry Press, 1985.

13. Coulton CJ: A study of person environment fit among the chronically ill. *Social Work Health Care* 5 (1979): 5–17.

14. Turnbull JE, and Nash KB. *A unifying model for medical and psychiatric social work.* Paper presented at the National Association of Social Workers annual meeting, New Orleans, March 1987.

15. Germaine CB: *Social work in practice in health care.* New York: Free Press Collier MacMillan Publishers, 1984.

16. Williams I, Earles A, and Pack B. Psychological considerations in sickle cell disease. *Nurse Clin North Am* 18 (1983): 215–229.

17. Johnson C. *Sickle cell disease, Handbook of severe disability,* ed. W Stolov and J Clowers. Rockville, MD: U.S. Department of Education, 1983.

18. Vavassur JW: Psychosocial aspects of chronic disease: cultural and ethnic implications. *Birth Defects* 23, no. 6 (1987): 144–152.

19. Hurtig AL, and White LS: Psychosocial adjustment in children and adolescents with sickle cell disease. *J Ped Psycho* 2, no. 3 (1986): 411–427.

20. Morgan SA, and Jackson J: Psychological and social concomitants of sickle cell anemia in adolescents. *J Ped Psycho* 2, no. 3 (1986): 429–440.

21. Nash KB: Ethnicity, race and the health care delivery system. In A Hutig and C Viera, eds.: *Sickle cell disease: psychological and psychosocial issues,* pp. 131–146. Chicago: University of Illinois Press, 1986.

22. Whitten CF, and Nishiura E: Sickle cell anemia. In N Hobbs and JM Perrin; eds.: *Issues in the care of children with chronic illness,* pp. 236–260. San Francisco: Jossey-Bass Publishers, 1985.

23. Abrams MR, Whitworth EA, Holmes MP, et al.: *Psychosocial adjustment of an adult population with sickle cell disease: A developmental perspective.* Unpublished manuscript, 1988.

24. Christ GH: A psychosocial assessment framework for cancer patients and their families. *Health Social Work* 8, no. 1 (1983): 57–64.

25. Doremus B. The four r's: Social diagnosis in health care. *Health Social Work* 1, no. 4 (Nov. 1976) 120–139.

26. Leahey M, and Wright LM: Intervening with families with chronic illness. *Fam Systems Med* 3, no. 1 (1985): 60–69.

27. Whitworth EA: *North Carolina SPRANS I: Evaluation of readiness for implementation.* Unpublished masters thesis, University of North Carolina, Chapel Hill, Public Administration Program, Political Science Department, 1989.

28. Moise JR: Toward a model of competence and coping. In A. Hurtig and C. Viera, eds.: *Sickle cell disease: Psychological and psychosocial issues*, pp. 7–23. Chicago: University of Illinois Press, 1986.
29. Briscoe G. *The psychosocial impact of sickle cell anemia: A review*. Unpublished manuscript, 1986.

Bibliography

Barner TW, Moore GW, and Hutchins GM: The liver in sickle cell anemia. *Am J Med* 69 (1980): 833–837.

Benjamin LJ, Berkowitz LR, Orringer E, et al.: A collaborative double-blind, randomized study of cetiedil citrate in sickle cell crisis. *Blood* 67 (1986): 1442–1447.

Bookchin RM, and Lew UL: Red cell membrane abnormalities in sickle cell anemia. In EB Brown, ed.; *Progress in hematology,* Vol. 13, pp. 1–18. New York: Grune and Stratton, 1983.

Buchanan GR, and Holtkamp CA: Plasma levels of platelet and vascular prostaglandin derivatives in children with sickle cell anemia. *Thromb Haemostasis* (Stuttgart) 54 (1985): 394–396.

Bunn HF, and Forget BG: *Hemoglobin: Molecular and genetic aspects.* Philadelphia: W. B. Saunders, 1986.

Burrington JD, and Smith MD: Elective and emergency surgery in children with sickle cell anemia. *Surg Clin N Amer* 56 (1976): 55–71.

Charache S, Scott JC, and Charache P: Acute chest syndrome in adults with sickle cell anemia. *Arch Intern Med* 139 (1979): 67–69.

Dean J, and Schechter AN: Sickle cell anemia: Molecular and cellular bases of therapeutic approaches. *N Engl J Med* 299 (1978): 752–763, 804–811, 863–870.

Diggs LW: Anatomic lesions in sickle cell disease. In HA Abramson, JF Bertles, and DL Wethers, eds.: *Sickle cell disease: Diagnosis, management, education and research,* pp. 199–229. St. Louis: C. V. Mosby, 1973.

——— Blood picture in sickle cell anemia. *Southern Med J* 25 (1932): 615–620.

Embury SH: The clinical pathophysiology of sickle cell disease. *Ann Rev Med* 37 (1986): 361–376.

Galacteros F, Kleman K, Caburi-Martin J, et al.: Blood screening of hemoglobin abnormalities by thin layer isoelectric focusing. *Blood* 5–6 (1980): 1068–1071.

Gaston MH, Verter J, Woods G, et al.: Prophylaxis with oral penicillin in children with sickle cell anemia: A randomized trial. *N Engl J Med* 314 (1986): 1593–1599.

Grenett HE, and Garver FA: Identification and quantitation of sickle cell hemoglobin with an enzyme-linked immunosorbent assay (ELISA). *J Lab Clin Med* 96 (1980): 597–605.

Hebbel RP: Beyond hemoglobin polymerization. The red blood cell membrane and sickle cell pathophysiology. *Blood* 77 (1991): 214–237.

Herrick JB: Peculiar elongated and sickle-shaped red blood corpuscles in a case of severe anemia. *Arch Intern Med* 6 (1910): 517–521.

Lehman H: Distribution of the sickle cell gene. *Eugen Rev* 46 (1954): 101–121.

Livingstone FB: Malaria and human polymorphisms. *Ann Rev Genet* 5 (1971): 33–64.

Lubin B, Chiu D, Roelofeen B, et al.: Abnormal membrane phospholipid asymmetry in sickle erythrocytes and its pathophysiologic significance. *Prog Clin Biol Res* 56 (1981): 171–193.

Mankad VN, Williams JP, Harper M, et al.: Magnetic resonance imaging of bone marrow in sickle cell disease: Clinical, hematologic and pathologic correlations. *Blood* 75; no. 1 (1990): 274–283.

Nagel RL, Fabry ME, Pagnier J, et al.: Hematologically and genetically distinct forms of sickle cell anemia in Africa. *N Engl J Med* 312, (1985): 880–884.

Nash KB: Ethnicity, race and health care delivery system. In AL Hurtig, and CT Viera, eds.: *Sickle cell disease: Psychological and psychosocial issues,* pp. 131–146. Urbana: University of Illinois Press, 1986.

Pauling L, Itano HA, Singer SJ, et al.: Sickle cell anemia: A molecular disease. *Science* 110 (1949): 543–548.

Payne R: Pain management in sickle cell disease: Rationale and techniques. In CF Whitten, and JF Bertles, eds.: *Sickle cell disease,* p. 565. New York: Annals of the New York Academy of Sciences; 1989.

Pearson HA, Gallapher D, Chilcote R, et al.: Developmental patterns of splenic dysfunction in sickle cell disorders. *Pediatrics* 76; no. 3 (1985): 392–397.

Platt OS, Fakone JF, and Lux SE: Molecular defect in sickle erythrocyte skeleton. Abnormal spectrin binding to sickle inside-out vesicles. *J Clin Invest* 75 (1985): 266–271.

Poncz M, Kane E, and Gill FM: Acute chest syndrome in sickle cell disease: Etiology and clinical correlates. *J Peds* 107 (1985): 861–866.

Powars D: Natural history of sickle cell disease, The first ten years. *Semin Hematol* 12 (1975): 267–285.

Powars D, Wilson B, Imbus C, et al.: The natural history of stroke in sickle cell disease. *Am J Med* 65 (1978): 461–471.

Reynolds J: *The roentgenological features of sickle cell disease and related hemoglobinopathies,* pp. 184–218. Springfield, Ill; Charles C. Thomas, 1965.

Rickles FR, and O'Leary DS: Role of coagulation system in pathophysiology of sickle cell disease. *Arch Intern Med* 133 (1974): 635–641.

Rogers BB, Wessels RA, Ou CN, et al.: High performance liquid chromatography in the diagnosis of hemoglobinopathies and thalassemias. *Am J Clin Pathol* 84 (1985): 671–674.

Sarnaik SA, and Lusher JM: Neurological complications of sickle cell anemia. *Am J Ped Hem Onc* 4, no. 4 (1982): 386–394.

Searle JF: Anesthesia in sickle cell states. *Anesthesia* 28 (1973): 48–58.

Seeler RA, and Shwiaki MZ: Acute splenic sequestration crises in young children with sickle cell anemia. *Clin Pediatr* 11 (1972): 701–704.

Serjeant GR: *Sickle cell disease*. New York: Oxford University Press, 1985.

Serjeant GR, Topley JM, Mason K, et al.: Outbreak of aplastic crisis in sickle cell anemia associated with parvovirus like agent. *Lancet* no. 2 (1981): 595–598.

Shapiro BS: The management of pain in sickle cell disease. *Ped Clin N Amer* 36, no. 4 (1989): 1029–1045.

Song YS: *Pathology of sickle cell disease*. Springfield, Ill: Charles C. Thomas, 1971.

Statius Van Eps LW, and DeJong PE: Psychosocial problems. In RW Schrier, VN Gottschalk, eds.: *Sickle cell disease of the kidney*, 4th ed., pp. 2561–2581. Boston: Little Brown, 1988.

United States Department of Health Services. Public Health Service Center for Disease Control. Division of Host Factors: *Laboratory methods for detecting hemoglobinopathies*, pp. 45–76. Atlanta: US Public Health Service, 1984.

United States. National Institutes of Health. Concensus Conference from the Office of Medical Applications of Research: Newborn screening for sickle cell disease and other hemoglobinopathies. *J Amer Med Assoc* 258 (1987): 1205–1209.

Whitten CF, and Bertles JF: *Sickle cell disease*. Vol. 565 of *Annals of the New York Academy of Science*. New York: New York Academy of Sciences, 1989.

Whitten CF, and Nishiwa E: Sickle cell anemia. In N Hobbs, and JM Perrin, eds.: *Issues in the care of children with chronic illness*, pp. 236–260. San Francisco: Jossey-Bass, 1985.

Zarkowsky H, Gallagher D, Gill F, et al.: Bacteremia in sickle hemoglobinopathies. *AJDC* 136 (1982): 543–547.

Index

About the Editors and Contributors

VIPUL N. MANKAD, M.D., a physician scientist and a pediatric hematologist-oncologist, is Professor of Pediatrics and Chairman of the Department of Pediatrics at the University of Kentucky. He was formerly the Louise Lenoir Locke Distinguished Professor and Vice Chairman of Pediatrics and Director of the Comprehensive Sickle Cell Center at the University of South Alabama College of Medicine.

R. BLAINE MOORE, Ph.D., a biochemist and a red cell scientist, is Associate Professor of Pediatrics and Biochemistry and Associate Director of the Comprehensive Sickle Cell Center at the University of South Alabama College of Medicine.

A. SEETHARAMA ACHARYA, Ph.D., is Associate Professor of Medicine at Albert Einstein College of Medicine.

LENNETTE J. BENJAMIN, M.D., is Assistant Professor of Medicine and Associate Director of the Comprehensive Sickle Cell Center at Albert Einstein College of Medicine and Montefiore Hospital.

SUSAN BRIGHAM, M.S., is a Senior Technologist at the Comprehensive Sickle Cell Center at the University of South Alabama College of Medicine.

B. GIL BROGDON, M.D., is Professor and Chairman of the Department of Radiology and Senior Scientist at the Comprehensive Sickle Cell Center at the University of South Alabama College of Medicine.

LEMUEL W. DIGGS, M.D., is Goodman Professor of Medicine, Emeritus, at the University of Tennessee Medical School.

PAUL R. DYKEN, M.D., is Professor and Chairman of the Department of Neurology and Senior Scientist at the Comprehensive Sickle Cell Center at the University of South Alabama College of Medicine.

JOHN J. FARRER, M.D., is Attending Urological Surgeon at Memorial Clinic, Olympia, Washington, and former Assistant Professor of Surgery at the University of South Alabama College of Medicine.

MARILYN H. GASTON, M.D., is Director of the Bureau of Health Care and Delivery and Assistant Surgeon General at the U.S. Department of Health and Human Services. She was formerly Deputy Chief of the Sickle Cell Disease Branch, National Heart, Lung and Blood Institute.

CHARLES HOFF, Ph.D., is Professor of Pediatrics and Consultant to the Comprehensive Sickle Cell Center at the University of South Alabama.

MYRON L. LECKLITNER, M.D., is Professor of Radiology at the University of South Alabama College of Medicine.

PAUL I. LIU, Ph.D., is a Senior Scientist and former Director of Core Laboratory, Comprehensive Sickle Cell Center; former Professor and Vice Chairman of Pathology at the University of South Alabama College of Medicine; and Director of Clinical Laboratories at Irvine Medical Center.

GESINA L. LONGENECKER, Ph.D., is Professor and Chairman of the Department of Biomedical Sciences and Senior Scientist at the Comprehensive Sickle Cell Center at the University of South Alabama College of Medicine.

BYRON C. MACHEN, M.D., is a former Assistant Professor of Radiology at the University of South Alabama College of Medicine.

APARNA V. MANKAD, M.D., is Director, Division of Obstetrical Anesthesia and Clinical Associate Professor of Anesthesiology at the University of South Alabama College of Medicine.

KERMIT B. NASH, Ph.D., is a Professor in the School of Social Work at the University of North Carolina, Chapel Hill.

CLARICE D. REID, M.D., is Chief of the Sickle Cell Disease Branch of the National Heart, Lung and Blood Institute.

CHARLES B. RODNING, M.D., is Associate Professor and Vice Chairman of the Departments of Surgery and Structural and Cellular Biology at the University of South Alabama College of Medicine.

JOHN P. SUTTON, M.D., is an Instructor in Surgery at the University of South Alabama College of Medicine.

JOHN POWELL WILLIAMS, M.D., is a Senior Scientist at the Comprehensive Sickle Cell Center and Professor of Radiology at the University of South Alabama College of Medicine.

YIH-MING YANG, M.D., is a Scientist at the Comprehensive Sickle Cell Center and Associate Professor of Pediatrics at the University of South Alabama College of Medicine.